HUMAN LABOR
AND BIRTH

fourth edition

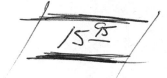

Harry Oxorn

B.A., M.D., C.M., F.R.C.S.(C.), F.A.C.O.G.

Professor of Obstetrics and Gynecology, University of Ottawa; Obstetrician-Gynecologist-in-Chief, Ottawa Civic Hospital, Ottawa, Canada; Honorary Attending Obstetrician and Gynecologist, Royal Victoria Hospital, Montreal, Canada

Illustrations by DOROTHY IRWIN

Additional illustrations for the Fourth Edition by VALERIE OXORN

HUMAN LABOR AND BIRTH

fourth edition

 APPLETON-CENTURY-CROFTS / New York

80 81 82 83 84 XXXX 10 9 8 7 6 5 4 3 2 1

Prentice-Hall International, Inc., London
Prentice-Hall of Australia, Pty. Ltd., Sydney
Prentice-Hall of India Private Limited, New Delhi
Prentice-Hall of Japan, Inc., Tokyo
Prentice-Hall of Southeast Asia (Pte.) Ltd., Singapore
Whitehall Books Ltd., Wellington, New Zealand

Library of Congress Cataloging in Publication Data
Oxorn, Harry.
   Human labor and birth.

   Includes bibliographies and index.
   1. Labor (Obstetrics) 2. Delivery (Obstetrics)
I. Foote, William R., joint author. II. Title.
RG651.09 1980   618.4   80-12352
ISBN 0-8385-7664-8

Text design: RFS Graphic Design, Inc.
Cover design: Gretczko Graphic Design, Inc.

PRINTED IN THE UNITED STATES OF AMERICA

Preface

THE REVISION of the material for the Fourth Edition of *Human Labor and Birth* is extensive, including much new information and over two dozen illustrations. The thrust of the book, however, remains the same. It deals with the mechanisms by which the fetus passes through the pelvis, the actual birth of the baby, and the management of the patient in the labor and delivery rooms in normal and abnormal situations.

Because this book deals with relatively common situations and does so in a straightforward manner, it should be particularly useful for personnel who work in the delivery room—nurses, midwives, house staff, family physicians, and practicing obstetricians. Medical students may find this book a useful adjunct to didactic lectures, cutting down on garbled note taking and increasing their readiness for practical demonstrations and discussions of problems.

Included in the revision are sections dealing with the positions for delivery, the supine hypotensive syndrome, meconium aspiration, hyperextension of the fetal head in breech presentation, investigation and management of breech presentation, the use of the vacuum extractor, abnormal attachments of the placenta, ultrasound, uterotonic agents, induction of labor, intrauterine growth retardation and prolonged pregnancy, preterm labor, and symphysiotomy. There is a new chapter on antepartum hemorrhage in the third trimester. The section dealing with the assessment of the fetus in utero has been re-written and expanded greatly.

One of the key problems in obstetrics is to keep advances in perspective. It is tempting, but frequently not wise, to utilize a new procedure simply because it is new. However, a non-invasive, non-surgical approach often can be as safe and efficacious as an aggressive one. In such cases, we freely opt for the conservative approach, and this attitude is reflected in the presentation of material in this edition.

A valid general principle is that, as long as the boundaries of medical safety are observed, every woman has the right to give birth to her baby in the manner she chooses. Only when a difficulty arises is interference justified.

For instance, continuous monitoring of the fetal heart rate and the uterine contractions has made immense contributions to our knowledge, and, by leading to timely intervention, has saved many babies from damage or death. Nevertheless, the majority of infants can be delivered safely without the use of electronic equipment; the latter is reserved for problem cases. Furthermore, since we are not always certain of the exact significance of the information provided by the machines, we must, by maintaining the priority of critical clinical judgment, guard against hasty and unnecessary interference.

So aggressive, impatient, and apprehensive have many North American obstetricians become, that it seems, sometimes, that the doctor is having the baby rather than the woman. Unless the baby falls out of the pelvis, cesarean section is performed. It is our opinion that, barring serious complications, vaginal birth is safer for both mother and child; that a posterior position of the occiput, to use one example, arrested at a station of +2, is delivered better by rotation and extraction than by cesarean section. The role of cesarean section has increased, and properly so. Abdominal delivery is far preferable, for both mother and child, to dragging a baby through a pelvis that is too small for it. However, the maternal mortality and morbidity rates are higher and the period of convalescence longer following cesarean section than after vaginal delivery. Repeated cesarean section is associated with the same problems as the primary procedure. We must not stretch the indications for cesarean section to the point where the danger to the mother is out of proportion to the fetal results.

Finally, we note the death, on the 25th of April 1973, of our collaborator and friend, William R. Foote.

Contents

CONTENTS

1.

Pelvis: Bones, Joints, Ligaments

PELVIC BONES

The pelvis is the bony basin in which the trunk terminates and through which the body weight is transmitted to the lower extremities. In the female it is adapted for childbearing. The pelvis consists of four bones: the two innominates, the sacrum, and the coccyx. These are united by four joints.

Innominate Bones

The innominate bones are placed laterally and anteriorly. Each is formed by the fusion of three bones (ilium, ischium, pubis) around the acetabulum.

ILIUM
The ilium is the upper bone: It has a body (which is fused with the ischial body) and an ala. Points of note concerning the ilium include:

1. The anterior superior iliac spine gives attachment to the inguinal ligament.
2. The posterior superior iliac spine marks the level of the second sacral vertebra. Its presence is indicated by a dimple in the overlying skin.
3. The iliac crest extends from the anterior superior iliac spine to the posterior superior iliac spine.

ISCHIUM
The ischium consists of a body in which the superior and inferior rami merge.

1. The body forms part of the acetabulum.
2. The superior ramus is behind and below the body.

1

3. The inferior ramus fuses with the inferior ramus of the pubis.
4. The ischial spine separates the greater sciatic from the lesser sciatic notch. It is an important landmark. Part of the levator ani muscle is attached to it.
5. The ischial tuberosity is the lower part of the ischium and is the bone on which humans sit.

PUBIS

The pubis consists of the body and two rami.

1. The body has a rough surface on its medial aspect. This is joined to the corresponding area on the opposite pubis to form the symphysis pubis. The levator ani muscles are attached to the pelvic aspect of the pubis.
2. The pubic crest is the superior border of the body.
3. The pubic tubercle, or spine, is the lateral end of the pubic crest. The inguinal ligament and conjoined tendon are attached here.
4. The superior ramus meets the body of the pubis at the pubic spine and the body of the ilium at the iliopectineal line. Here it forms a part of the acetabulum.
5. The inferior ramus merges with the inferior ramus of the ischium.

Landmarks can be identified:

1. The iliopectineal line extends from the pubic tubercle back to the sacroiliac joint. It forms the greater part of the boundary of the pelvic inlet.
2. The greater sacrosciatic notch is between the posterior inferior iliac spine above and the ischial spine below.
3. The lesser sacrosciatic notch is bounded by the ischial spine superiorly and the ischial tuberosity inferiorly.
4. The obturator foramen is delimited by the acetabulum, the ischial rami, and the pubic rami.

Sacrum

The sacrum is a triangular bone with the base above and the apex below. It consists of five vertebrae fused together; rarely, there are four or six. The sacrum lies between the innominate bones and is attached to them by the sacroiliac joints.

The upper surface of the first sacral vertebra articulates with the lower surface of the fifth lumbar vertebra. The anterior (pelvic) surface of the sacrum is concave, and the posterior surface convex.

The sacral promontory is the anterior superior edge of the first sacral vertebra. It protrudes slightly into the cavity of the pelvis, reducing the anteroposterior diameter of the inlet.

Coccyx

The coccyx (tail bone) is composed of four rudimentary vertebrae. The superior surface of the first coccygeal vertebra articulates with the lower surface of the fifth sacral vertebra to form the sacrococcygeal joint. Rarely, there is fusion between the sacrum and coccyx, with resultant limitation of movement.

The coccygeus muscle, the levator ani muscles, and the sphincter ani externus are attached to the coccyx from above downward.

PELVIC JOINTS AND LIGAMENTS

The sacrum, coccyx, and two innominate bones are linked by four joints: (1) the symphysis pubis, (2) the sacrococcygeal, and (3) the two sacroiliac synchondroses (Fig. 1).

Sacroiliac Joint

The sacroiliac joint lies between the articular surfaces of the sacrum and the ilium. Through it the weight of the body is transmitted to the pelvis and thence to the lower limbs. It is a synovial joint and permits a small degree of movement. The capsule is weak, and stability is maintained especially by the muscles around it as well as by four primary and two accessory ligaments.

PRIMARY LIGAMENTS

1. The anterior sacroiliac ligaments are short and transverse, runing from the preauricular sulcus on the ilium to the anterior aspect of the ala of the sacrum.
2. The interosseus sacroiliac ligaments are short, strong transverse bands that extend from the rough part behind the auricular surface on the ilium to the adjoining area on the sacrum.
3. The short posterior sacroiliac ligaments are strong transverse bands that lie behind the interosseus ligaments.

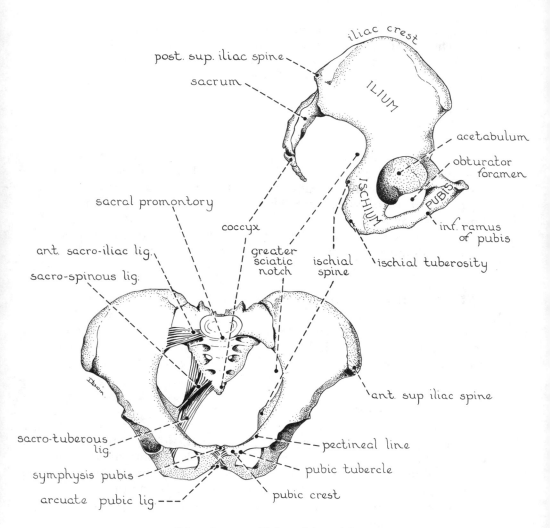

FIG. 1. Bones and joints of the pelvis.

4. The long posterior sacroiliac ligaments are each attached to the posterosuperior spine on the ilium and to the tubercles on the third and fourth sacral vertebrae.

ACCESSORY LIGAMENTS

1. The sacrotuberous ligaments are attached on one side to the posterior superior iliac spine; posterior inferior iliac spine; tubercles on the third, fourth, and fifth sacral vertebrae; and lateral border

of the coccyx. On the other side the sacrotuberous ligaments are attached to the pelvic aspect of the ischial tuberosity.

2. The sacrospinous ligament is triangular. The base is attached to the lateral parts of the fifth sacral and first coccygeal vertebrae, and the apex is attached to the ischial spine.

Sacrococcygeal Joint

The sacrococcygeal is a synovial hinge joint between the fifth sacral and the first coccygeal vertebrae. It allows both flexion and extension. Extension, by increasing the anteroposterior diameter of the outlet of the pelvis, plays an important role in parturition. Overextension during delivery may break the small cornua by which the coccyx is attached to the sacrum. This joint has a weak capsule, which is reinforced by anterior, posterior, and lateral sacrococcygeal ligaments.

Symphysis Pubis

The symphysis pubis is a cartilaginous joint with no capsule and no synovial membrane. Normally there is little movement. The posterior and superior ligaments are weak. The strong anterior ligaments are reinforced by the tendons of the rectus abdominis and the external oblique muscles. The strong inferior ligament in the pubic arch is known as the arcuate pubic ligament. It extends between the rami and leaves a small space in the subpubic angle.

MOBILITY OF PELVIS

During normal pregnancy, under the influence of progesterone and relaxin, there is increased flexibility of the sacroiliac joints and the symphysis pubis. Hyperemia and softening of the ligaments around the joints takes place also. The pubic bones may separate by 1 to 12 mm. Excessive mobility of the symphysis pubis leads to pain and difficulty in walking.

MALE AND FEMALE PELVIS

At birth there is no difference between the male and female pelvis. Sexual dimorphism does not take place until puberty. A female pelvis develops in offspring born with no gonads. Thus, ovaries and estrogen are not necessary for the formation of the female-type pelvis, but the presence of a testis that is producing androgen is essential for development of the male pelvis.

ADOLESCENCE

The pelvis of the gravid adolescent is smaller than that of the mature woman. Not only does the pelvis grow during adolescence, but it changes from an anthropoid to a gynecoid configuration. Fetopelvic disproportion occurs with greater frequency in teenaged girls than in their older counterparts.

BIBLIOGRAPHY

Aiman J: X-ray pelvimetry of the pregnant adolescent. Obstet Gynecol 48:281, 1976.

2.

Floor of the Pelvis

The pelvic floor (Fig. 1) is a muscular diaphragm that separates the pelvic cavity above from the perineal space below. It is formed by the levator ani and coccygeus muscles and is covered completely by parietal fascia.

The urogenital hiatus is an anterior gap through which the urethra and vagina pass. The rectal hiatus is posterior, and the rectum and anal canal pass through it.

PELVIC FLOOR FUNCTIONS

1. In humans it supports the pelvic viscera.
2. To build up effective intraabdominal pressure, the muscles of

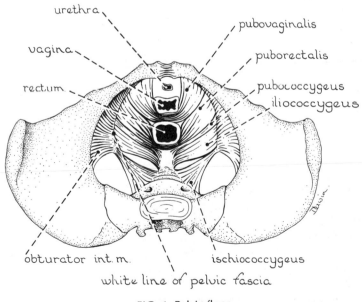

FIG. 1. Pelvic floor.

7

the diaphragm, abdominal wall, and pelvic floor must contract together.
3. The pelvic floor helps the anterior rotation of the presenting part and directs it downward and forward along the birth passage.

PELVIC FLOOR MUSCLES

1. Levators ani, each composed of two muscles:
   a. Pubococcygeus, which has three divisions: pubovaginalis, puborectalis, pubococcygeus proper
   b. Iliococcygeus
2. Coccygeus (ischiococcygeus)

Levator Ani Muscle

The levator ani muscle has a lateral origin and a central insertion, where it joins with the corresponding muscle from the other side. The direction of the muscle from origin to insertion is downward and medial. The origin of each levator ani is from the:

1. Posterior side of the pubis
2. Arcuate tendon of the pelvic fascia (the white line of the pelvic fascia)
3. Pelvic aspect of the ischial spine.

The insertion, from front to back, is into:

1. Vaginal walls
2. Central point of the perineum
3. Anal canal
4. Anococcygeal body
5. Lateral border of the coccyx

PUBOCOCCYGEUS

The pubococcygeus is the most important, most dynamic, and most specialized part of the pelvic floor. It lies in the midline; is perforated by the urethra, vagina, and rectum; and is often damaged during delivery. It originates from the posterior side of the pubis and from the part of the white line of the pelvic fascia in front of the obturator canal. The muscle passes backward and medially in three sections: (1) pubovaginalis, (2) puborectalis, and (3) pubococcygeus proper.

Pubovaginalis Muscle   The most medial section of the pubococcygeus, this muscle is shaped like a horseshoe and is open anteriorly. The fibers make contact and blend with the muscles of the urethral wall, after which they form a loop around the vagina. They insert into the sides and back of the vagina and into the central point of the perineum.

The principal function of the pubovaginalis is to act as a sling for the vagina. Since the vagina helps to support the uterus and appendages, bladder and urethra, and rectum, this muscle is the main support of the female pelvic organs. Tearing or overstretching predisposes to prolapse, cystocele, and rectocele. The muscle also functions as the vaginal sphincter, and when it goes into spasm the condition is called *vaginismus*.

Puborectalis Muscle   The intermediate part of the pubococcygeus, this muscle forms a loop around the anal canal and rectum. The insertion is into the lateral and posterior walls of the anal canal between the sphincter ani internus and externus, with whose fibers the puborectalis joins. It inserts also in the anococcygeal body.

The puborectalis suspends the rectum, but since this organ does not support the other pelvic viscera, the puborectalis plays a small role in holding up the pelvic structures. The main work of this muscle is in controlling the descent of the feces, and in so doing it acts as an auxiliary sphincter for the anal canal. When the anococcygeal junction is pulled forward, the puborectalis increases the anorectal flexure and retards the descent of feces.

Pubococcygeus Proper   This muscle is composed of the most lateral fibers of the pubococcygeus muscle. It has a Y-shaped insertion into the lateral margins of the coccyx. When it contracts it pulls the coccyx forward, increasing the anorectal juncture. Thus, in combination with the external sphincter ani it helps control the passage of feces.

ILIOCOCCYGEUS

The iliococcygeus muscles arise from the white line of the pelvic fascia behind the obturator canal. They join with the pubococcygeus muscle proper and insert into the lateral margins of the coccyx. These are less dynamic than the pubovaginalis and act more like a musculo-fascial layer.

Ischiococcygeus

The ischiococcygeus or coccygeus muscles originate from the ischial spines and insert into the lateral borders of the coccyx and the fifth sacral vertebra. These muscles supplement the levators ani and occupy most of the posterior portion of the pelvic floor.

PELVIC FLOOR DURING PARTURITION

When the presenting part has reached the proper level during the second stage of labor, the central point of the perineum becomes thin. The levator ani muscles and the anal sphincter relax, and the muscles of the pelvic floor are drawn over the advancing head. Tearing and overstretching these muscles weaken the pelvic floor and may cause extensive and irreparable damage.

3.

Perineum

The perineum is a diamond-shaped space that lies below the pelvic floor (Fig. 1). Its boundaries are as follows:

1. Superiorly: the pelvic floor, made up of the levator ani muscles and the coccygei
2. Laterally: the bones and ligaments that make up the pelvic outlet; from front to back, these are the subpubic angle, ischiopubic rami, ischial tuberosities, sacrotuberous ligaments, coccyx
3. Inferiorly: the skin and fascia

This area is divided into two triangles: anteriorly, the urogenital

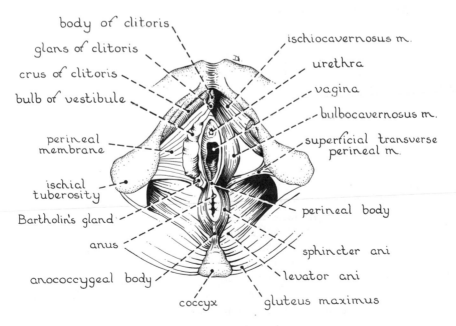

body of clitoris

glans of clitoris

crus of clitoris

bulb of vestibule

perineal membrane

ischial tuberosity

Bartholin's gland

anus

anococcygeal body

coccyx

ischiocavernosus m.

urethra

vagina

bulbocavernosus m.

superficial transverse perineal m.

perineal body

sphincter ani

levator ani

gluteus maximus

FIG. 1. Perineum.

11

triangle; posteriorly, the anal triangle. These are separated by a transverse band composed of the transverse perineal muscles and the base of the urogenital diaphragm.

UROGENITAL TRIANGLE

The urogenital triangle is bounded:

1. In front: by the subpubic angle
2. At the sides: by the ischiopubic rami and the ischial tuberosities
3. Behind: by the transverse perineal muscles and the base of the urogenital diaphragm

The urogenital triangle contains:

1. Opening of the vagina
2. Terminal part of the urethra
3. Crura of the clitoris with the ischiocavernosus muscles
4. Vestibular bulbs (erectile tissue) covered by the bulbocavernosus muscles
5. Bartholin glands and their ducts
6. Urogenital diaphragm
7. Muscles that constitute the central point of the perineum (perineal body)
8. Perineal pouches, superficial and deep
9. Blood vessels, nerves, and lymphatics

Urogenital Diaphragm

The urogenital diaphragm (triangular ligament) lies in the anterior triangle of the perineum. It is composed of muscle tissue covered by fascia.

1. The two muscles are the deep transverse perineal and the sphincter of the membranous urethra.
2. The superior layer of fascia is thin and weak.
3. The inferior fascial layer is a strong fibrous membrane. It extends from a short distance beneath the arcuate pubic ligament to the ischial tuberosities. The fascial layers fuse superiorly and form the transverse perineal ligament. Inferiorly, they join in the central point of the perineum.

The deep dorsal vein of the clitoris lies in a small space between the apex of the urogenital diaphragm and the arcuate pubic ligament. Through the diaphragm pass the urethra, the vagina, blood vessels, lymphatics, and nerves.

Superficial Perineal Pouch

The superficial perineal pouch is a space that lies between the inferior layer of the urogenital diaphragm and Colles' fascia.

SUPERFICIAL TRANSVERSE PERINEAL MUSCLES
The superficial transverse perineal muscles are the superficial parts of the deep muscles and have the same origin and insertion. These are outside the urogenital diaphragm. Sometimes they are entirely lacking.

ISCHIOCAVERNOSUS MUSCLES
The ischiocavernosus muscles cover the clitoral crura. The origin of each is the inferior ramus of the pubis, and they insert at the lateral aspect of the crus. These muscles compress the crura, and by blocking the venous return cause the clitoris to become erect.

BULBOCAVERNOSUS MUSCLE
The bulbocavernosus muscle surrounds the vagina. With the external anal sphincter it makes a figure eight around the vagina and rectum. It is also called the bulbospongiosus. It originates from the central point of the perineum and inserts into the dorsal aspect of the clitoral body. The muscle passes around the orifice of the vagina and surrounds the bulb of the vestibule.

The bulbocavernosus muscle compresses the erectile tissue around the vaginal orifice (bulb of the vestibule) and helps in the clitoral erection by closing its dorsal vein. It acts as a weak vaginal sphincter. The real sphincter of the vagina is the pubovaginalis section of the levator ani.

Deep Perineal Pouch

The deep perineal pouch lies between the two fascial layers of the urogenital diaphragm.

SPHINCTER OF THE MEMBRANOUS URETHRA
The sphincter of the membranous urethra lies between the fascial layers of the urogenital diaphragm. It is also called the compressor of the urethra.

The voluntary fibers have their origin from the inferior rami of the ischium and pubis. They join with the deep transverse perineal muscles. Their action is to expel the last drops of urine.

The involuntary fibers surround the urethra and act as its sphincter.

DEEP TRANSVERSE PERINEAL MUSCLES

The deep transverse perineal muscles lie between the layers of fascia of the urogenital diaphragm. They blend with the sphincter of the membranous urethra. The origin is the ischiopubic ramus on each side, and they insert at the central point of the perineum (perineal body).

ANAL TRIANGLE

The anal triangle is bounded:

1. Anteriorly: by the transverse perineal muscles and the base of the urogenital diaphragm
2. Laterally: by the ischial tuberosities and the sacrotuberous ligaments
3. Posteriorly: by the coccyx

The anal triangle contains the following:

1. Lower end of the anal canal and its sphincters
2. Anococcygeal body
3. Ischiorectal fossa
4. Blood vessels, lymphatics, and nerves

SPHINCTER ANI EXTERNUS

The sphincter ani externus has two parts.

1. The superficial portion surrounds the anal orifice. Its fibers are voluntary and act during defecation or in an emergency. The origin is the tip of the coccyx and the anococcygeal body. Insertion is in the central point of the perineum.
2. The deep part is an involuntary muscle that surrounds the lower part of the anal canal and acts as a sphincter for the anus. It blends with the levators ani and the internal anal sphincter. When inactive, the deep circular fibers are in a state of tonus, occluding the anal orifice.

ANOCOCCYGEAL BODY

The anococcygeal body is composed of muscle tissue (levators ani and external sphincter ani) and fibrous tissue. It is located between the tip of the coccyx and the anus.

PERINEAL BODY

The central point of the perineum or perineal body lies between the posterior angle of the vagina in front and the anus behind. In obstetrics it is referred to as the perineum. It is often torn at delivery. The following muscles meet to form this structure:

1. Sphincter ani externus
2. Two levator ani muscles
3. Superficial and deep transverse perineal muscles
4. Bulbocavernosus muscle

4.

Uterus and Vagina

UTERUS

The normal uterus is a small muscular organ in the female pelvis. It is composed of three layers:

1. An outer, covering, serous peritoneal layer—the perimetrium
2. A thick middle layer made up of muscle fibers—the myometrium
3. An inner mucous layer of glands and supporting stroma—the endometrium—which is attached directly to the myometrium

The *myometrium* is made up of three layers of muscle:

1. An outer layer of mainly longitudinal fibers.
2. An inner layer whose fibers run, for the most part, in a circular direction.
3. A thick middle layer, whose fibers are arranged in an interlacing pattern and through which the blood vessels course. When these fibers contract and retract after the products of conception have been expelled, the blood vessels are kinked and constricted. In this way postpartum bleeding is controlled.

Uterine Shape

In the nonpregnant condition and at the time of implantation the uterus is pear-shaped. By the third month of gestation the uterus is globular. From the seventh month to term the contour is again pyriform.

Uterine Size

The uterus grows from the nonpregnant dimensions of about 7.5 × 5.0 × 2.5 cm to 28 × 24 × 21 cm. The weight rises from 30 to 60 g to

1000 g at the end of pregnancy. The uterus changes from a solid organ in the nullipara to a large sac, the capacity increasing from almost nil to 4000 ml.

Uterine Location

Normally the uterus is entirely in the pelvis. As it enlarges it gradually rises, and by the fourth month of gestation it extends into the abdominal region.

Uterine Divisions

1. The fundus (Fig. 1) is the part above the openings of the fallopian tubes.
2. The body (corpus) is the main part; it has thick walls, lies between the tubal openings and the isthmus, and is the main contractile portion. During labor the contractions force the baby downward, distend the lower segment of the uterus, and dilate the cervix.
3. The isthmus is a small constricted region of the uterus. It is about 5 to 7 mm in length and lies above the internal os of the cervix.

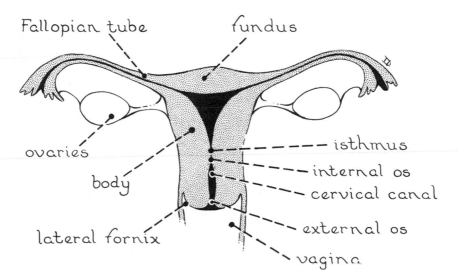

FIG. 1. Uterus, cervix, vagina.

4. The cervix (Fig. 2) is composed of a canal with an internal os in its upper portion, separating the cervix from the uterine cavity, and an external os below, which closes off the cervix from the vagina. The cervix is about 2.5 cm in length. The lower part pierces the anterior wall of the vagina, and its tissue blends with that of the vagina.

MYOMETRIUM

Most of the uterine growth takes place in the myometrium of the body and fundus. During the first half of pregnancy the main factor in uterine growth is hyperplasia (formation of new muscle fibers). In the second half hypertrophy predominates (enlargement of existing myometrial cells). Individual myometrial fibers increase tenfold during pregnancy from a nonpregnant length of 50–100 μ to 500–800 μ during pregnancy. At term the estimated number of cells is 200 billion. The myometrial fibers are composed of four major proteins: myosin, actin, tropomysin, and troponin. The main stimulus to growth is provided by 17 β-estradiol, although some myometrial hypertrophy occurs in response to stretch.

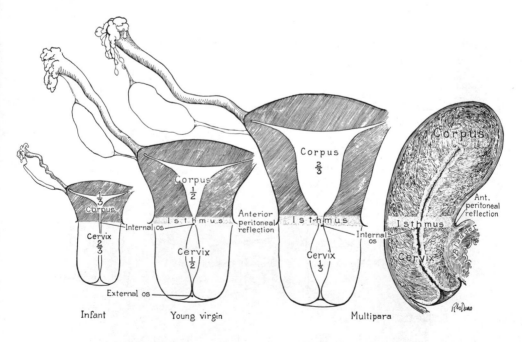

FIG. 2. Normal uterus and cervix. (From Eastman and Hellman. *Williams Obstetrics*, 14th ed, 1971. Courtesy of Appleton-Century-Crofts.)

There is also an increase in the number and size of the blood vessels and lymphatics, as well as a marked overgrowth of connective tissue.

During early pregnancy the uterine walls are thicker than in the nonpregnant woman. As gestation continues the lumen becomes larger and the walls thinner. At the end of the fifth month they are 3 to 5 mm thick and remain so until term. Thus, during late pregnancy the uterus is a large muscular sac with thin, soft, easily compressible walls. This makes the corpus indentable and enables the fetus to be palpated. The walls of the uterus are so malleable that the uterus changes shape easily and markedly to accommodate to changes in fetal size and position.

ISTHMUS

The isthmus lies between the body of the uterus and the cervix. In the human its boundaries are not well defined, and it is important as a physiologic rather than as an anatomic entity. In the nonpregnant uterus it is 5 to 7 mm long. It differs from the corpus in that it is free of mucus-secreting glands. The upper limit of the isthmus corresponds to a constriction in the lumen of the uterus which marks the lower boundary of the body of the uterus (the anatomic internal os of Aschoff). The lower limit is the site of transition from the mucosa of the isthmus to the endocervical mucous membrane (histologic internal os).

While the isthmus is of small moment in the normal state, in pregnancy it plays an important role. As the uterus grows, the isthmus increases in length (Fig. 3) to about 25 mm and becomes soft and compressible. Hegar's sign of early pregnancy depends upon palpation of the soft isthmus between the body of the uterus above and the cervix below.

The ovum implants, in the great majority of cases, in the upper part of the uterus. At about the third month the enlarging embryo grows into the isthmus, which unfolds and expands to make room for it. As this process continues, the isthmus is incorporated gradually into the general uterine cavity, and the shape of the uterus changes from pyriform to globular. The expanded isthmus forms part of the lower uterine segment of the uterus during labor. The histologic internal os becomes the internal os of pregnancy, while the anatomic internal os becomes the physiologic retraction ring of normal labor (and pathologic retraction ring of obstructed labor).

The unfolding of the isthmus continues until it has reached the firm cervix, where it stops. After the seventh month most of the enlargement takes place in the body and fundus, and the uterus becomes pear-shaped once more. At the onset of labor the lower uterine segment comprises about one-third of the whole uterus. While this area is not the passive part it was once thought to be, its contractions during normal labor are extremely weak when compared with those of the body.

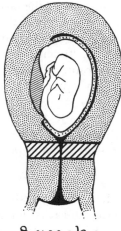

8 weeks

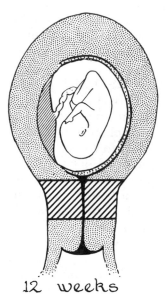

12 weeks

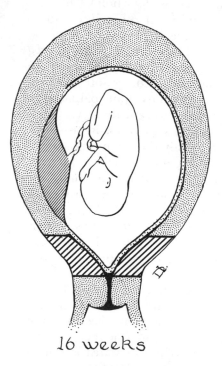

16 weeks

FIG. 3. Isthmus of pregnant uterus.

CERVIX

The cervix is composed mostly of connective tissue interspersed with muscle fibers. It feels hard and fibrous in the nonpregnant state. During pregnancy the cervix becomes progressively softer. This is caused by increased vascularity, general edema, and hyperplasia of the glands. The compound tubular glands become overactive and produce large quantities of mucus. The secretion accumulates in the cervical canal and thickens to form the so-called mucous plug. This inspissated mucus effectively seals off the canal from the vagina and prevents the ascent of bacteria and other substances into the uterine cavity. This plug is expelled early in labor.

At the end of gestation and during labor the internal os gradually disappears, and the cervical canal also becomes part of the lower uterine segment, leaving only the external os.

VAGINA

The vagina is a fibromuscular membranous tube surrounded by the vulva below, the uterus above, the bladder in front, and the rectum behind. Its direction is obliquely upward and backward. The cervix uteri enters the vagina through the anterior wall, and for this reason the anterior wall of the vagina (6 to 8 cm) is shorter than the posterior wall (7 to 10 cm). The protrusion of the cervix into the vagina divides the vaginal vault into four fornices: an anterior, a posterior, and two lateral fornices. The posterior fornix is much deeper than the others.

The wall of the vagina is made up of four layers:

1. The mucosa is the epithelial layer.
2. The submucosa is rich in blood vessels.
3. The muscularis is the third layer.
4. The outer connective tissue layer connects the vagina to the surrounding structures.

Even in the normal condition the vagina is capable of great distention, but in pregnancy this ability is increased many times. In the pregnant state there is greater vascularity, thickening and lengthening of the walls, and increased secretion, so that most women have varying quantities of vaginal discharge during the period of gestation.

5.

Obstetric Pelvis

The pelvis is made up of the two innominate bones (which occupy the front and sides) and the sacrum and coccyx (which are behind). The bones articulate through four joints. The sacroiliac joint is the most important, linking the sacrum to the iliac part of the innominate bones. The symphysis of the pubis joins the two pubic bones. The sacrococcygeal joint attaches the sacrum to the coccyx.

The *false pelvis* lies above the true pelvis, superior to the linea terminalis. Its only obstetric function is to support the enlarged uterus during pregnancy. Its boundaries are:

1. Posteriorly: lumbar vertebrae
2. Laterally: iliac fossae
3. Anteriorly: anterior abdominal wall

The *true pelvis* (Fig. 1A) lies below the pelvic brim, or linea terminalis, and is the bony canal through which the baby must pass. It is divided into three parts: (1) the inlet, (2) the pelvic cavity, and (3) the pelvic outlet.

The *inlet* (pelvic brim) is bounded:

1. Anteriorly: by the pubic crest and spine
2. Laterally, by the iliopectineal lines on the innominate bones
3. Posteriorly, by the anterior borders of the ala and promontory of the sacrum

The *pelvic cavity* (Fig. 1B) is a curved canal.

1. The anterior wall is straight and shallow. The pubis is 5 cm long.
2. The posterior wall is deep and concave. The sacrum is 10 to 15 cm long.
3. The ischium and part of the body of the ilium are found laterally.

The *pelvic outlet* is diamond-shaped. It is bounded:

1. Anteriorly: by the arcuate pubic ligament and the pubic arch

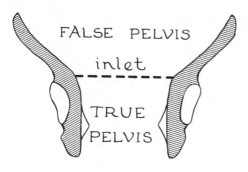

A. True pelvis.

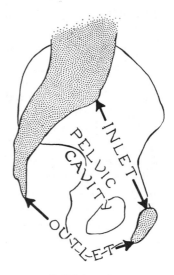

B. Pelvic cavity.

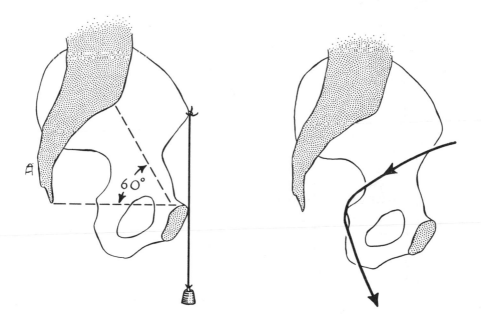

C. Pelvic inclination.

D. Axis of birth canal.

FIG. 1. Pelvic cavity.

2. Laterally: by the ischial tuberosity and the sacrotuberous ligament
3. Posteriorly: by the tip of the sacrum

The *pelvic inclination* (Fig. 1C) is assessed when the woman is in the upright position. The plane of the pelvic brim makes an angle of about 60° with the horizontal. The anterior superior iliac spine is in the same vertical plane as the pubic spine.

The *axis of the birth canal* (Fig. 1D) is the course taken by the presenting part as it passes through the pelvis. At first it moves downward and backward to the level of the ischial spines, which is the area of the bony attachment of the pelvic floor muscles. Here the direction changes and the presenting part proceeds downward and forward.

The *pelvic planes* (Fig. 2) are imaginary flat surfaces passing across the pelvis at different levels. They are used for the purposes of description. The important ones are as follows:

1. The plane of the inlet is also called the superior strait.
2. The pelvic cavity has many planes, two of which are the plane of greatest dimensions and the plane of least dimensions.
3. The plane of the outlet is also called the inferior strait.

The *diameters* are distances between given points. Important ones are the following:

1. Anteroposterior diameters.
2. Transverse diameters.
3. Left oblique: Oblique diameters are designated left or right according to their posterior terminal.
4. Right oblique.
5. Posterior sagittal diameter: This is the back part of the anteroposterior diameter, extending from the intersection of the transverse and anteroposterior diameters to the posterior limit of the latter.
6. Anterior sagittal diameter: This is the front part of the anteroposterior diameter, extending from the intersection of the transverse and anteroposterior diameter to the anterior limit of the latter.

OBSTETRIC PELVIS

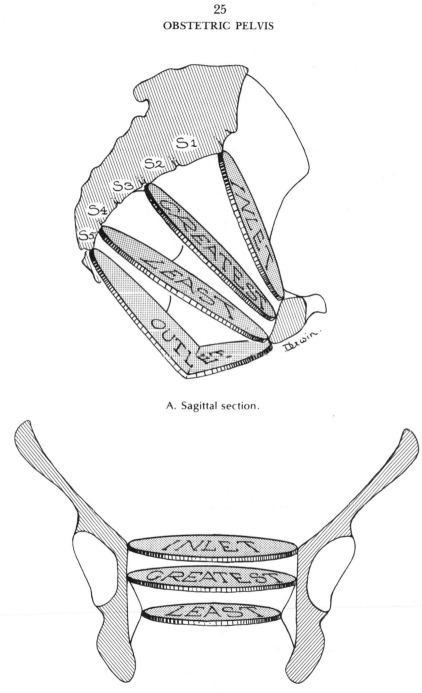

A. Sagittal section.

B. Coronal section.

FIG. 2. Pelvic planes.

PELVIC INLET

Plane of Obstetric Inlet

The plane of the obstetric inlet is bounded:

1. Anteriorly: by the posterior superior margin of the pubic symphysis
2. Laterally: by the iliopectineal lines
3. Posteriorly: by the promontory and ala of the sacrum

Diameters of Inlet

The diameters of the inlet are as follows:

1. Anteroposterior diameters:
   a. The anatomic conjugate (Fig. 3) extends from the middle of the sacral promontory to the middle of the pubic crest (superior surface of the pubis). It measures 11.5 cm. It has no obstetric significance.
   b. The obstetric conjugate extends from the middle of the sacral promontory to the posterior superior margin of the pubic symphysis. This point on the pubis, which protrudes back into the cavity of the pelvis, is about 1 cm below the pubic crest. The obstetric conjugate is about 11.0 cm in length. This is the important anteroposterior diameter, since it is the one through which the fetus must pass.
   c. The diagonal conjugate extends from the subpubic angle to the middle of the sacral promontory. It is 12.5 cm in length. This diameter can be measured manually in the patient. It is of clinical significance because by subtracting 1.5 cm an approximate length of the obstetric conjugate can be obtained.
2. Transverse diameter is the widest distance between the iliopectineal lines and is 13.5 cm.
3. Left oblique diameter extends from the left sacroiliac joint to the right iliopectineal eminence and is about 12.5 cm.
4. Right oblique diameter extends from the right sacroiliac joint to the left iliopectineal eminence and is about 12.5 cm.
5. Posterior sagittal extends from the intersection of the anteroposterior and transverse diameters to the middle of the sacral promontory and is about 4.5 cm long.

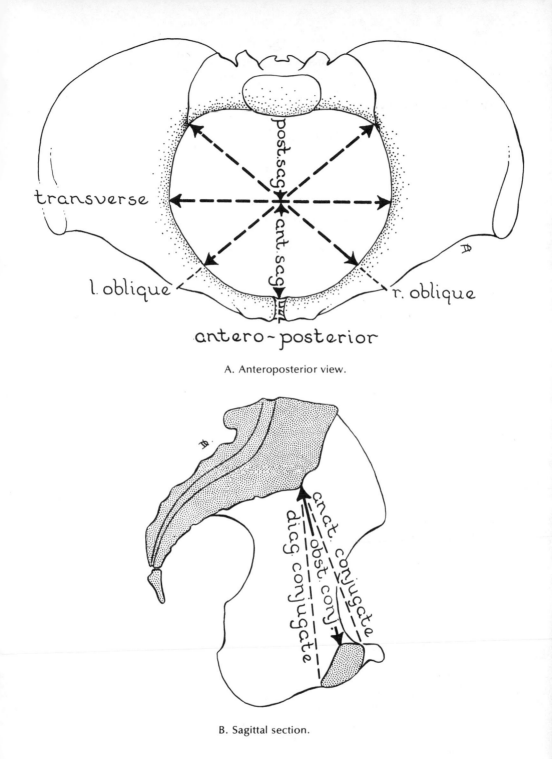

A. Anteroposterior view.

B. Sagittal section.

FIG. 3. Pelvic inlet.

PELVIC CAVITY

The pelvic cavity extends from the inlet to the outlet.

Plane of Greatest Dimensions

This is the roomiest part of the pelvis and is almost circular. Its obstetric significance is small. Its boundaries are:

1. Anteriorly: midpoint of the posterior surface of the pubis
2. Laterally: upper and middle thirds of the obturator foramina
3. Posteriorly: the junction of the second and third sacral vertebrae

The diameters of importance are:

1. The anteroposterior diameter extends from the midpoint of the posterior surface of the pubis to the junction of the second and third sacral vertebrae and measures 12.75 cm.
2. The transverse diameter is the widest distance between the lateral aspects of the plane and is 12.5 cm.

Plane of Least Dimensions

This is the most important plane of the pelvis (Fig. 4). It has the least room, and it is here that most instances of arrest of progress take place. This plane extends from the apex of the subpubic arch, through the ischial spines, to the sacrum, usually at or near the junction of the fourth and fifth sacral vertebrae. The boundaries are, from front to back:

1. Lower border of the pubic symphysis
2. White line on the fascia covering the obturator foramina
3. Ischial spines
4. Sacrospinous ligaments
5. Sacrum

The diameters of importance are:

1. Anteroposterior diameter, extending from the lower border of the pubic symphysis to the junction of the fourth and fifth sacral vertebrae and measuring 12.0 cm
2. Transverse diameter, lying between the ischial spines and measuring 10.5 cm

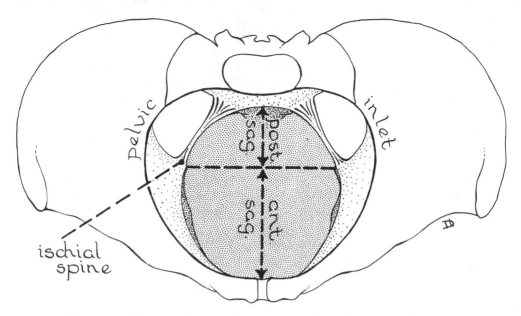

A. Anteroposterior view showing the anteroposterior and transverse diameters.

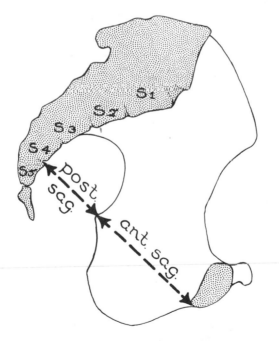

B. Sagittal section showing the anteroposterior diameter.

FIG. 4. Pelvic cavity: the plane of least dimensions.

3. Posterior sagittal diameter, extending from the bispinous diameter to the junction of the fourth and fifth sacral vertebrae and measuring 4.5 to 5.0 cm

PELVIC OUTLET

The outlet is made up of two triangular planes, having as their common base and most inferior part the transverse diameter between the ischial tuberosities (Fig. 5).

Anterior Triangle

The anterior triangle has the following boundaries:

1. The base is the bituberous diameter (transverse diameter).
2. The apex is the subpubic angle.
3. The sides are the pubic rami and ischial tuberosities.

Posterior Triangle

The posterior triangle has the following boundaries:

1. The base is the bituberous diameter.
2. The obstetric apex is the sacrococcygeal joint.
3. The sides are the sacrotuberous ligaments.

Diameters of the Outlet

1. The anatomic anteroposterior diameter is from the inferior margin of the pubic symphysis to the tip of the coccyx. It measures about 9.5 cm. The obstetric anteroposterior diameter is from the inferior margin of the pubic symphysis to the sacrococcygeal joint. This measures 11.5 cm. Because of the mobility at the sacrococcygeal joint, the coccyx is pushed out of the way by the advancing presenting part, increasing the available space.
2. The transverse diameter is the distance between the inner surfaces of the ischial tuberosities and measures about 11.0 cm.
3. The posterior sagittal diameter extends from the middle of the transverse diameter to the sacrococcygeal junction and is 9.0 cm.
4. The anterior sagittal diameter extends from the middle of the transverse diameter to the subpubic angle and measures 6.0 cm.

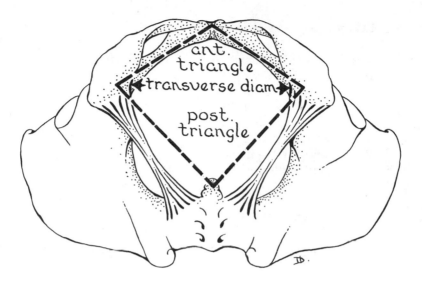

A. Inferior view.

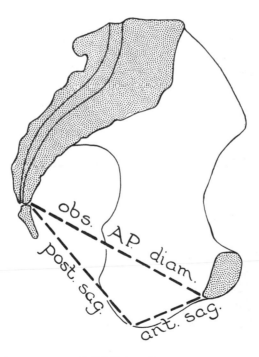

B. Sagittal section.

FIG. 5. Pelvic outlet.

IMPORTANT MEASUREMENTS

In assessing the obstetric capacity of the pelvis the most important measurements are the following:

1. Obstetric conjugate of the inlet
2. Distance between the ischial spines
3. Subpubic angle and bituberous diameter
4. Posterior sagittal diameters of the three planes
5. Curve and length of the sacrum

CLASSIFICATION OF THE PELVIS

Variations in the female pelvis and in the planes of any single pelvis are so great that a rigid classification is not possible. A pelvis of the female type in one plane may be predominantly male in another. Many pelves are mixed in that the various planes do not conform to a single parent type.

For the purpose of classification the pelvis is named on the basis of the inlet, and mention is made of nonconforming characteristics. For example, a pelvis may be described as a female type with male features at the outlet.

We prefer the classification of Caldwell and Moloy (Table 1 and Figs. 6 through 8).

TABLE 1. Classification of Pelvis (Caldwell and Moloy)

	Gynecoid	Android	Anthropoid	Platypelloid
INLET				
Sex type	Normal female	Male	Ape-like	Flat female
Incidence	50 percent	20 percent	25 percent	5 percent
Shape	Round or transverse oval; transverse diameter is a little longer than the anteroposterior	Heart or wedge shaped	Long antero-posterior oval	Transverse oval
Anteroposterior diameter	Adequate	Adequate	Long	Short
Transverse diameter	Adequate	Adequate	Adequate, but relatively short	Long
Posterior sagittal diameter	Adequate	Very short and inadequate	Very long	Very short
Anterior sagittal diameter	Adequate	Long	Long	Short

TABLE 1. (cont.)

	Gynecoid	Android	Anthropoid	Platypelloid
Posterior segment	Broad, deep, roomy	Shallow; sacral promontory indents the inlet and reduces its capacity	Deep	Shallow
Anterior segment	Well rounded forepelvis	Narrow, sharply angulated forepelvis	Deep	Shallow

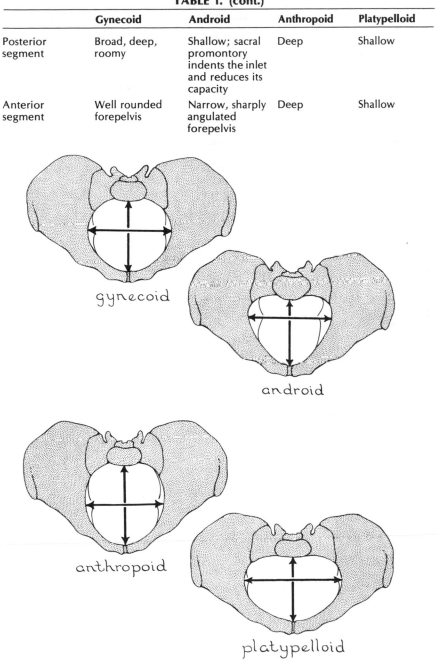

FIG. 6. Pelvic inlet (Caldwell-Moloy classification).

TABLE 1. (cont.)

	Gynecoid	Android	Anthropoid	Platypelloid
PELVIC CAVITY: MIDPELVIS				
Anteroposterior diameter	Adequate	Reduced	Long	Shortened
Transverse diameter	Adequate	Reduced	Adequate	Wide
Posterior sagittal diameter	Adequate	Reduced	Adequate	Shortened
Anterior sagittal diameter	Adequate	Reduced	Adequate	Short
Sacrum	Wide, deep curve; short; slopes backward; light bone	Flat; inclined forward; long; narrow; heavy	Inclined backward; narrow; long	Wide, deep curve; often sharply angulated with enlarged sacral fossa
Sidewalls	Parallel, straight	Convergent; funnel pelvis	Straight	Parallel
Ischial spines	Not prominent	Prominent	Variable	Variable
Sacrosciatic notch	Wide; short	Narrow; long; high arch	Wide	Short
Depth: iliopectineal eminence to tuberosities	Average	Long	Long	Short
Capacity	Adequate	Reduced in all diameters	Adequate	Reduced

CLASSIFICATION OF THE PELVIS

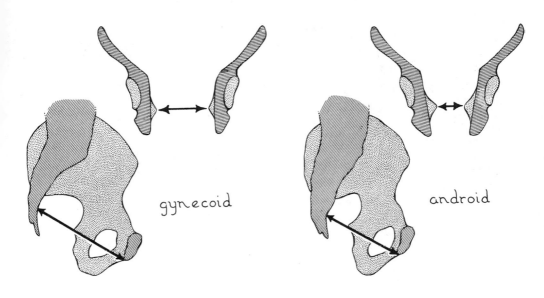

gynecoid

android

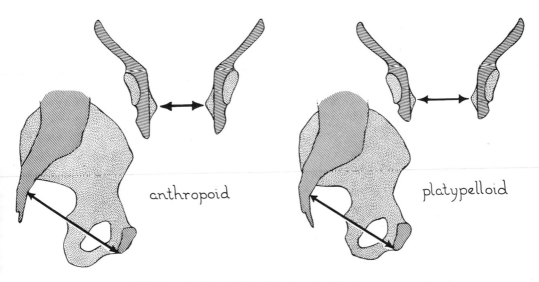

anthropoid

platypelloid

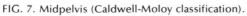

FIG. 7. Midpelvis (Caldwell-Moloy classification).

TABLE 1. (cont.)

	Gynecoid	Android	Anthropoid	Platypelloid
OUTLET				
Anteroposterior diameter	Long	Short	Long	Short
Transverse diameter (bituberous)	Adequate	Narrow	Adequate	Wide
Pubic arch	Wide and round; 90°	Narrow; deep; 70°	Normal or relatively narrow	Very wide
Inferior pubic rami	Short; concave inward	Straight; long	Long; relatively narrow	Straight; short
Capacity	Adequate	Reduced	Adequate	Inadequate
EFFECT ON LABOR				
Fetal head	Engages in transverse or oblique diameter in slight asynclitism; good flexion; OA is common	Engages in transverse or posterior diameter in asynclitism; extreme molding	Engages in anteroposterior or oblique; often occiput posterior	Engages in transverse diameter with marked asynclitism
Labor	Good uterine function; early and complete internal rotation; spontaneous delivery; wide pubic arch reduces perineal tears	Deep transverse arrest is common; arrest as OP with failure of rotation; delivery is often by difficult forceps application, rotation, and extraction; the narrow pubic arch may lead to major perineal tears	Delivery and labor usually easy; birth face to pubis is common	Delay at inlet
Prognosis	Good	Poor	Good	Poor; disproportion; delay at inlet; labor often terminated by cesarean section

CLASSIFICATION OF THE PELVIS

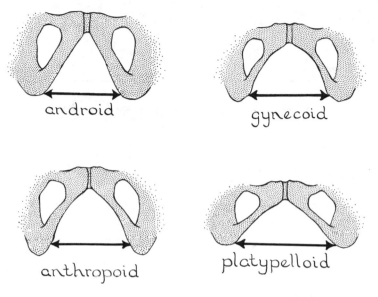

FIG. 8. Pelvic outlet (Caldwell-Moloy classification).

The Passenger: Fetus

GENERAL CONSIDERATIONS

1. Resemblance to the adult human form may be perceptible at the end of 8 weeks and is obvious at the end of 12 weeks.
2. By the end of 12 weeks, and sometimes sooner, the sexual differences in the external genitalia may be recognized in abortuses.
3. Growth is greatest during the sixth and seventh months of intrauterine life.
4. Quickening (the perception by the pregnant woman of fetal movements in utero) occurs between the 16th and 20th weeks of pregnancy. The time of quickening is too variable to be of value in determining the expected date of confinement or when term has been reached. Active intestinal peristalsis is the most common phenomenon mistaken for quickening.
5. The fetal heart is audible by the 18th or 20th week.
6. The average length of the fetus at term is 50 cm.
7. Within wide variations the average male (7.5 pounds or 3400 g) is a little heavier at birth than the female (7.0 pounds or 3150 g).
8. In premature babies the circumference of the head is relatively large as compared with the shoulders. As the fetus matures the body grows faster than the head, so that at term the circumferences of the head and the shoulders are nearly the same.

FETAL OVOIDS

In its passage through the pelvis the fetus presents two oval parts, movable on each other at the neck. The oval of the head is longer in its anteroposterior diameter, while that of the shoulders and body is longer transversely. Thus, the two ovoids are perpendicular to each other.

FETAL HEAD

From the obstetric standpoint the fetal head (Fig. 1) is the most important part of the fetus. It is the largest, the least compressible, and the most

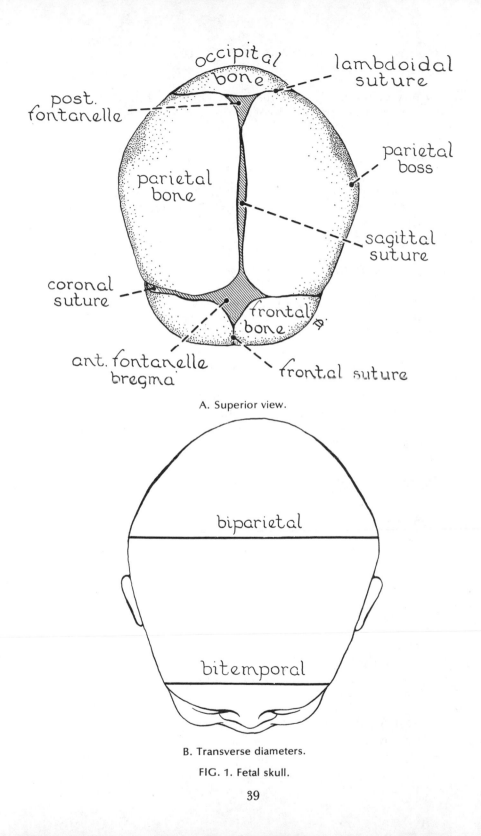

A. Superior view.

B. Transverse diameters.

FIG. 1. Fetal skull.

frequently presenting part of the baby. Once the head has been born, rarely is there delay or difficulty with the remainder of the body.

Base of Skull

The bones of the base of the skull are large, ossified, firmly united, and not compressible. Their function is to protect the vital centers in the brain stem.

Vault of Skull: Cranium

The cranium is made up of several bones. Important ones are the occipital bone posteriorly, the two parietal bones on the sides, and the two temporal and the two frontal bones anteriorly. The bones of the cranial vault are laid down in membrane. At birth they are thin, poorly ossified, easily compressible, and joined only by membrane. This looseness of union of the bones (actually there are spaces between them) permits their overlapping under pressure. In this way the head can change its shape to fit the maternal pelvis, an important function known as *molding*. The top of the skull is wider posteriorly (biparietal diameter) than anteriorly (bitemporal diameter).

Sutures of Skull

Sutures are membrane-occupied spaces between the bones. They are useful in two ways:

1. Their presence makes molding possible.
2. By identifying the sutures on vaginal examination, the position of the baby's head can be diagnosed. The important sutures include the following.

SAGITTAL SUTURE
The sagittal suture lies between the parietal bones. It runs in an anteroposterior direction between the fontanelles and divides the head into left and right halves.

LAMBDOIDAL SUTURES
The lambdoidal sutures extend transversely from the posterior fontanelle and separate the occipital bone from the two parietals.

CORONAL SUTURES
The coronal sutures extend transversely from the anterior fontanelle and lie between the parietal and frontal bones (Fig. 1).

FRONTAL SUTURE
The frontal suture is between the two frontal bones and is an anterior continuation of the sagittal suture. It extends from the glabella to the bregma.

Fontanelles

Where the sutures intersect are the membrane-filled spaces known as fontanelles. Two are important: the anterior and the posterior. These areas are useful clinically in two ways:

1. Their identification helps in diagnosing the position of the fetal head in the pelvis.
2. The large fontanelle is examined in assessing the condition of the child after birth. In dehydrated infants the fontanelle is depressed below the surface of the bony skull. When the intracranial pressure is elevated, the fontanelle is bulging, tense, and raised above the level of the skull.

ANTERIOR FONTANELLE
The anterior fontanelle (bregma) is at the junction of the sagittal, frontal, and coronal sutures. It is by far the larger of the two, measuring about 3 × 2 cm, and is diamond-shaped. It becomes ossified by 18 months of age. The anterior fontanelle facilitates molding. By remaining patent long after birth it plays a part in accommodating the remarkable growth of the brain.

POSTERIOR FONTANELLE
The posterior fontanelle (lambda) is located where the sagittal suture meets the two lambdoidals. The skull is not truly deficient at this point, and the area is a meeting point of the sutures rather than a true fontanelle. It is much smaller than the anterior one. The intersection of the sutures makes a Y with the sagittal suture as the base and the lambdoidals as the arms. This fontanelle closes at 6 to 8 weeks of age.

Landmarks of Skull

From posterior to anterior certain areas are identified (Fig. 2A).

1. Occiput: the area of the back of the head occupied by the occipital bone. It is behind and inferior to the posterior fontanelle and the lambdoidal sutures.
2. Posterior fontanelle.
3. Vertex: the area between the two fontanelles. It is the top of the skull and is bounded laterally by the parietal bosses.
4. Bregma or large anterior fontanelle.
5. Sinciput (or brow): the region bounded superiorly by the bregma and the coronal sutures, inferiorly by the glabella and the orbital ridges.
6. Glabella: the elevated area between the orbital ridges.
7. Nasion: the root of the nose.
8. Parietal bosses: two eminences, one on the side of each parietal bone. The distance between them is the widest transverse diameter of the fetal head.

Diameters of Fetal Skull

The diameters are distances between given points on the fetal skull (Fig. 2B). Their size varies, and the particular anteroposterior diameter that presents to the maternal pelvis depends on the degree of flexion or extension of the fetal head.

1. The biparietal diameter (Fig. 1B) is between the parietal bosses. It is the largest transverse diameter and measures 9.5 cm.
2. The bitemporal diameter lies between the temporal bones. It is 8.0 cm in length and is the shortest transverse diameter.
3. The suboccipitobregmatic diameter extends from the under surface of the occipital bone, where it meets the neck, to the center of the bregma. It is 9.5 cm long. It is the anteroposterior diameter that presents when the head is flexed well.
4. The occipitofrontal diameter presents in the military attitude, neither flexion nor extension. It extends from the external occipital protuberance to the glabella and is 11.0 cm long.
5. The verticomental diameter is involved in brow presentations (halfway extension of the head). It runs from the vertex to the chin, measures 13.5 cm, and is the longest anteroposterior diameter of the head.
6. The submentobregmatic is the diameter in face presentations

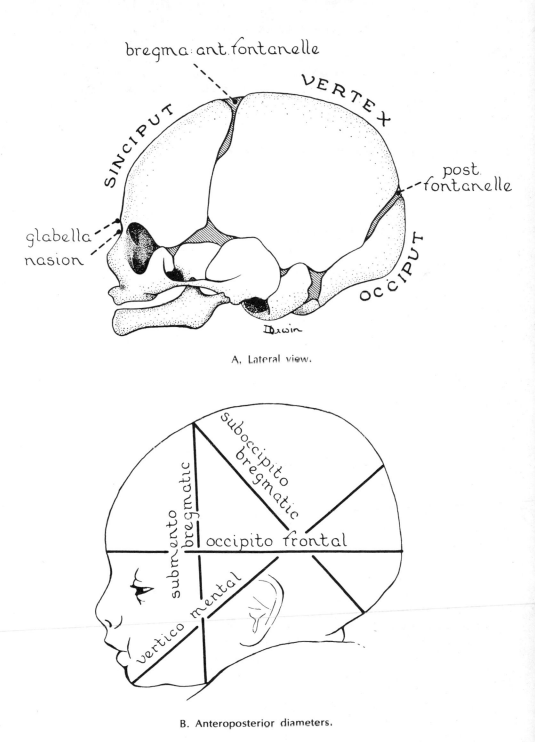

A. Lateral view.

B. Anteroposterior diameters.

FIG. 2. Landmarks and diameters of fetal skull.

43

(complete extension of the head). Reaching from the junction of the neck and lower jaw to the center of the bregma, it is 9.5 cm long.

Circumferences of Fetal Skull and Shoulders

1. In the occipitofrontal plane the circumference of the head is 34.5 cm.
2. In the suboccipitobregmatic plane it is 32 to 34 cm.
3. At term the bisacromial diameter of the shoulders is 33 to 34 cm.

Molding

Molding is the ability of the fetal head to change its shape and so adapt itself to the unyielding maternal pelvis (Fig. 3). This property is of the greatest value in the progress of labor and descent of the head through the birth canal.

The fetal bones are joined loosely by membranes so that actual spaces exist between the edges of the bones. This permits the bones to alter their relationships to each other as pressure is exerted on the head by the bony pelvis; the bones can come closer to each other or move apart. The side-to-side relationships of the bones are changeable, and one bone is able to override the other. When such overlapping takes place, the frontal and occipital bones pass under the parietal bones. The posterior parietal bone is subjected to greater pressure by the sacral promontory; therefore it passes beneath the anterior parietal bone. A contributing factor to molding is the softness of the bones.

Compression in one direction is accompanied by expansion in another, and hence the actual volume of the skull is not reduced. Provided that molding is not excessive and that it takes place slowly, no damage is done to the brain.

Alteration of the shape of the head is produced by compression of the presenting diameter, with resultant bulging of the diameter that is at right angles. For example, in the occipitoanterior position the suboccipitobregmatic is the presenting diameter. The head therefore is elongated in the verticomental diameter, with bulging behind and above.

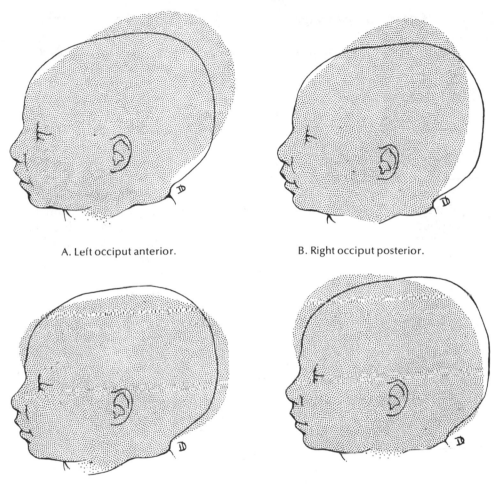

A. Left occiput anterior.

B. Right occiput posterior.

C. Face presentation.

D. Brow presentation.

FIG. 3. Molding.

Caput Succedaneum

The caput succedaneum is a localized swelling of the scalp formed by the effusion of serum (Fig. 4). Pressure of the cervical ring causes obstruction of the venous return, so that the part of the scalp that lies within the cervix becomes edematous. The caput forms during labor and after the membranes have been ruptured. It is absent if the baby is dead, the contractions are poor, or the cervix is not applied closely to the head.

The location of the caput varies with the position of the head. In occipitoanterior (OA) positions the caput forms on the vertex, to the right of the sagittal suture in left (L)OA, and to the left in right (R)OA. As flexion becomes more pronounced during labor, the posterior part of the vertex becomes the presenting part and the caput is found in that region, a little to the right or left as before. Thus, when the position is LOA the caput is on the posterior part of the right parietal bone, and in ROA on the posterior part of the left parietal bone.

The size of the caput succedaneum is an indication of the amount of pressure that has been exerted against the head. A large one suggests strong pressure from above and resistance from below. A small caput is present when the contractions have been weak or the resistance feeble. The largest are found in contracted pelves after long, hard labor. In the presence of prolonged labor a large caput suggests disproportion or occipitoposterior position, while a small one indicates uterine inertia.

In performing rectal or vaginal examinations during labor one must take care to distinguish between the station of the caput and that of the skull. The enlarging caput may make the accoucheur believe that the head is descending, when in reality it means that advancement of the head is delayed or arrested. A growing caput is an indication for reassessing the situation.

The caput is present at birth, begins to disappear immediately afterward, and is usually gone after 24 to 36 hours.

Cephalhematoma

Cephalhematoma is a hemorrhage under the periosteum of one or more of the bones of the skull (Fig. 4D). It is situated on one or, rarely, both parietal bones and is similar in appearance to a caput succedaneum. A cephalhematoma is caused by trauma to the skull, including:

1. Prolonged pressure of the head against the cervix, perineum, or pubic bones
2. Damage from forceps blades

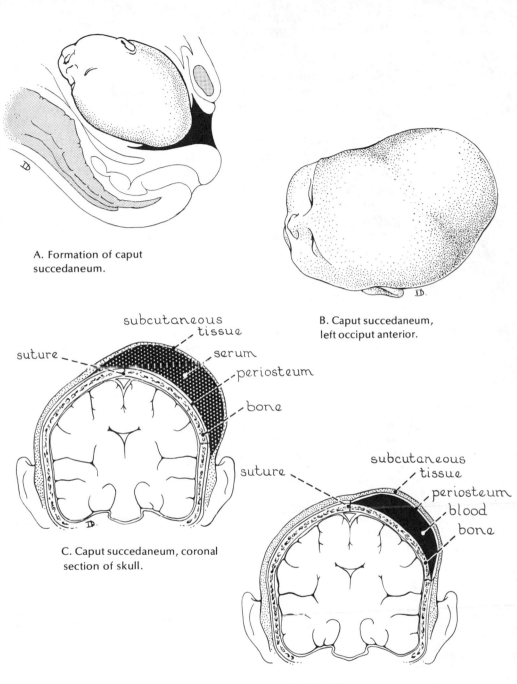

A. Formation of caput succedaneum.

B. Caput succedaneum, left occiput anterior.

subcutaneous tissue

suture

serum

periosteum

bone

C. Caput succedaneum, coronal section of skull.

suture

subcutaneous tissue

periosteum

blood

bone

D. Cephalhematoma, coronal section of skull.

FIG. 4. Caput succedaneum (CS) and cephalhematoma.

3. Difficult manual rotation of the head
4. Rapid compression and relaxation of the forces that act on the fetal head, as in precipitate births

This injury may occur also during normal spontaneous delivery.

Since the hemorrhage is under the periosteum, the swelling is limited to the affected bone and does not cross the suture lines; this is one way of distinguishing it from a caput succedaneum. The swelling appears within a few hours of birth, and since absorption is slow it takes 6 to 12 weeks to disappear. The blood clots early at the edges and remains fluid to the center. Rarely, ossification takes place in the clot and may cause a permanent deformity of the skull. The health of the child is not affected, and the brain is not damaged.

The prognosis is good. No local treatment is indicated. Vitamin K may be given to reduce further bleeding. The area should be protected from injury, but no attempt is made to evacuate the blood. Rarely, infection ensues with formation of an abscess that must be drained. The differential diagnosis of caput succedaneum and cephalhematoma includes these criteria:

Caput succedaneum	Cephalhematoma
Present at birth	May not appear for several hours
Soft, pits on pressure	Soft, does not pit
Diffuse swelling	Sharply circumscribed
Lies over and crosses the sutures	Limited to individual bones, does not cross suture lines
Movable on skull, seeks dependent portions	Fixed to original site
Is largest at birth and immediately begins to grow smaller, disappearing in a few hours	Appears after a few hours, grows larger for a time, and disappears only after weeks or months

Meningocele

A meningocele is a hernial protrusion of the meninges. It is a serious congenital deformity and must be distinguished from caput succedaneum and cephalhematoma. The meningocele always lies over a suture or a fontanelle and becomes tense when the baby cries.

7.

Fetopelvic Relationships

DEFINITIONS

LIE   Relationship of the long axis of the fetus to the long axis of the mother.

PRESENTATION   The part of the fetus that lies over the inlet. The three main presentations are cephalic (head first), breech (pelvis first), and shoulder.

PRESENTING PART   The most dependent part of the fetus, lying nearest the cervix. During vaginal or rectal examination it is the area with which the finger makes contact first.

ATTITUDE   Relation of fetal parts to each other. The basic attitudes are flexion and extension. The fetal head is in flexion when the chin approaches the chest and in extension when the occiput nears the back. The typical fetal attitude in the uterus is flexion, with the head bent in front of the chest, the arms and legs folded in front of the body, and the back curved forward slightly.

DENOMINATOR   An arbitrarily chosen point on the presenting part of the fetus used in describing position. Each presentation has its own denominator.

POSITION   Relationship of the denominator to the front, back, or sides of the maternal pelvis.

LIE

The two lies are: (1) longitudinal, when the long axes of the fetus and mother are parallel; and (2) transverse, or oblique, when the long axis of the fetus is perpendicular or oblique to the long axis of the mother.

All terms of direction refer to the mother in the standing position. Upper means toward the maternal head, and lower toward the feet. Anterior, posterior, right, and left refer to the mother's front, back, right, and left, respectively.

Longitudinal Lies

Longitudinal lies are grouped into: (1) cephalic, when the head comes first; and (2) breech, when the buttocks or lower limbs lead the way (Table 1).

CEPHALIC PRESENTATIONS

Cephalic presentations are classified into four main groups, according to the attitude of the fetal head:

1. Flexion is present when the baby's chin is near its chest (Fig. 1A). The posterior part of the vertex is the presenting part, and the occiput is the denominator.
2. The position with neither flexion nor extension is called the military attitude or the median vertex presentation (Fig. 1B). The

TABLE 1. Fetopelvic Relationships According to Fetal Position

Presentation	Attitude	Presenting Part	Denominator
Longitudinal lie (99.5%)			
Cephalic (96 to 97%)	Flexion	Vertex (posterior part)	Occiput (O)
	Military	Vertex (median part)	Occiput (O)
	Partial extension	Brow	Forehead (frontum) (Fr)
	Complete extension	Face	Chin (mentum) (M)
Breech (3 to 4%)			
Complete	Flexed hips, knees	Buttocks	Sacrum (S)
Frank	Flexed hips, extended knees	Buttocks	Sacrum (S)
Footling: single, double	Extended hips, knees	Feet	Sacrum (S)
Kneeling: single, double	Extended hips; flexed knees	Knees	Sacrum (S)
Transverse or oblique lie (0.5%)			
Shoulder	Variable	Shoulder, arm, trunk	Scapula (Sc)

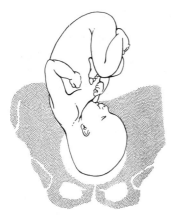

A. Flexion of head.

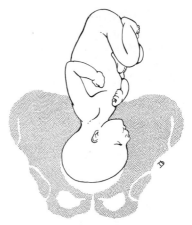

B. Military attitude.

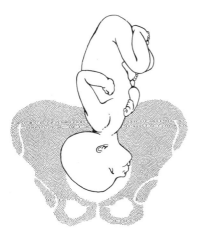

C. Brow presentation, partial
extension.

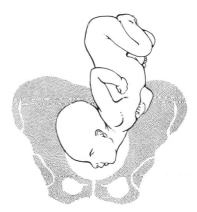

D. Face presentation, complete
extension.

FIG. 1. Attitude.

    vertex (area between the two fontanelles) presents, and the occiput
is the denominator.
3. In brow presentation (Fig. 1C) there is halfway extension. The
frontum (forehead) leads the way and is also the denominator.
4. When extension is complete the presenting part is the face (Fig.
1D), and the denominator is the mentum (chin).

BREECH PRESENTATIONS

Breech or pelvic presentations are classified according to the attitudes at the hips and knees (Fig. 2).

1. The breech is complete when there is flexion at both hips and knees. The buttocks are the presenting part.
2. Flexion at the hips and extension at the knees change it to a frank breech. The lower limbs lie anterior to the baby's abdomen. The buttocks lead the way.
3. When there is extension both at the hips and at the knees we have a footling breech—single if one foot is presenting, and double if both feet are down.
4. Extension at the hips and flexion at the knees make it a kneeling breech, single or double. Here the knees present.

In all variations of breech presentation the sacrum is the denominator.

Transverse or Oblique Lie

Transverse or oblique lie (Fig. 3) exists when the long axis of the fetus is perpendicular or oblique to the long axis of the mother. Most often the shoulder is the presenting part, but it may be an arm or some part of the trunk, such as the back, abdomen, or side. The scapula is the denominator. The position is anterior or posterior depending on the situation of the scapulas, and right or left according to the location of the head.

POSITION

Position is the relationship of the denominator to the front, back, or sides of the mother's pelvis. The pelvic girdle has a circumference of 360°. The denominator can occupy any part of the circumference. In practice, eight points, 45° from each other, are demarcated, and the position of the fetus is described as the relationship between the denominator and one of these landmarks.

Three sets of terms are used to describe position: the *denominator;* *right* or *left,* depending upon which side of the maternal pelvis the denominator is in; and *anterior, posterior,* or *transverse,* according to whether the denominator is in the front, in the back, or at the side of the pelvis.

With the patient lying in the lithotomy position, the pubic symphysis is anterior and the sacrum posterior. Starting at the symphysis and moving

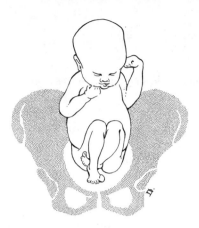

A. Complete breech.

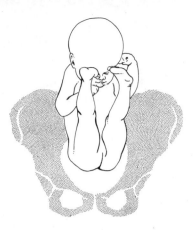

B. Frank breech.

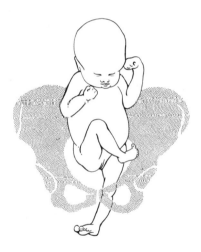

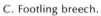

C. Footling breech.

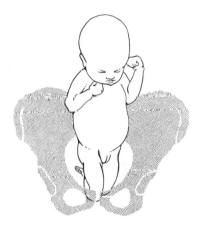

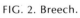

D. Kneeling breech.

FIG. 2. Breech.

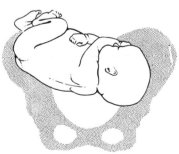

FIG. 3. Transverse lie.

in a clockwise direction, eight positions are described in succession, each 45° from the preceding one (Fig. 4A).

1. Denominator anterior (DA): The denominator is situated directly under the pubic symphysis.
2. Left denominator anterior (LDA): The denominator is in the anterior part of the pelvis, 45° to the left of the midline.
3. Left denominator transverse (LDT): The denominator is on the left side of the pelvis, 90° from the midline, at 3 o'clock.
4. Left denominator posterior (LDP): The denominator is now in the posterior segment of the pelvis and is 45° to the left of the midline.
5. Denominator posterior (DP): The denominator has rotated a total of 180° and is now in the posterior part of the pelvis, directly in the midline and directly above the sacrum.
6. Right denominator posterior (RDP): The denominator is in the posterior part of the pelvis, 45° to the right of the midline.
7. Right denominator transverse (RDT): The denominator is on the right side of the pelvis, 90° from the midline, at 9 o'clock.
8. Right denominator anterior (RDA): The denominator is in the anterior segment of the pelvis, 45° to the right of the midline.

Further rotation of 45° completes the circle of 360°, and the denominator is back under the symphysis pubis in the denominator anterior position.

This method of describing position is used for every presentation. Each presentation has its own denominator, but the basic descriptive terminology is the same.

Figure 4A demonstrates the various positions in which the vertex is the presenting part. The occiput (back of the head) is the denominator, and the eight positions (moving clockwise) are: OA—LOA—LOT—LOP—OP—ROP—ROT—ROA—OA.

In face presentations (Fig. 4B) the chin (mentum) is the denominator, and the sequence of positions is: MA—LMA—LMT—LMP—MP—RMP—RMT—RMA—MA.

A further example would be in breech presentations where the sacrum is the denominator (Fig. 4C). Here the eight positions are: SA—LSA—LST—LSP—SP—RSP—RST—RSA—SA.

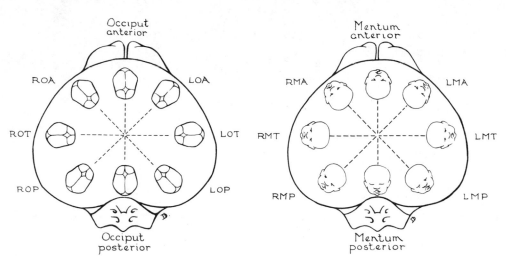

A. Occiput.

B. Face.

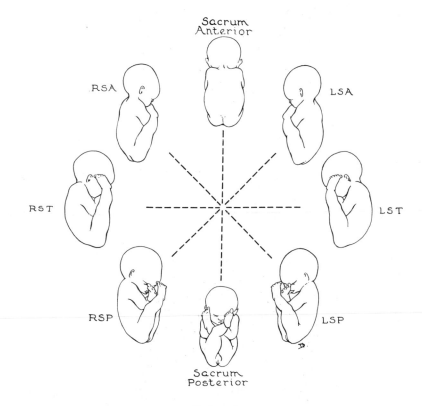

C. Breech.

FIG. 4. Position.

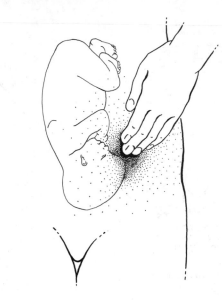

A. Flexion.

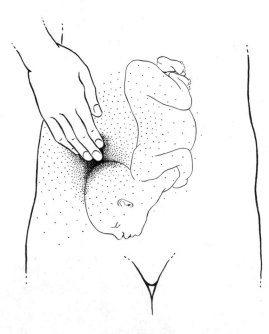

B. Extension.

FIG. 5. Cephalic prominence.

CEPHALIC PROMINENCE

The cephalic prominence is produced by flexion or extension (Fig. 5). When the head is well flexed, the occiput is lower than the sinciput and the forehead is the cephalic prominence. When there is extension, the occiput is higher than the sinciput and the occiput or back of the head is the cephalic prominence. The cephalic prominence can be palpated through the abdomen by placing both hands on the sides of the lower part of the uterus and moving them gently toward the pelvis. When there is a cephalic prominence, the fingers abut against it on that side and on the other side meet little or no resistance. The location of the cephalic prominence aids in diagnosing attitude. When the cephalic prominence and the back are on opposite sides, the attitude is flexion. When the cephalic prominence and the back are on the same side, there is extension. When no cephalic prominence is palpable, there is neither flexion nor extension and the head is in the military attitude.

LIGHTENING

Lightening is the subjective sensation felt by the patient as the presenting part descends during the latter weeks of pregnancy. It is not synonymous with engagement, although both may take place at the same time. Lightening is caused by the tonus of the uterine and abdominal muscles and is part of the adaptation of the presenting part to the lower uterine segment and to the pelvis. Symptoms include:

1. Less dyspnea
2. Decreased epigastric pressure
3. A feeling that the child is lower
4. Increased pressure in the pelvis
5. Low backache
6. Urinary frequency
7. Constipation
8. Initial appearance or aggravation of already present hemorrhoids and varicose veins of the lower limbs
9. Edema of the legs and feet
10. More difficulty in walking

GRAVIDITY AND PARITY

Gravidity

1. A *gravida* is a pregnant woman.
2. The word *gravida* refers to a pregnancy regardless of its duration.
3. A woman's *gravidity* relates to the total number of her pregnancies, regardless of their duration.
4. A *primigravida* is a woman pregnant for the first time.
5. A *secundagravida* is a woman pregnant for the second time.
6. A *multigravida* is a woman who has been pregnant several times.

Parity

1. The word *para* alludes to past pregnancies that have reached viability.
2. *Parity* refers to the number of past pregnancies that have gone to viability and have been delivered, regardless of the number of children involved. (For example, the birth of triplets increases the parity by only one.)
3. A *primipara* is a woman who has delivered one pregnancy in which the child has reached viability, without regard to the child's being alive or dead at the time of birth. Some authors consider that the designation of primipara includes women in the process of giving birth to their first child.
4. A *multipara* is a woman who has had two or more pregnancies that terminated at the stage when the children were viable.
5. A *parturient* is a woman in labor.

Gravida and Para

1. A woman pregnant for the first time is a primigravida and is described as gravida 1, para 0.
2. If she aborts before viability she remains gravida 1, para 0.
3. If she delivers a fetus that has reached viability she becomes a primipara, regardless of whether the child is alive or dead. She is now gravida 1, para 1.
4. During a second pregnancy she is gravida 2, para 1.
5. After she delivers the second child she is gravida 2, para 2.
6. A patient with two abortions and no viable children is gravida 2,

para 0. When she becomes pregnant again she is gravida 3, para 0. When she delivers a viable child she is gravida 3, para 1.

7. Multiple births do not affect the parity by more than one. A woman who has viable triplets in her first pregnancy is gravida 1, para 1.

TPAL

A different way of describing the patient's obstetrical situation is as follows:

1. Term pregnancies
2. Premature births
3. Abortions
4. Living children

8.

Engagement, Synclitism, Asynclitism

ENGAGEMENT

By definition engagement (Fig. 1C) has taken place when the widest diameter of the presenting part has passed through the inlet. In cephalic presentations this diameter is the biparietal, between the parietal bosses. In breech presentation it is the intertrochanteric.

In most women, once the head is engaged the bony presenting part (not the caput succedaneum) is at or nearly at the level of the ischial spines. Radiologic studies have shown that this relationship is not constant and that in women with deep pelves the presenting part may be as much as a centimeter above the spines even though engagement has occurred.

The presence or absence of engagement is determined by abdominal, vaginal, or rectal examination. In primigravidas engagement usually takes place 2 to 3 weeks before term. In multiparas engagement may occur any time before or after the onset of labor. Engagement tells us that the pelvic inlet is adequate. It gives no information as to the midpelvis or the outlet. While failure of engagement in a primigravida is an indication for careful examination to rule out disproportion, abnormal presentation, or some condition blocking the birth canal, it is no cause for alarm. The occurrence of engagement in normal cases is influenced by the tonus of the uterine and abdominal muscles.

When the presenting part is entirely out of the pelvis and is freely movable above the inlet, it is said to be floating (Fig. 1A).

When the presenting part has passed through the plane of the inlet but engagement has not occurred, it is said to be dipping (Fig. 1B).

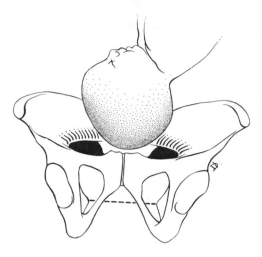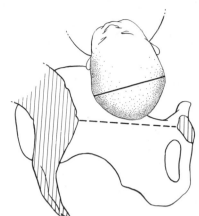

A. Floating.

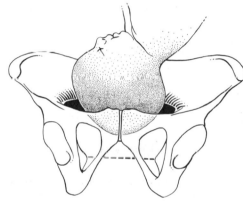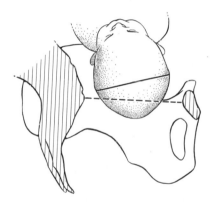

B. Dipping.

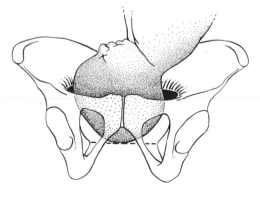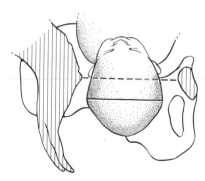

C. Engaged.

FIG. 1. Process of engagement.

STATION

Station is the relationship of the presenting part to an imaginary line drawn between the ischial spines (Fig. 2). The location of the buttocks in breech presentations or the bony skull (not the caput succedaneum) in cephalic presentations at the level of the spines indicates that the station is zero. Above the spines the station is minus one, minus two, and so forth, depending on how many centimeters above the spines the presenting part is. At spines minus five it is at the inlet. Below the spines it is plus one, plus two, and so forth. There are various relationships between station and the progress of labor.

1. In nulliparas entering labor with the fetal head well below the spines, further descent is often delayed until the cervix is fully dilated.
2. In nulliparas beginning labor with the head deep in the pelvis, descent beyond the spines often takes place during the first stage of labor.
3. An unengaged head in a nullipara at the onset of labor may indicate disproportion and warrants investigation. This condition is not rare, however, and in many cases descent and vaginal delivery take place.
4. The incidence of disproportion is more common when the head is high at the onset of labor.
5. Patients who start labor with high fetal heads usually have lesser degrees of cervical dilatation. There is a tendency for lower stations to be associated with cervices that are more effaced and dilated, both at the onset of labor and at the beginning of the active phase.
6. Other factors being equal, the higher the station the longer the labor.
7. Dysfunctional labor is more frequent when the station is high.
8. The high head that descends rapidly is usually not associated with abnormal labor.

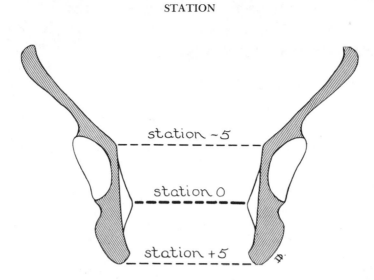

A. Anteroposterior view.

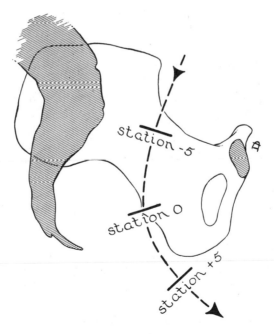

B. Lateral view.

FIG. 2. Station of the presenting part.

SYNCLITISM AND ASYNCLITISM

Engagement in Synclitism

In cephalic presentations engagement has occurred when the biparietal diameter has passed through the inlet of the pelvis. The fetal head engages most frequently with its sagittal suture (the anteroposterior diameter) in the transverse diameter of the pelvis. Left occiput transverse is the commonest position at engagement.

When the biparietal diameter of the fetal head is parallel to the planes of the pelvis, the head is in *synclitism.* The sagittal suture is midway between the front and the back of the pelvis. When this relationship does not obtain, the head is in *asynclitism.*

Engagement in synclitism takes place when the uterus is perpendicular to the inlet and the pelvis is roomy (Fig. 3). The head enters the pelvis with the plane of the biparietal diameter parallel to the plane of the inlet, the sagittal suture lies midway between the pubic symphysis and the sacral promontory, and the parietal bosses enter the pelvis at the same time.

Posterior Asynclitism (Litzmann's Obliquity)

In most women the abdominal wall maintains the pregnant uterus in an upright position and prevents it from lying perpendicular to the plane of the pelvic inlet. As the head approaches the pelvis, the posterior parietal bone is lower than the anterior parietal bone, the sagittal suture is closer to the symphysis pubis than to the promontory of the sacrum, and the biparietal diameter of the head is in an oblique relationship to the plane of the inlet. This is posterior asynclitism (Fig. 4). It is the usual mechanism in normal women and is more common than engagement in synclitism or anterior asynclitism.

As the head enters the pelvis, the posterior parietal bone leads the way, and the posterior parietal boss (eminence) descends past the sacral promontory. At this point the anterior parietal boss is still above the pubic symphysis and has not entered the pelvis. Uterine contractions force the head downward and into a movement of lateral flexion. The posterior parietal bone pivots against the promontory, the sagittal suture moves posteriorly toward the sacrum, and the anterior parietal boss descends past the symphysis and into the pelvis. This brings the sagittal suture midway between the front and back of the pelvis, and the head is now in synclitism.

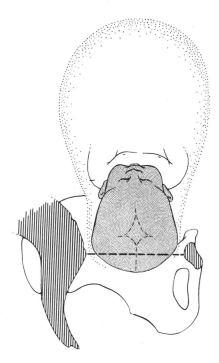

FIG. 3. Synclitism at the inlet.

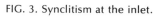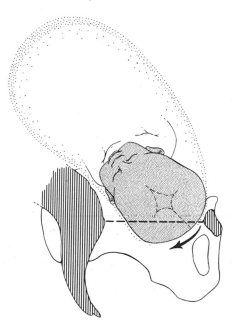

FIG. 4. Posterior asynclitism.

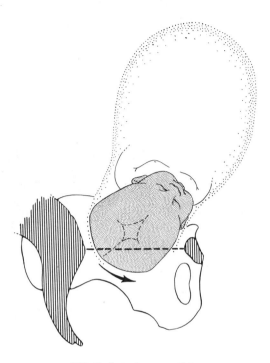

FIG. 5. Anterior asynclitism.

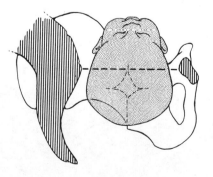

FIG. 6. Synclitism in the pelvis.

Anterior Asynclitism (Nägele's Obliquity)

When the woman's abdominal muscles are lax and the abdomen is pendulous so that the uterus and baby fall forward, or when the pelvis is abnormal and prevents the more common posterior asynclitism, the head enters the pelvis by anterior asynclitism (Fig. 5). In this mechanism the anterior parietal bone descends first, the anterior parietal boss passes by the pubic symphysis into the pelvis, and the sagittal suture lies closer to the sacral promontory than to the pubic symphysis. When the anterior parietal bone becomes relatively fixed behind the symphysis, a movement of lateral flexion takes place so that the sagittal suture moves anteriorly toward the symphysis and the posterior parietal boss squeezes by the sacral promontory and into the pelvis. The mechanism of engagement in anterior asynclitism is the reverse of that with posterior asynclitism.

There is a mechanical advantage to the head's entering the pelvis in asynclitism. When the two parietal bosses enter the pelvic inlet at the same time (synclitism), the presenting diameter is the biparietal of 9.5 cm. In asynclitism the bosses come into the pelvis one at a time, and the diameter is the subsuperparietal of 8.75 cm. Thus, engagement in asynclitism enables a larger head to pass through the inlet than would be possible if the head entered with its biparietal diameter parallel to the plane of the inlet (Fig. 6).

Whenever there is a small pelvis or a large head, asynclitism plays an important part in enabling engagement to take place. Marked and persistent asynclitism, however, is abnormal. When asynclitism is maintained until the head is deep in the pelvis, it may prevent normal internal rotation.

BIBLIOGRAPHY

Weekes ARL, Flynn MJ: Engagement of fetal head in primigravidas and its relationship to duration of gestation. Br J Obstet Gynaecol 82:7, 1975

Examination of the Patient

ABDOMINAL INSPECTION AND PALPATION

The position of the baby in utero is determined by inspecting and palpating the mother's abdomen, with these questions in mind:

1. Is the lie longitudinal, transverse, or oblique?
2. What presents at or in the pelvic inlet?
3. Where is the back?
4. Where are the small parts?
5. What is in the uterine fundus?
6. On which side is the cephalic prominence?
7. Has engagement taken place?
8. How high in the abdomen is the uterine fundus?
9. How big is the baby?

The patient lies on her back with the abdomen uncovered (Fig. 1). In order to help relax the abdominal wall muscles the shoulders are raised a little and the knees are drawn up slightly. If the patient is in labor the examination is carried out between contractions.

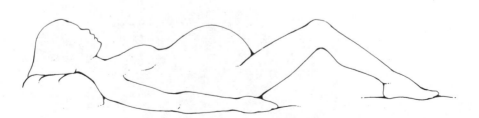

FIG. 1. Position of patient for abdominal palpation.

68

First Maneuver: What is the Presenting Part?

The examiner stands at the patient's side and grasps the lower uterine segment between the thumb and fingers of one hand to feel the presenting part (Fig. 2A). The other hand may be placed on the fundus to steady the uterus. This maneuver should be performed first. Since the head is the part of the fetus that can be identified with the most certainty, and since it is at or in the pelvis in 90 percent of cases, the logical thing to do first is to look for the head in its most frequent location. Once it has been established that the head is at the inlet, two important facts are known: (1) that the lie is longitudinal, and (2) that the presentation is cephalic.

An attempt is made to move the head from side to side to see whether it is outside the pelvis and free (floating) or in the pelvis and fixed (engaged). In contrast to the breech, the head is harder, smoother, more globular, and easier to move. A groove representing the neck may be felt between the head and the shoulders. The head can be moved laterally without an accompanying movement of the body. When the head is in the fundus and when there is sufficient amniotic fluid, the head can be ballotted. When a floating rubber ball is forced under water, it returns to the surface as soon as it is released; so the fetal head can be pushed posteriorly in the amniotic fluid, but as soon as the pressure on it is relaxed it rises back and abuts against the examining fingers.

Second Maneuver: Where is the Back?

The examiner stands at the patient's side facing her head. The hands are placed on the sides of the abdomen, using one hand to steady the uterus while the other palpates the fetus (Fig. 2B). The location of the back and of the small parts is determined.

The side on which the back is located feels firmer and smoother and forms a gradual convex arch. Resistance to the palpating fingers (as pressure is exerted toward the umbilicus) is even in all regions.

On the other side the resistance to pressure is uneven, the fingers sinking deeper in some areas than they do in others. The discovery of moving limbs is diagnostic.

Third Maneuver: What is the Fundus?

The hands are moved up the sides of the uterus and the fundus is palpated (Fig. 2C). In most cases the breech is here. It is a less definite structure than the head and is not identified as easily. The breech is softer,

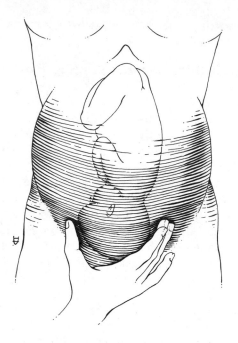

A. First maneuver: What is the Presenting Part?

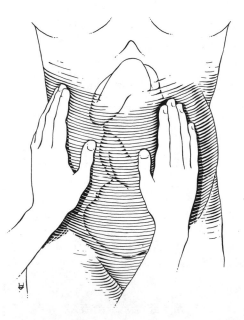

B. Second maneuver: Where is the Back?

FIG. 2. Abdominal palpation.

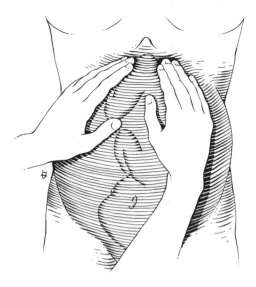

C. Third maneuver: What is the Fundus?

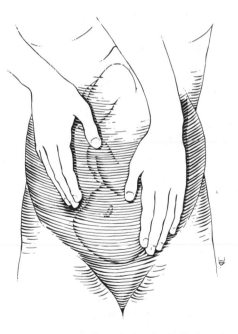

D. Fourth maneuver: Where is the Cephalic Prominence?

FIG. 2. (cont.). Abdominal palpation.

more irregular, less globular, and not as mobile as the head. It is continuous with the back, there being no intervening groove. When the breech is moved laterally the body moves as well. Finding moving small parts in the vicinity of the breech strengthens the diagnosis.

Fourth Maneuver: Where is the Cephalic Prominence?

The examiner turns and faces the patient's feet. Gently the fingers are moved down the sides of the uterus toward the pubis (Fig. 2D). The cephalic prominence is felt on the side where there is greater resistance to the descent of the fingers into the pelvis. In attitudes of flexion the forehead is the cephalic prominence. It is on the opposite side from the back. In extension attitudes the occiput is the cephalic prominence and is on the same side as the back. In addition it is noted whether the head is free and floating or fixed and engaged.

Relationship of Head to Pelvis

1. The floating head lies entirely above the symphysis pubis, so that the examining fingers can be placed between the head and the pubis. The head is freely movable from side to side.
2. When the head is engaged, the biparietal diameter has passed the inlet and only a small part of the head may be palpable above the symphysis. The head is fixed and cannot be moved laterally. Sometimes it is so low in the pelvis that it can barely be felt through the abdomen.
3. The head may be midway between the previous two locations. Part of it is felt easily above the symphysis. It is not freely movable but is not fixed; nor is it engaged. The head is described as lying in the brim of the pelvis, or dipping. (See Chapter 8 under *Engagement* and Figures 1A, 1B, and 1C.)

AUSCULTATION OF FETAL HEART

The fetal heart should be auscultated every 15 minutes during the first stage of labor, and every 3 to 5 minutes in the second stage. It is heard best by using a fetoscope (Fig. 3). Information gained by listening to the fetal heart falls into two main groups. It tells us something about (1) the general health of the baby in utero, and (2) the presentation and position of the fetus.

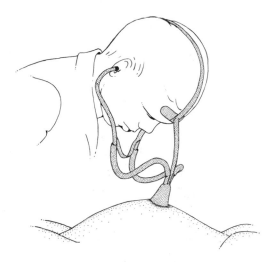

FIG. 3. Auscultation of the fetal heart beat.

General Health of the Fetus

The general health of the fetus can be estimated by observing the rate and rhythm of its heart.

1. The presence of the fetal heart sound indicates that the baby is alive.
2. The normal heart rate is 120 to 160 beats/minute. The fetal heart becomes slower at the height of a uterine contraction and speeds up after the contraction has worn off. A fetal heart rate of less than 100 or more than 160/minute with the uterus at rest suggests fetal distress. A slow rate has a greater significance than a rapid one.
3. The rhythm is regular and of a "tic toc" quality. Irregularity is a sign of fetal embarrassment.
4. The loudness of the fetal heart, contrary to popular belief, is not a sign of fetal vigor. It depends upon the following:
   a. The relationship between the fetal back and the mother's abdomen. When the baby's back is near the anterior abdominal wall, the fetal heart is strong and near. This is so in anterior positions. In posterior positions, on the other hand, the fetal heart gives the impression of being far away.
   b. In obese women with thick abdominal walls the fetal heart is not heard clearly.

    c. An excessive amount of amniotic fluid muffles the fetal heart tones.

5. Other sounds may be heard:
    a. The funic souffle, which is synchronous with the fetal heart, is caused by the blood rushing through the umbilical arteries.
    b. The uterine (maternal) souffle pulses at the same speed as the maternal pulse and results from the blood passing through the large blood vessels of the uterus.

6. Failure to hear the fetal heart may result from one of the following:
    a. Too early in the pregnancy. The fetal heart is heard only rarely before the 18th week.
    b. Fetal death. Inability to hear the baby's heart in a patient in whom it has been audible previously is a suggestion of fetal death. Usually fetal activity has ceased.
    c. Maternal obesity.
    d. Polyhydramnios (an excessive amount of amniotic fluid).
    e. A loud maternal souffle that obscures the fetal heart tones, making it difficult or impossible to identify them.
    f. Posterior position of the occiput, where the fetal back is away from the anterior abdominal wall.
    g. At the height of a strong uterine contraction.
    h. Defective stethoscope.
    i. An excessive amount of noise in the room.

In some instances one observer is unable to find the fetal heart tones, while another listener can hear them clearly.

Presentation and Position

In most cases there is a constant relationship between the location of the baby's heart and the fetal position in the uterus. In attitudes of flexion the fetal heart sound is transmitted through the scapula and the back of the shoulder. It is therefore heard loudest in that area of the mother's abdomen to which the fetal back is closest. In attitudes of extension the fetal heart beat is transmitted through the anterior chest wall of the baby.

In cephalic presentations the fetal heart beat is loudest below the umbilicus; in anterior positions it is clearest in one or the other lower quadrant of the mother's abdomen. The relationship of the fetal back and the fetal heart to the midline of the maternal abdomen is similar. As the one comes nearer to or moves away from the midline, so does the other. In posterior positions the fetal heart is loudest in the maternal flank on the side to which the back is related. In breech presentation the point of maximum intensity of the baby's heart sound is above the umbilicus.

The position of the fetal heart changes with descent and rotation. As the baby descends, so does the fetal heart. The anterior rotation of an occipitoposterior position can be followed by listening to the fetal heart as it moves gradually from the maternal flank toward the midline of the abdomen.

The location of the fetal heart (Fig. 4) may be used to check, but should not be relied upon to make, the diagnosis of presentation and position. Occasionally the point of maximum intensity of the fetal heart beat is not in the expected location for a given position. For example, it is not unusual in breech presentations for the fetal heart to be heard loudest below the umbilicus, instead of above it. The diagnosis made by careful abdominal palpation is the more reliable finding. Finding the fetal heart sound in an unexpected place is an indication for reexamination. If the findings on palpation are confirmed, the fetal heart sound should be disregarded.

The Role of Continuous Electronic Fetal Heart Monitoring

The achievements of electronic monitoring of the fetal heart rate have been impressive. Unfortunately, excessive reliance has been placed on the

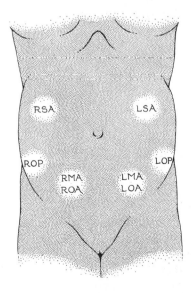

FIG. 4. Location of the fetal heart beat in relation to the various positions.

machinery and clinical judgment denigrated. Good clinical evaluation encompassing all factors and data must be the final arbiter in selecting the optimal management for the particular patient.

It has been shown that for almost all normal cases, and even for some high-risk pregnancies, intermittent human auscultation of the fetal heart rate is almost as effective as continuous monitoring. To achieve this degree of excellence it is necessary that an almost one-to-one relationship exist between the patient and nurse, that the auscultator be experienced, and that the fetal heart be evaluated rigidly every 15 minutes in the first stage and every 5 minutes in the second stage of labor. Auscultation of the fetal heart every 1 to 2 hours, not infrequently seen on a busy obstetrical service, is inadequate.

INDICATIONS FOR FETAL HEART MONITORING

1. Clinically detected abnormalities of the FHR
2. Meconium in the amniotic fluid
3. Stimulation of labor by oxytocin
4. Preterm labor
5. Slow progress in labor
6. Patients at high risk for utero-placental insufficiency including those with:
   a. Previous stillbirth
   b. Hypertension and preeclampsia
   c. Intrauterine growth retardation
   d. Postterm pregnancy
   e. Abnormal presentation
   f. Rh affected infant
   g. Diabetes
   h. Premature rupture of the membranes
   i. Multiple gestation

RECTAL EXAMINATION

Because some obstetricians believe that there is danger of infection during vaginal examinations, the course of labor in normally progressing cases is followed by rectal examinations. During pregnancy and especially during labor the muscles of the pelvic floor soften and are more easily dilated, so that rectal examination is easier to perform. However, rectal examination is painful and should be done only as often as is necessary for the safe conduct of labor.

Rectal examination during labor has several drawbacks:

1. It is less accurate than vaginal examination and must not be relied on in problem cases.
2. The condition and dilatation of the cervix is often difficult to determine, especially when a bag of waters is present.
3. The caput succedaneum may be mistaken for the skull, resulting in erroneous diagnoses of station.
4. It is unreliable in breech presentation.
5. During examination the posterior wall of the vagina is pushed against the cervix, bringing the vaginal bacteria into direct contact with the cervix.
6. Rectal examination is painful and aggravates hemorrhoids.

VAGINAL EXAMINATION

Several recent studies demonstrated that there is no greater danger of infection with vaginal than with rectal examination. Points in favor of the vaginal examination in the management of labor are as follows:

1. Vaginal examination is more accurate than rectal examination in determining the condition and dilatation of the cervix, station and position of the presenting part, and relationship of the fetus to the pelvis.
2. Vaginal examination takes less time, requires less manipulation, and gives more information than the rectal approach.
3. Cultures taken during the puerperium from women whose vaginas were sterile on admittance to hospital showed no higher incidence of positive results in those who had vaginal examinations during labor than those who had only rectal evaluations.
4. Clinical studies have shown that maternal morbidity is no higher following vaginal than following rectal examinations.
5. Vaginal examination causes less pain.
6. Vaginaphobia leads to the dangerous attitude of always waiting a little longer before doing a necessary vaginal examination during labor.
7. Prolapse of the umbilical cord can be diagnosed early, as can compound presentations.
8. It is important to remember that a clean or sterile glove is different from the contaminated finger of Semmelweis's time, when doctors went from infected surgical cases to the maternity ward without using aseptic precautions.

The examination must be done gently, carefully, thoroughly, and under aseptic conditions. Sterile gloves should be used. We prefer the lithotomy or dorsal position, finding the examination and orientation easier. It is the best position for determining proportion between the presenting part and the pelvis.

Palpation of Cervix

1. Is the cervix soft or hard?
2. Is it thin and effaced or thick and long?
3. Is it easily dilated or is it resistant?
4. Is it closed or open? If it is open, estimate the length of the diameter of the cervical ring.

Presentation

1. What is the presentation—breech, cephalic, shoulder?
2. Is there a caput succedaneum, and is it small or extensive?
3. What is that station? What is the relationship of the presenting part (not the caput succedaneum) to a line between the ischial spines? If it is above the spines it is –1, –2, or –3 cm. If it is below the spines it is +1, +2, or +3 cm.

Position

1. If it is a breech, where is the sacrum? Are the legs flexed or extended?
2. With a cephalic presentation, identify the sagittal suture (Fig. 5A). What is its direction? Is it in the anteroposterior, oblique, or transverse diameter of the pelvis?
3. Is the sagittal suture midway between the pubis and the sacrum (synclitism); is it near the sacral promontory (anterior asynclitism); or is it near the pubic symphysis (posterior asynclitism)?
4. Is the bregma right or left, anterior or posterior? (It is diamond-shaped and is the meeting point of four sutures.) (Fig. 5A.)
5. Where is the posterior fontanelle (Fig. 5B)? (It is Y-shaped and has three sutures.)
6. Is the head in flexion (occiput lower than sinciput) or is there extension (sinciput lower than occiput)?
7. In cases where there is difficulty in identifying the sutures, palpation of an ear (Fig. 5D) helps establish the direction of the sagittal suture and thus the anteroposterior diameter of the long axis of the head. The tragus points to the face.

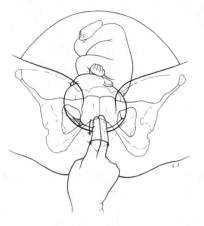 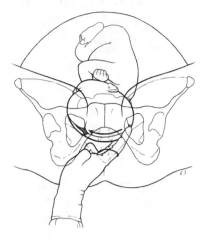

A. Determining the station and palpation of the sagittal suture.

B. Identification of the posterior fontanelle.

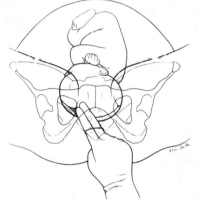

C. Identification of the anterior fontanelle.

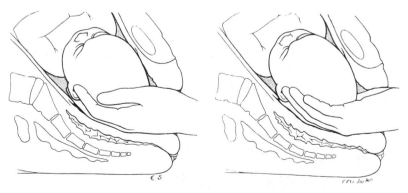

D. Palpation of the posterior ear.

FIG. 5. Diagnosis of station and position. (From Douglas and Stromme. *Operative Obstetrics,* 2nd ed., 1965. Courtesy of Appleton-Century-Crofts.)

Membranes

Feeling the bag of waters is evidence that the membranes are intact. The drainage of fluid, passage of meconium, and grasping of fetal hair in a clamp indicate that the membranes have ruptured.

General Assessment of Pelvis

1. Can the sacral promontory be reached? The diagonal conjugate can be measured clinically. It extends from the inferior margin of the pubic symphysis to the middle of the sacral promontory, and its average length is 12.5 cm. During the vaginal examination the promontory is palpated. When the distal end of the finger reaches the middle of the promontory, the point where the proximal part of the finger makes contact with the subpubic angle is marked (Figs. 6A, B, and C). The fingers are withdrawn from the vagina, and the distance between these two points is measured. By deducting 1.5 cm. from the diagonal conjugate (Fig. 6C), the approximate length of the obstetric conjugate can be obtained. In many women the promontory cannot be reached, and this is accepted as evidence that the anteroposterior diameter of the inlet is adequate. If the promontory can be felt, the obstetric conjugate may be short.
2. Is the pelvic brim symmetrical?
3. Are the ischial spines prominent and posterior?
4. Is the sacrum long and straight or short and concave?
5. Are the sidewalls parallel or convergent?
6. Is the sacrosciatic notch wide or narrow?
7. Is there any bony or soft tissue encroachment into the cavity of the pelvis?
8. How wide is the subpubic angle? The distance between the ischial tuberosities (average 10.5 cm) can be measured roughly by placing a fist between them (Fig. 6D). If this can be done the transverse diameter of the outlet is considered adequate.
9. Are the soft tissues and the perineum relaxed and elastic or hard and rigid?

Fetopelvic Relationship

1. How does the presenting part fit the pelvis?
2. If engagement has not taken place, can the presenting part be pushed into the pelvis by fundal and suprapubic pressure?
3. Does the presenting part ride over the pubic symphysis?

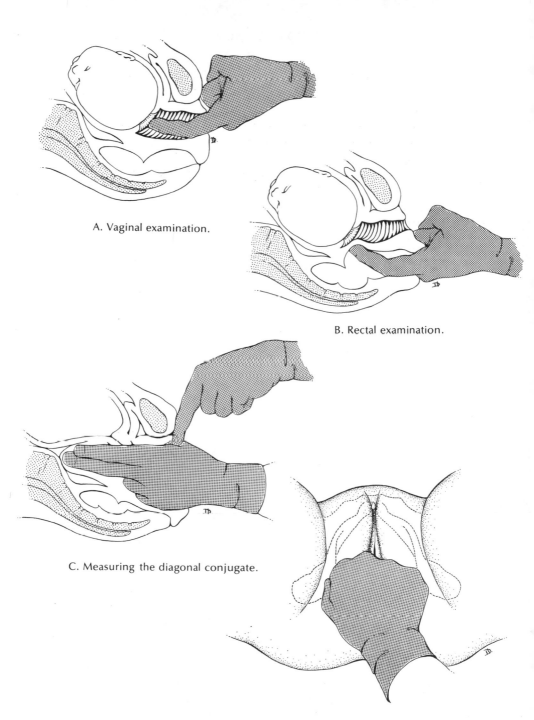

A. Vaginal examination.

B. Rectal examination.

C. Measuring the diagonal conjugate.

D. Measuring the bituberous diameter.

FIG. 6. Pelvic assessment.

X-RAY EXAMINATION

In some problem cases radiologic pelvimetry can provide valuable information about the following:

1. Shape and type of pelvis
2. Internal measurements of pelvis
3. Presentation, position, and station of fetus
4. Relationship of fetus to pelvis
5. Estimate of fetal size

10.

Anterior Positions of the Occiput and the Normal Mechanism of Labor

LEFT OCCIPUT ANTERIOR: LOA

LOA is a common longitudinal cephalic presentation (Fig. 1). The attitude is flexion, the presenting part is the posterior part of the vertex and the posterior fontanelle, and the denominator is the occiput (O).

Diagnosis of Position: LOA

ABDOMINAL EXAMINATION

1. The lie is longitudinal. The long axis of the fetus is parallel to the long axis of the mother.
2. The head is at or in the pelvis.
3. The back is on the left and anterior and is palpated easily except in obese women.
4. The small parts are on the right and are not felt clearly.
5. The breech is in the fundus of the uterus.
6. The cephalic prominence (in this case the forehead) is on the right. When the attitude is flexion, the cephalic prominence and the back are on opposite sides. The reverse is true in attitudes of extension.

ANTERIOR POSITIONS OF THE OCCIPUT

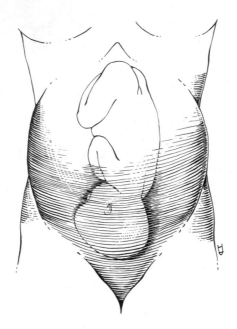

A. Abdominal view.

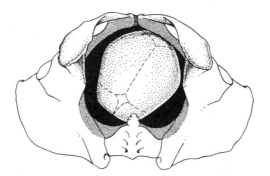

B. Vaginal view.

FIG. 1. Left occiput anterior.

FETAL HEART

The fetal heart is heard loudest in the left lower quadrant of the mother's abdomen. In attitudes of flexion the fetal heart rate is transmitted through the baby's back. The point of maximum intensity varies with the degree of rotation. As the child's back approaches the midline of the maternal abdomen, so does the point where the fetal heart is heard most strongly. Therefore in a left anterior position it is heard below the umbilicus and somewhere to the left of the midline, depending on the exact situation of the back.

VAGINAL EXAMINATION

1. The station of the head is noted—whether it is above, at, or below the ischial spines.
2. If the cervix is dilated, the suture lines and the fontanelles of the baby's head can be felt. In the LOA position the sagittal suture is in the right oblique diameter of the pelvis.
3. The small posterior fontanelle is anterior and to the mother's left.
4. The bregma is posterior and to the right.
5. Since the head is probably flexed, the occiput is a littler lower than the brow.

Normal Mechanism of Labor: LOA

The mechanism of labor as we know it today was described first by William Smellie during the 18th century. It is the way the baby adapts itself to and passes through the maternal pelvis. There are six movements, with considerable overlapping. The following description is for left anterior positions of the occiput.

DESCENT
Descent, which includes engagement in the right oblique diameter of the pelvis, continues throughout normal labor as the baby passes through the birth canal. The other movements are superimposed on it. In primigravidas considerable descent should have taken place before the onset of labor (Fig. 2A and B) in the process of engagement, provided there is no disproportion and the lower uterine segment is well formed. In multiparas engagement may not take place until good labor has set in. Descent is brought about by the downward pressure of the uterine contractions, aided in the second stage by the bearing-down efforts of the patient, and to a minimal extent by gravity.

FLEXION
Partial flexion exists before the onset of labor, since this is the natural attitude of the fetus in utero. Resistance to descent leads to increased flexion. The occiput descends in advance of the sinciput, the posterior fontanelle is lower than the bregma, and the baby's chin approaches its chest (Figs. 3A and B). This usually takes place at the inlet, but it may not be complete until the presenting part reaches the pelvic floor. The effect of flexion is to change the presenting diameter from the occipitofrontal of 11.0 cm to the smaller and rounder suboccipitobregmatic of 9.5 cm. Since the fit between fetal head and maternal pelvis may be snug, the reduction of 1.5 cm in the presenting diameter is important.

LEFT OCCIPUT ANTERIOR: LOA

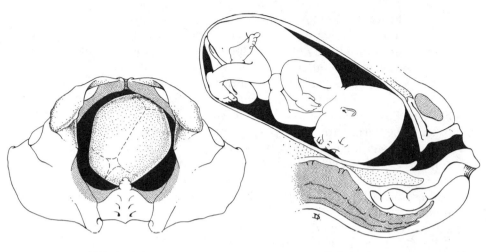

A. Vaginal view.   B. Lateral view.

FIG. 2. Mechanism of labor: LOA. Onset of labor.

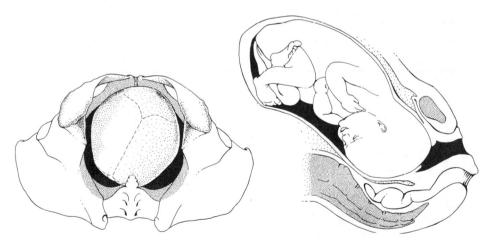

A. Vaginal view.   B. Lateral view.

FIG. 3. Descent and flexion of the head.

INTERNAL ROTATION

In the majority of pelves the inlet is a transverse oval. The anteroposterior diameter of the midpelvis is a little longer than the transverse diameter. The outlet is an anteroposterior oval, as is the fetal head. The long axis of the fetal head must fit into the long axis of the maternal pelvis. Hence the head, which entered the pelvis in the transverse or oblique diameter, must rotate internally to the anteroposterior diameter in order to be born. This is the purpose of internal rotation (Fig. 4).

The occiput now leads the way to the midpelvis, where it makes contact with the pelvic floor (the levator ani muscles and fascia). Here the occiput rotates 45° to the right (toward the midline). The sagittal suture turns from the right oblique diameter to the anteroposterior diameter of the pelvis: LOA to OA. The occiput comes to lie near the pubic symphysis and the sinciput near the sacrum.

The head rotates from the right oblique diameter to the anteroposterior diameter of the pelvis. The shoulders, however, remain in the left oblique diameter. Thus the normal relationship of the long axis of the head to the long axis of the shoulders is changed, and the neck undergoes a twist of 45°. This situation is maintained as long as the head is in the pelvis.

We do not know accurately why the fetal head, which entered the pelvis in the transverse or oblique diameter, rotates so that the occiput turns anteriorly in the great majority of cases and posteriorly in so few. One explanation is based on pelvic architecture. Both the bones and the soft tissues play a part. The ischial spines extend into the pelvic cavity. The sidewalls of the pelvis anterior to the spines curve forward, downward, and medially. The pelvic floor, made up of the levator ani muscles and fascia, slopes downward, forward, and medially. The part of the head that reaches the pelvic floor and ischial spines first is rotated anteriorly by these structures. In most cases the head is well flexed when it reaches the pelvic floor, and the occiput is lower than the sinciput. Hence the occiput strikes the pelvic floor first and is rotated anteriorly under the pubic symphysis.

This does not explain why some well flexed heads in the LOT and ROT positions (proved by x-ray) do not rotate posteriorly. Nor do the theories based upon pelvic architecture explain the situation in which, in the same patient, the head rotates anteriorly during one labor and posteriorly in another. In truth we do not know the exact reasons internal rotation takes place in the way it does. In most labors internal rotation is complete when the head reaches the pelvic floor, or soon after. Early internal rotation is frequent in multiparas and in patients having efficient uterine contractions. Internal rotation takes place mainly during the second stage of labor.

LEFT OCCIPUT ANTERIOR: LOA

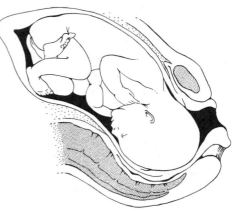

A. Lateral view.

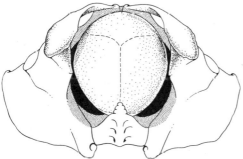

B. Vaginal view.

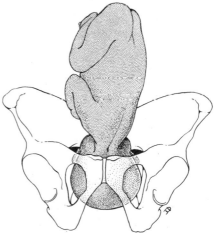

C. Anteroposterior view.

FIG. 4. Internal rotation: LOA to OA.

EXTENSION

Extension (Fig. 5) is basically the result of two forces: (1) uterine contractions exerting downward pressure and (2) the pelvic floor offering resistance. It must be pointed out that the anterior wall of the pelvis (the pubis) is only 4 to 5 cm long, while the posterior wall (the sacrum) is 10 to 15 cm. Hence the sinciput has a greater distance to travel than the occiput. As the flexed head continues its descent there is bulging of the perineum followed by crowning. The occiput passes through the outlet slowly, and the nape of the neck pivots in the subpubic angle. Then by a rapid process of extension the sinciput sweeps along the sacrum, and the bregma, forehead, nose, mouth, and chin are born in succession over the perineum.

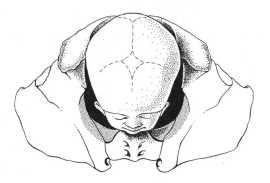

A. Vaginal view.

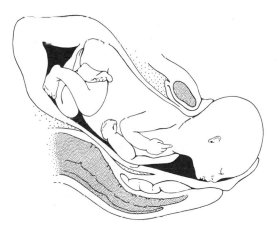

B. Lateral view.

FIG. 5. Extension of the head: birth.

RESTITUTION

When the head reaches the pelvic floor the shoulders enter the pelvis (Fig. 6). Since the shoulders remain in the oblique diameter while the head rotates anteriorly, the neck becomes twisted. Once the head is born and is free of the pelvis, the neck untwists and the head restitutes back 45° (OA to LOA) to resume the normal relationship with the shoulders and its original position in the pelvis.

LEFT OCCIPUT ANTERIOR: LOA

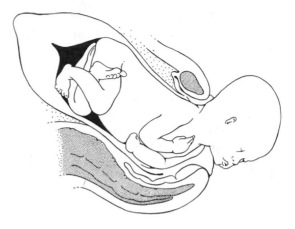

A. Lateral view.

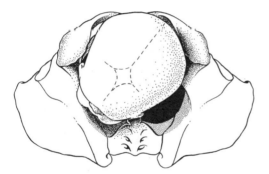

B. Vaginal view.

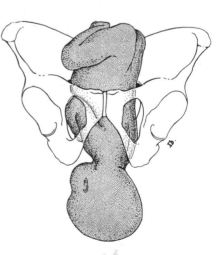

C. Anteroposterior view.

FIG. 6. Restitution: OA to LOA.

EXTERNAL ROTATION

External rotation of the head is really the outward manifestation of internal rotation of the shoulders. As the shoulders reach the pelvic floor the lower anterior shoulder is rotated forward under the symphysis, and the bisacromial diameter turns from the left oblique to the anteroposterior diameter of the pelvis. In this way the long diameter of the shoulders can fit the long diameter of the outlet. The head, which had already restituted 45° to resume its normal relationship to the shoulders, now rotates another 45° to maintain it: LOA to LOT (Fig. 7).

A summary of the mechanism of labor to this point is seen in Figure 8.

LEFT OCCIPUT ANTERIOR: LOA

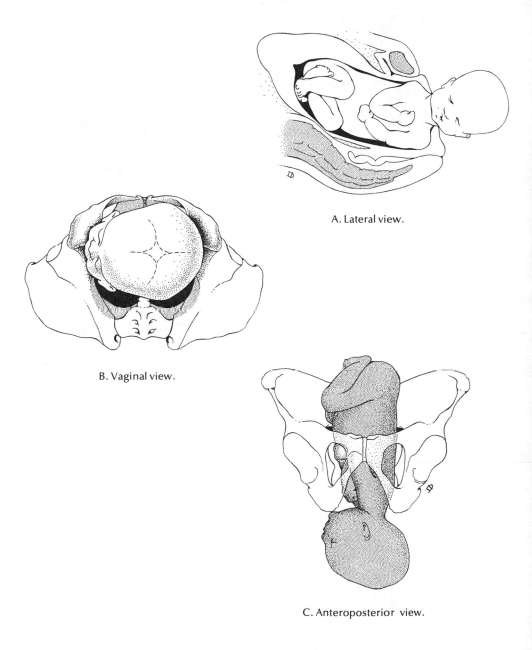

A. Lateral view.

B. Vaginal view.

C. Anteroposterior view.

FIG. 7. External rotation: LOA to LOT.

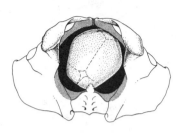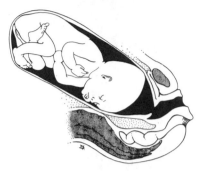

A. Onset of labor.

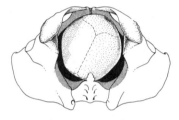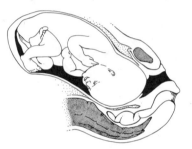

B. Descent and flexion.

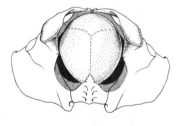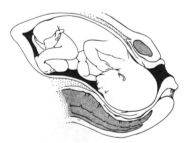

C. Internal rotation: LOA to OA.

FIG. 8. Summary of mechanism of labor: LOA.

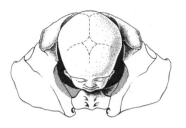
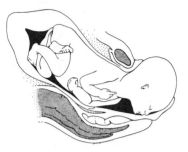

D. Extension.

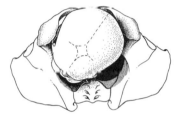
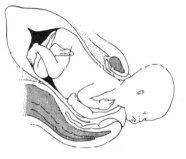

E. Restitution: OA to LOA.

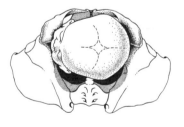
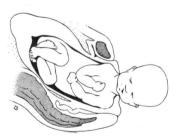

F. External rotation: LOA to LOT.

FIG. 8 (cont.). Summary of mechanism of labor: LOA.

Mechanism of Shoulders

When the head appears at the outlet, the shoulders enter the inlet. They engage in the oblique diameter opposite that of the head. For example, in LOA, when the head engages in the right oblique diameter of the inlet the shoulders engage in the left oblique.

The uterine contractions and the bearing-down efforts of the mother force the baby downward. The anterior shoulder reaches the pelvic floor first and rotates anteriorly under the symphysis. Anterior rotation of the shoulders takes place in a direction opposite to that of anterior rotation of the head. The anterior shoulder is born under the pubic symphysis and pivots there (Fig. 9A). Then the posterior shoulder slides over the perineum by a movement of lateral flexion (Fig. 9B).

Birth of Trunk and Extremities

Once the shoulders have been born the rest of the child is delivered by the mother's forcing down, with no special mechanism, and with no difficulty.

Molding

In LOA the presenting suboccipitobregmatic diameter is diminished, and the head is elongated in the verticomental diameter (Fig. 10).

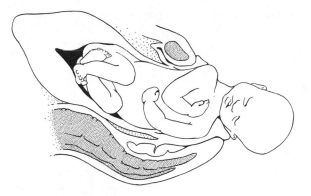

A. Birth of anterior shoulder.

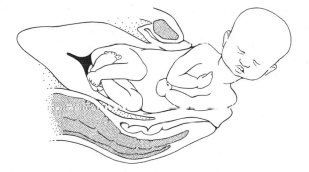

B. Birth of posterior shoulder.

FIG. 9. Birth of the shoulders.

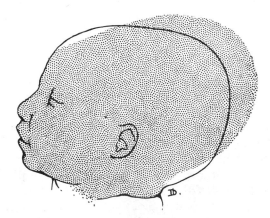

FIG. 10. Molding: LOA.

BIRTH OF PLACENTA

Separation of Placenta

Within a few minutes of delivery of the child the uterine contractions begin again. Because the fetus is no longer in the uterus, the extent of the retraction of the upper segment is larger than during the first and second stages. This retraction decreases greatly the area where the placenta is attached (Fig. 11A). The size of the placenta itself, however, is not reducible. The resultant disparity between the size of the placenta and its area of attachment leads to a cleavage in the spongy layer of the decidua, and in this way the placenta is separated from the wall of the uterus (Fig. 11B). During the process of separation blood accumulates between the placenta and uterus. When the detachment is complete the blood is released and gushes from the vagina.

Expulsion of Placenta

Soon after the placenta has separated it is expelled into the vagina by the uterine contractions. From here it is delivered by the bearing-down efforts of the patient. Two methods of expulsion have been described. In the Duncan method the lower edge of the placenta comes out first, with the maternal and fetal surfaces appearing together, and the rest of the organ slides down. In the Schultze method the placenta comes out like an inverted umbrella, the shiny fetal side appearing first, and the membranes trailing after. Although the Schultze mechanism suggests fundal implantation, while the Duncan method intimates that the placenta was attached to the wall of the uterus, the exact birth mechanism of the placenta is of little practical significance.

Control of Hemorrhage

The blood vessels that pass through the myometrium are tortuous and angular. The muscle fibers are arranged in an interlacing network through which the blood vessels pass. After the placenta has separated, retraction leads to a permanent shortening of the uterine muscle fibers. This compresses, kinks, twists, and closes the arterioles and venules in the manner of living ligatures. The blood supply to the placental site is effectively shut off, and bleeding is controlled. If the uterus is atonic and fails to retract properly after separation of the placenta, the vessels are not closed off, and severe postpartum hemorrhage may take place.

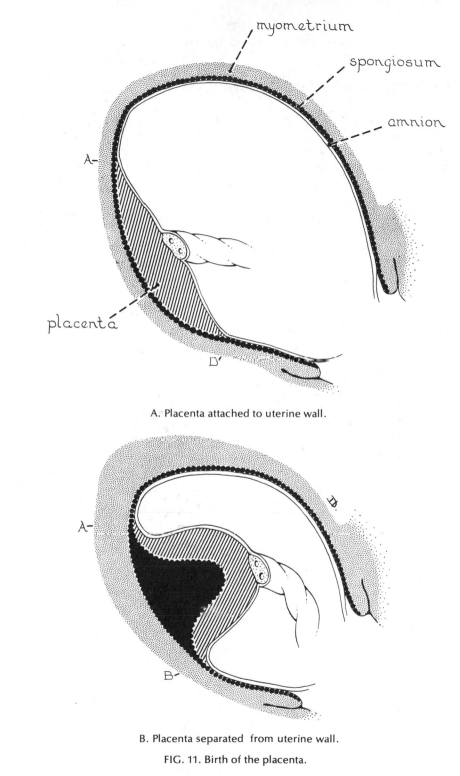

A. Placenta attached to uterine wall.

B. Placenta separated from uterine wall.

FIG. 11. Birth of the placenta.

CLINICAL COURSE OF LABOR: LOA

Almost always an LOA turns 45° to bring the occiput under the pubic arch, from where spontaneous delivery takes place. Occasionally, because of minor degrees of disproportion, a rigid perineum, or generalized fatigue, the patient may not be able to complete the second stage.

Arrests may take place in two positions:

1. It can occur after rotation to occiput anterior (OA) is complete, so that the sagittal suture is in the anteroposterior diameter.
2. Rotation may fail, the fetal head remaining in the original LOA position, with the sagittal suture in the right oblique diameter of the pelvis.

Management of arrested occipitoanterior positions consists of the following steps:

1. If rotation to OA has occurred, the forceps are applied to the sides of the baby's head, which is then extracted. (See Chapter 25 for details of technic.)
2. If rotation has failed, the forceps are applied to the sides of the baby's head. First the head is rotated with the forceps from LOA to OA and then it is extracted. (See Chapter 25 for details of technic.)

RIGHT OCCIPUT ANTERIOR: ROA

ROA is less common than LOA. The physical findings and the mechanism of labor are similar but opposite to LOA. The difference lies in the fact that in ROA the occiput and back of the fetus are on the mother's right side, while the small parts are on the left.

BIBLIOGRAPHY

Woodling BA, Kroener JM, Puffer HW, et al: Gross examination of the placenta. Clin Obstet Gynecol 19:21, 1976

11.

Clinical Course of Normal Labor

DEFINITIONS

LABOR   A function of the female by which the products of conception (fetus, amniotic fluid, placenta, and membranes) are separated and expelled from the uterus through the vagina into the outside world.

PRETERM LABOR   The onset of regular uterine contractions accompanied by cervical effacement and/or dilatation and fetal descent in a gravid woman whose period of gestation is less than 37 completed weeks (less than 259 days) from the first day of the last menstrual period.

EUTOCIA   Normal labor. Labor is considered normal when the child presents by the vertex of the head, when there are no complications, and when the labor is completed by the natural efforts of the mother. It should take no longer than 24 hours.

DYSTOCIA   Abnormal labor.

EXPECTED DATE OF CONFINEMENT   On an average this is 280 days from the first day of the last menstrual period or 267 days from conception. It is calculated by going back 3 months from the first day of the last menses and adding 7 days.

ONSET OF LABOR

Causes of Onset of Labor

We do not know the exact reason for the onset of labor, or why it takes place at about 40 weeks' gestation. Several theories have evolved to explain this phenomenon:

1. It is suggested that labor begins when the uterus is stretched to a certain degree. The early onset of labor in the case of twins and in patients with polyhydramnios is thus explained.

103

2. Pressure of the presenting part on the cervix and the lower uterine segment, as well as on the nerve plexuses around the cervix and vagina, stimulates the initiation of labor.

3. Placental aging, either by an alteration in the production of existing hormones or by the secretion of a new substance, leads to the onset of labor.

4. Hippocrates' concept that the fetus determines the time of its birth has been proven in some animals. In human beings there is evidence that the fetus plays a part in initiating labor, the adrenal cortex being the main organ concerned. In anencephalic fetuses, in whom there is absence of the hypothalamus, hypoplasia of the pituitary, and secondary hypoplasia of the adrenal cortex, there is a tendency for pregnancy to be prolonged and the onset of labor to be delayed. In primary adrenal hypoplasia, with normal hypothalamus and pituitary, gestation is also prolonged. Patients with Cushing's disease often go into premature labor. However, large doses of corticosteroids, effective in some animals, fail to bring on labor in pregnant women.

Phenomena Preliminary to the Onset of Labor

1. Lightening occurs 2 to 3 weeks before term and is the subjective sensation felt by the mother as the baby settles into the lower uterine segment.

2. Engagement takes place 2 to 3 weeks before term in primigravidas.

3. Vaginal secretions increase in amount.

4. Loss of weight is caused by the excretion of body water.

5. The mucous plug is discharged from the cervix.

6. Bloody show is noted.

7. The cervix becomes soft and effaced.

8. Persistent backache is present.

9. False labor pains occur with variable frequency.

TRUE AND FALSE LABOR

Signs of True Labor

1. Uterine contractions occur at regular intervals. Coming every 20 or 30 minutes at the beginning, the contractions get closer together. As labor proceeds the contractions increase in duration and severity.

2. The uterine systoles are painful.

3. Hardening of the uterus is palpable.

4. Pain is felt both in the back and in the front of the abdomen.
5. True labor is effective in dilating the cervix.
6. The presenting part descends.
7. The head is fixed between pains.
8. Bulging of the membranes is a frequent result.

False Labor Pains

False labor pains are inefficient contractions of the uterus or painful spasms of the intestines, bladder, and abdominal wall muscles. They appear a few days to a month before term. They are sometimes brought on by a digestive upset or a strong laxative. Usually they start on their own. They are irregular and short, and are felt more in the front than in the back.

There may be either no accompanying uterine contraction at all, or one that lasts only a few seconds. The uterus does not become stony hard and can be indented with the finger. These contractions are inefficient in pushing down the presenting part and do not bring about progressive effacement and dilatation of the cervix.

False labor pains can have the harmful effect of tiring the patient, so that when true labor does begin she is in poor condition, both mentally and physically. The treatment is directed to the cause if there is one, or the physician can prescribe an efficient sedative that stops the false labor pains but does not interfere with true labor.

True Labor	False Labor
Pains at regular intervals	Irregular
Intervals gradually shorten	No change
Duration and severity increase	No change
Pain starts in back and moves to front	Pain mainly in front
Walking increases the intensity	No change
Association between the degree of uterine hardening and intensity of pain	No relationship
Bloody show often present	No show
Cervix effaced and dilated	No change in cervix
Descent of presenting part	No descent
Head is fixed between pains	Head remains free
Sedation does not stop true labor	Efficient sedative stops false labor pains

STAGES OF LABOR

First Stage From the onset of true labor to complete dilatation of the cervix. It lasts 6 to 18 hours in a primigravida, and 2 to 10 hours in a multipara.

Second Stage   From complete dilatation of the cervix to the birth of the baby. It takes 30 minutes to 3 hours in a primigravida, and 5 to 30 minutes in the multipara. The median duration is slightly under 20 minutes in multiparas, and just under 50 minutes for primigravidas.

Third Stage   From the birth of the baby to delivery of the placenta. It takes 5 to 30 minutes.

Fourth Stage   From the birth of the placenta until the postpartum condition of the patient has become stabilized.

First Stage of Labor

The first stage of labor lasts from the onset of true labor to full dilatation of the cervix. The contractions are intermittent and painful, and the uterine hardening is felt easily by a hand on the abdomen. The pains become more frequent and more severe as labor proceeds. As a rule they begin in the back and pass to the front of the abdomen and the upper thighs.

EFFACEMENT AND DILATATION OF THE CERVIX

During most of pregnancy the cervix uteri is about 2.5 cm in length and closed. Toward the end of the period of gestation progressive changes occur in the cervix, including softening, effacement (shortening), dilatation, and movement from a posterior to an anterior position in the vagina. The internal os starts to disappear as the cervical canal becomes part of the lower segment of the uterus. The extent to which these changes have taken place correlates with the proximity of the onset of labor and with the success of attempts to induce labor.

Ideally the cervix should be ripe at the onset of labor. A ripe cervix is one that is soft, less than 1.3 cm in length, admits a finger easily, and is dilatable. When the cervix is ripe, it is a sign that the uterus is ready to begin labor. When these conditions are present, induction of labor is feasible. During labor the cervix shortens further, and the external os dilates. When the os has opened enough (average 10 cm) to permit passage of the fetal head it is said to be fully dilated (Fig. 1).

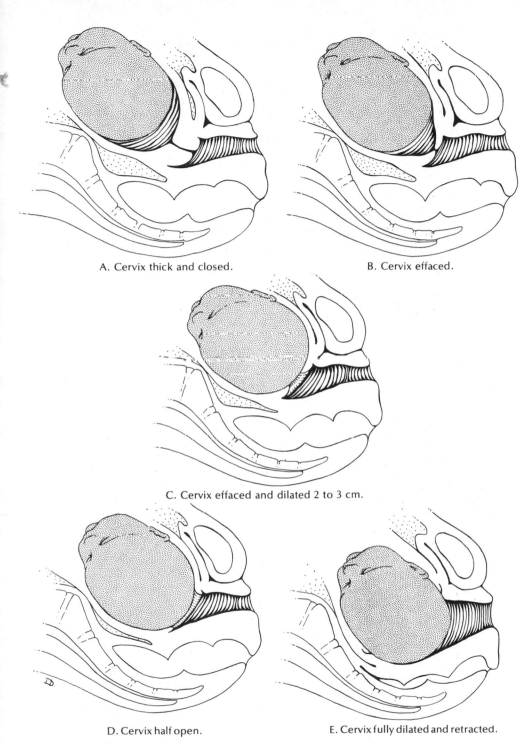

A. Cervix thick and closed.

B. Cervix effaced.

C. Cervix effaced and dilated 2 to 3 cm.

D. Cervix half open.

E. Cervix fully dilated and retracted.

FIG. 1. Dilatation of the cervix.

BAG OF WATERS: MEMBRANES

The fetus lies in a sac with an inner layer of amnion and an outer covering of chorion. The sac is filled with the amniotic fluid. As labor proceeds and the internal os becomes effaced and opens, the membranes separate from the lower uterine segment. The lower pole of the membranes bulges a little with each contraction and may adopt various shapes:

1. The protruding part may have the shape of a watch glass (Fig. 2A) containing a small amount of amniotic fluid. This is called the forewaters.
2. In other cases the membranes point into the cervix like a cone (Fig. 2B).
3. Still again, the bag may hang into the vagina (Fig. 2C).
4. In some cases the membranes are applied so tightly to the fetal head that no bag forms (Fig. 2D).

Frequently the membranes rupture near the end of the second stage, but this event can take place at any time during or before labor. When the membranes rupture, the fluid may come away with a gush or may dribble away. On occasion it is difficult to know whether the membranes are ruptured or intact. Methods of determining whether the bag of waters has ruptured include:

1. Seeing the fluid escaping from the vagina spontaneously or by pressure on the fundus.
2. Putting a speculum in the vagina and seeing whether fluid is coming from the cervix. The amount may be increased by pressure on the fundus of the uterus.
3. Grasping the fetal scalp with a forceps. If hair is seen in the forceps, it is proof that the membranes have ruptured.
4. The passage of meconium.
5. Use of Nitrazine paper to determine the pH of the vaginal fluid. The vagina, normally acidic, becomes neutral or alkaline when contaminated with alkaline amniotic fluid. Hence an alkaline pH in the vagina suggests that the membranes are ruptured.
6. Use of special staining of vaginal fluid, followed by microscopic search for components of amniotic fluid, including lanugo hairs, * fetal squamous cells, and fat. Quinaldine blue stains fetal cells only faintly, while vaginal squamous cells become dark.
7. The arborization test depends on the property of dried amniotic fluid to form crystals in an arborization pattern. A few drops of vaginal fluid are aspirated from the vagina by a bulb syringe and are placed on a clean, dry glass slide. After waiting 5 to 7 min-

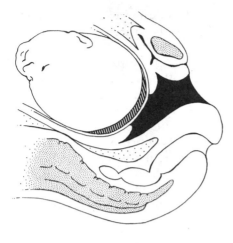

A. Forewaters: watchglass shape.

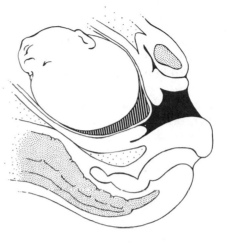

B. Forewaters: cone into the cervix.

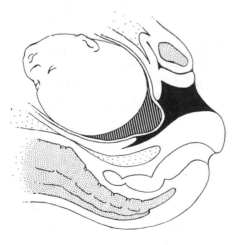

C. Bag of waters in the vagina.

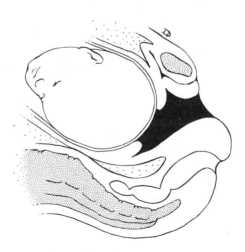

D. No forewaters.

FIG. 2. The membranes.

utes for drying to take place, the slide is examined under the low power microscope for identification of the arborization pattern.

A bag of waters that hangs into the vagina is of little or no help in dilating the cervix; it may impede labor by filling the vagina and preventing descent of the fetal head. The intact bag of amniotic fluid does little to help labor progress. In normal cases after the membranes have ruptured (spontaneously or artificially) the uterine contractions are more efficient and labor progresses faster. In dysfunctional labor, however, or in the presence of an unripe cervix (one that is thick, hard, and closed), amniotomy is ineffectual in shortening labor and may complicate the situation by introducing an irreversible factor.

Several conditions should be present before amniotomy is perperformed:

1. Labor is in progress, as indicated by observed change in the cervix.
2. The cervix is at least 3 cm dilated.
3. The head is fixed in the pelvis and applied to the cervix.

MANAGEMENT: FIRST STAGE OF LABOR

1. As long as the patient is healthy, the presentation normal, the presenting part engaged, and the fetus in good condition, the parturient may walk about or may be in bed, as she wishes. There is evidence to suggest that uterine action is more efficient, the duration of labor shorter, the need for analgesia less, and the necessity of augmenting labor by oxytocin less in women who are ambulatory during labor as compared with those who remain in bed.
2. The patient's condition and progress is checked periodically. The pulse, temperature, and blood pressure are measured every 4 hours or more often if necessary.
3. The fetal heart is auscultated every 15 minutes if normal and more frequently if irregular or slow.
4. The progress of labor is followed by abdominal, rectal, or vaginal examination to note the position of the baby, station of the presenting part, and dilatation of the cervix. These examinations should be done only often enough to ensure safe conduct of labor.
5. The patient is given an enema. This cleans the rectum and stimulates contractions.
6. Overdistention of the bladder is obviated by urging the patient to pass urine every few hours. If she is not able to do so, catheterization may be necessary, since a full bladder impedes progress.

7. Adequate amounts of fluid and nourishment are essential. In most normal labors sugared drinks or clear soups can be taken by mouth. Since solid foods remain in the stomach during labor, tend to be vomited, and increase the danger of aspiration, they should not be given. If the patient is unable to take enough orally, an intravenous infusion of glucose in water is given.

8. The patient must rest and maintain her self-restraint. This is important, for lost control is difficult to regain. The attendants can help the patient by continual reassurance, frequent encouragement, and judicious sedation. Such relaxation helps the patient rest, assists her in keeping control, and accelerates the progress of labor. When the pains are severe an analgesic preparation may be given. Since there is a limit to the amount of drugs that can be administered without harming the baby or interfering with labor, these must be given in logical dosage and sequence. (It has been said that the best sedative for a woman in labor is to see her doctor at the side of the bed.)

9. During the first stage the patient is impressed continually with the importance of relaxing with the contractions. Bearing down must be avoided, as it does nothing to improve progress. Bearing down comes into its own use when the cervix is fully dilated and not before. During the first stage it has only bad effects:
   a. It delays cervical dilatation.
   b. It tires the patient needlessly.
   c. It forces down the uterus and stretches the supporting ligaments, predisposing to later prolapse.

10. Measures to improve the character and the efficiency of the contractions include:
    a. Hot soapsuds enema
    b. Walking, which increases stimulation of the cervix and reflexly intensifies the uterine contractions.
    c. Artificial rupture of the membranes
    d. Oxytocin

11. While an intravenous infusion of 5 percent glucose in water is often useful in normal labor, it is mandatory in the complicated case for these reasons:
    a. Fluids and nourishment can be given without provoking emesis. The woman who cannot take adequate fluids by mouth or who is nauseated or vomiting can be maintained in a state of good hydration.
    b. Analgesics in small amounts can be administered for rapid effect.

    c. When uterine action is inefficient pitocin added to the solution improves labor.

    d. When there is excessive bleeding in the third or fourth stages, oxytocic agents can be given quickly.

    e. Blood and plasma expanders may be infused without delay.

    f. Once hypotension has occurred the veins often collapse and it is difficult to insert a needle. Having an infusion already underway obviates this problem.

PASSAGE OF MECONIUM IN CEPHALIC PRESENTATIONS

The passage per vaginam of meconium or meconium-stained amniotic fluid in a cephalic presentation is a sign of fetal distress. It is believed to result from relaxation of the rectal sphincter and increased peristalsis as a consequence of anoxia. Etiologic factors include cord entanglements, prolonged labor, and toxemia of pregnancy. In most cases no cause is found.

The incidence of meconium staining is around 5 percent. The occurrence of stillbirth, when this is the only sign, is low, but the number of newborns requiring resuscitation is higher than the overall incidence.

When meconium is passed the fetal heart must be observed closely. Should there be a significant alteration in the rate and rhythm of the fetal heart, immediate delivery may be needed to save the child. Operative delivery is not indicated on the basis of meconium staining alone, however.

In breech presentations the passage of meconium is caused by pressure of the uterine contractions on the fetal intestines and is not accepted as a sign of anoxia or fetal distress.

Second Stage of Labor

The second stage of labor lasts from the end of the first stage, when the cervix has reached full dilatation, to the birth of the baby. As the patient passes through the end of the first stage and into the second stage, the contractions become more frequent and are accompanied by some of the worst pain of the whole labor. Once the second stage is achieved the discomfort is less.

There are clinical indications that the second stage has started:

1. There is an increase in bloody show.
2. The patients wants to bear down with each contraction.
3. She feels pressure on the rectum accompanied by the desire to defecate.

4. Nausea and retching occur frequently as the cervix reaches full dilatation.

These signs are not infallible, and the condition of the cervix and station of the presenting part must be confirmed by rectal examination.

POSITION FOR DELIVERY

The adaptability of the human female has led to a wide variation of the delivery positions used by various cultures. There is no single correct position; each has its good and bad features.

During the second and third stages of labor the expulsive powers include (1) involuntary uterine contractions, (2) voluntary efforts of the abdominal, thoracic, and diaphragmatic muscles, and (3) action of the levator ani muscles.

Positions for giving birth may be grouped:

Upright or Vertical This position includes the standing, sitting, squatting, and upright-kneeling positions. Studies have indicated that the woman can create 30 percent more intraabdominal pressure in the vertical than in the horizontal position. Benefits include a reduction in the length of labor, fewer complications, a lower incidence of forceps deliveries, and a decreased need for anesthesia. The parturient female seems to prefer the vertical position.

Horizontal or Semihorizontal In this group are the lateral, prone, semi-recumbent, knee-elbow, and dorsal ·positions. These were developed by obstetricians with the aim of achieving ease and efficiency in dealing with complications and administering drugs to relieve pain. However, they may not be best for normal deliveries.

Modern obstetrics has employed the horizontal plus the lithotomy, head-down (Trendelenburg), hanging-leg (Walcher), and lateral-prone (Sims) positions.

ADVANTAGES AND DISADVANTAGES OF VARIOUS POSITIONS

Squatting Position This posture has the advantages of enlarging the pelvic outlet a little and of enabling the patient to use her expulsive forces to the greatest advantage. The drawbacks are that it is difficult for the accoucheur to control the birth and to manage complications, and it is impossible to administer sedatives and analgesics in labor.

Lateral Position   Advantages of this posture include:

1. Ease, convenience, and comfort for the woman.
2. Relaxation of pelvic muscles, which facilitates descent of the fetal head.
3. Ease in controlling the head as it advances over the perineum, with fewer lacerations occurring.
4. Natural drainage of secretions or vomitus from the pharynx.
5. Absence of pressure by the pregnant uterus on the inferior vena cava, thus precluding the supine hypotensive syndrome.

This is not, however, a good position in which to handle complicated forceps deliveries. Lacerations of the vagina and cervix are awkward to repair. Complications of the third stage are difficult to manage.

Dorsal (Supine) Position   The woman lies on her back with the knees flexed. The dorsal position is advantageous for those multiparas who do not need an episiotomy, as they can be delivered without having to put their legs in stirrups. Episiotomy and forceps operations are not performed easily. The dorsal position is potentially harmful to the fetus during labor and delivery. Should the supine hypotensive syndrome occur, fetal hypoxia and bradycardia may result. A firm wedge placed under the patient's right side will, by producing a 15° left tilt, reduce the incidence of hypotension.

Lithotomy Position   Here the woman lies on her back, her legs in stirrups, and her buttocks close to the lower edge of the table. Advantages include:

1. Asepsis is more complete.
2. The fetal heart can be auscultated without change of position.
3. Anesthesia can be provided efficiently—general, conduction, and local.
4. The perineum can be protected and lacerations prevented.
5. This is a good position for the use of forceps, for the repair of episiotomy and lacerations, and for conduction of the third stage of labor.

Disadvantages include:

1. Risk of the supine hypotensive syndrome.
2. The use of stirrups or leg supports may lead to sacroiliac or lumbosacral strain, thrombosis in the veins of the lower limbs, and damage to the nerves, especially the peroneal, as a result of prolonged pressure.
3. There is danger of aspiration of vomitus.

Semisitting Position An adjustable backrest can be used on a standard delivery table during the second and third stages of labor. Women are most comfortable with their backs raised at an angle of between 30° and 45° from the horizontal, which places them in a modified sitting posture. The efficiency of the expulsive forces are increased by directing them toward the pelvis and by making use of the forces of gravity. For the obstetrician this position is compatible with modern methods of obstetric care.

SUPINE HYPOTENSIVE SYNDROME

The clinical picture is one of hypotension when, in the late stages of pregnancy, the woman lies on her back; there is rapid recovery when she turns on her side. Other symptoms include nausea, shortness of breath, faintness, pallor, tachycardia, and increased femoral venous pressure.

When the pregnant, near-term woman lies on her back, the flaccid uterus bulges over the vertebral column and compresses the inferior vena cava. This leads to an increased volume of blood in the lower limbs, but a decreased return to the heart, lowered pressure in the right atrium, diminished cardiac output, and hypotension. Reduced perfusion of the uterus and placenta leads to fetal hypoxia and changes in the fetal heart rate. During a uterine contraction the uterus sits on the spine and does not press on the large blood vessels. Complete relief of symptoms occurs when the baby has been delivered.

BEARING DOWN BY THE PATIENT

During the first stage, labor progresses faster and the patient feels less pain if she breathes slowly and deeply during each uterine contraction and avoids bearing down. The more effective the relaxation, the more rapid the cervical dilatation. In the second stage, on the other hand, the patient has to work hard. She must force down with each contraction and rest between them. The more effectively she bears down, the shorter the second stage. During the early part of the second stage the abdominal muscles, which are responsible for the bearing-down efforts, are under the patient's complete control. Later she sometimes finds it impossible to stop bearing down even if she wants to. This action is more efficient if the patient braces herself against a solid object. On delivery tables hand bars are provided. When the contraction comes on the patient takes one or two deep breaths and then holds her breath to fix the diaphragm. She then pulls on the hand bars, and at the same time bears down as hard and for as long a period as she can. This is shown in Fig. 3C. With each contraction the pressure on the perineum and rectum stimulates the patient to move toward the head of the table and out of the best position. Shoulder braces prevent this.

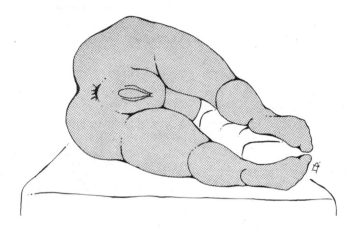

A. Left lateral position.

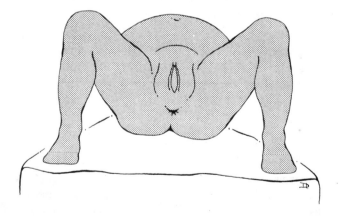

B. Dorsal position.

FIG. 3. Positions for delivery.

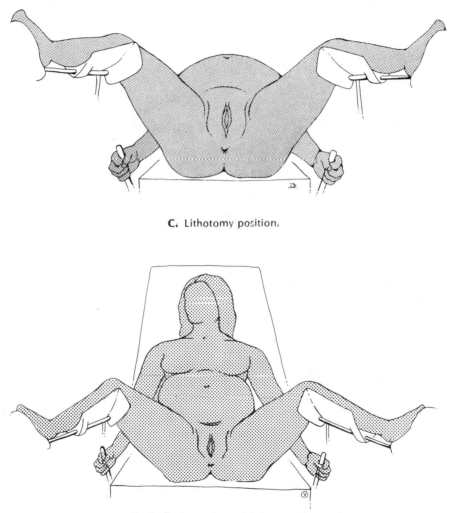

C. Lithotomy position.

D. Back elevated: semisitting position.

FIG. 3. (cont.) Positions for delivery.

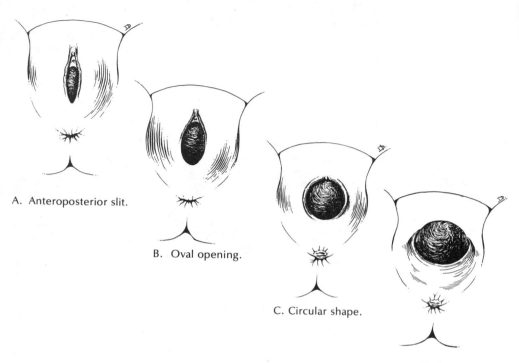

A. Anteroposterior slit.

B. Oval opening.

C. Circular shape.

D. Crowning.

DESCENT, CROWNING, AND SPONTANEOUS BIRTH OF THE HEAD

With each contraction the head advances and then recedes as the uterus relaxes. Each time a little ground is gained. The introitus becomes an anteroposterior slit, then an oval, and finally a circular opening (Figs. 4A–C). The pressure of the head thins out the perineum. Feces may be forced out of the rectum. As the anus opens, the anterior wall of the rectum bulges through. With descent the occiput comes to lie under the pubic symphysis. The head continues to advance and recede with the contractions, until a strong one forces the largest diameter of the head through the vulva (crowning), as seen in Figure 4D. Once this has occurred there is no going back, and by a process of extension (Fig. 4E) the head is born, as the bregma, forehead, nose, mouth, and chin appear over the perineum (Fig. 4F). At the stage where the head is passing through the introitus, the patient has the sensation of being torn apart. Laceration of the vulva sometimes occurs.

The head then falls back toward the anus. Once it is out of the vagina it restitutes (Fig. 4G) as the neck untwists. After a few moments, external rotation takes place (Fig. 4H) as the shoulders move from the oblique to the anteroposterior diameter of the pelvis.

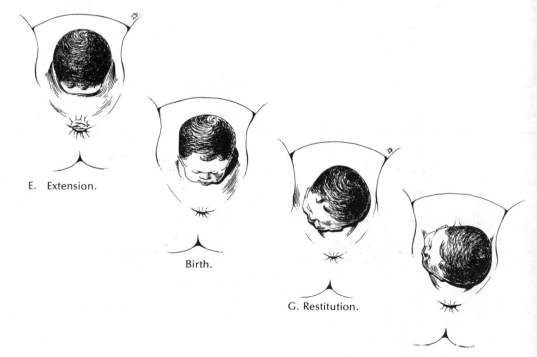

E. Extension.

Birth.

G. Restitution.

H. External rotation.

FIG. 4. Dilatation of the introitus and birth of the head.

ASSISTED DELIVERY OF HEAD

Many women can deliver their babies spontaneously in bed without assistance. There are advantages, however, of having an accoucheur in attendance and of having the patient on a delivery table. (1) Should an unexpected complication arise, immediate action can be carried out. (2) The obstetrician is able to assist the patient so that the incidence of large and uncontrolled lacerations is reduced.

Controlled Birth of Head Procedures designed to promote leisurely egress of the fetal head should be performed. Slow, gradual birth of the head reduces the incidence of lacerations. The attendant must guard against a sudden bursting out of the head, as this leads to large and jagged lacerations, which in the extreme may extend through the anal sphincter and into the rectum.

1. Management of bearing-down efforts: Correct management of the bearing-down efforts of the parturient is important. The two forces responsible for birth of the child are uterine contractions and bearing-down forces. The uterine contractions are involuntary, but the bearing-down forces can be controlled. During the first part of the second stage the patient must bear down during the uterine contractions to expedite progress. However, during the actual delivery too rapid emergence of the fetal head can be slowed by the patient's panting rapidly through the open mouth during the contraction. When the patient breathes in and out rapidly, the diaphragm moves, making it impossible for effective intraabdominal pressure to be built up, and so the power to bear down is lost.
2. Manual pressure: in most cases the speed of delivery can be reduced by gentle manual pressure against the baby's head. Occasionally the propulsive force is so great that it is impossible, or even dangerous, to try slowing the birth. The head should never be held back forcibly.
3. Ritgen maneuver: The objective of this maneuver is to encourage extension of the fetal head and thus expedite its birth. This procedure is performed ideally between uterine contractions. During this interval the head can be delivered slowly, gradually, and under the obstetrician's complete control. Further, the soft tissues are more relaxed and tissue damage is less. The maneuver cannot be carried out before the occiput has come under the symphysis. It is done when the suboccipitofrontal diameter is ready to be born.

   The operator's hand, covered with a towel or a pad, is placed so that the fingers are behind the maternal anus (Fig. 5A).

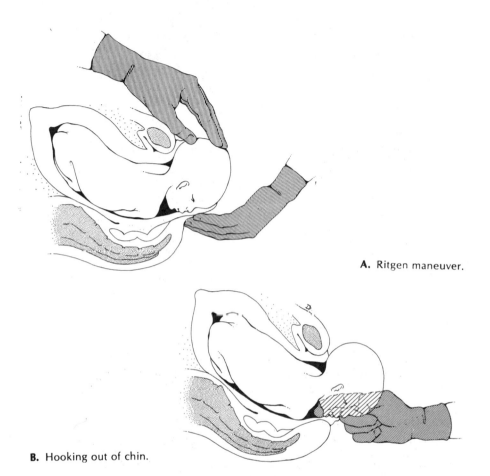

A. Ritgen maneuver.

B. Hooking out of chin.

FIG. 5. Birth of head.

Extension of the fetal head is furthered by pressing against the baby's face, preferably the chin, through the rectum. The bregma, forehead, and face are born in that order. The other hand is placed against the baby's head to control the speed of its delivery. Sometimes fundal pressure is needed to deliver the head, or if the patient is awake she can bear down gently.

4. Hooking out the chin: Occasionally the chin gets stuck against the perineum. It is extracted by inserting the fingers into the vagina, over the cheek and under the chin, which is then brought out over the perineum (Fig. 5B).

5. Episiotomy: When large lacerations seem inevitable it is better to make an incision into the perineum (episiotomy). In this way the direction and size of the cut can be controlled, and tears into the rectum can be obviated.

Following Delivery of Head

1. The head should be supported as it restitutes and rotates externally.
2. The face should be wiped gently and mucus aspirated from the mouth and throat by a small, soft, rubber bulb syringe.
3. The region of the neck is explored for coils of umbilical cord. If the cord is around the neck loosely it can be slipped over the head. If it is coiled around the neck tightly, it must be clamped doubly, cut between the clamps, and then unwound.
4. Meconium aspiration syndrome must be prevented. When thick meconium has been passed there is a danger that the fetus will aspirate it during the first deep postnatal breath. Therefore, in cases where meconium is present the following steps should be taken:
   a. As soon as the head is born, and before the baby breathes, the nostrils, nasopharynx, mouth, and hypopharynx are suctioned thoroughly.
   b. After the delivery is complete the laryngoscope is employed to see whether there is meconium at or below the level of the vocal cords.
   c. If there is, all the meconium should be suctioned out before any resuscitative measures, such as positive pressure breathing, are performed.

BIRTH OF BODY

Shoulders By the time the shoulders are ready for delivery, restitution has occurred and external rotation is taking place. During a uterine contraction the patient is asked to bear down. If the patient is anesthetized or unable to force down, pressure is exerted by an attendant on the fundus of the uterus. At the same time the head of the baby is grasped with the hands on the parietal bones or with one hand over the face and the other on the occiput (Fig. 6A); the head is then depressed toward the rectum. This enables the anterior shoulder to emerge under the symphysis pubis. (Fig. 6B). When this has been achieved the head is raised so that the posterior shoulder can be born over the perineum (Fig. 6C). It must be emphasized that the operator merely lowers and lifts the baby's head to facilitate birth of the shoulders. He does not exert great traction, as this carries with it the danger of damaging the nerve plexus in the neck. The force that actually pushes out the shoulder is provided by the bearing-down efforts of the mother is she is awake, or by pressure on the fundus by an assistant if the mother is asleep.

Trunk and Lower Limbs Once the head and shoulders have been

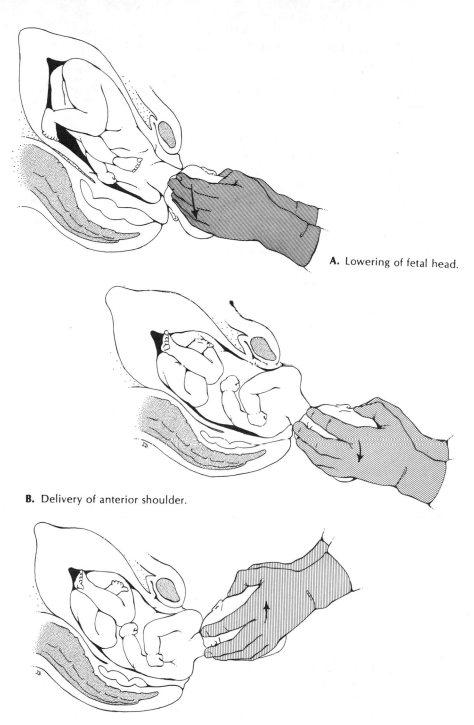

A. Lowering of fetal head.

B. Delivery of anterior shoulder.

C. Delivery of posterior shoulder.

FIG. 6. Delivery of the shoulders.

123

delivered, the rest of the body slips out easily, usually with a gush of amniotic fluid.

IMMEDIATE CARE OF BABY

Once the infant is born it should be held head down for a few moments to promote drainage of mucus. The best way of holding the baby is to place it with the back on the attendant's forearm; one leg is tucked between the doctor's arm and his side to prevent the infant from rolling off; the neck is between the third and fourth fingers; the shoulders rest on the palmar surfaces of the fingers; and the baby's head is below the operator's hand (Fig. 7). The advantages of this method are:

1. The infant is held securely and cannot slip between the fingers.
2. The head is maintained in slight extension, straightening the trachea and helping drainage.
3. The baby is held in a fixed position so that the trachea can be milked down, the mucus aspirated from the mouth and throat, and any other needed procedure carried out without the infant's swinging like a pendulum, as it does when held by the ankles.

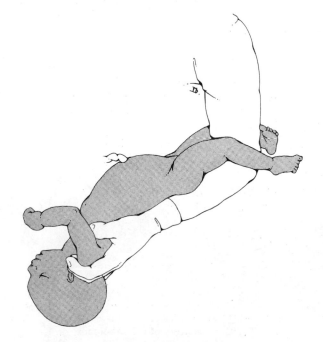

FIG. 7. Holding the baby.

The baby is then placed on the mother's abdomen. Further suction is carried out as needed. The umbilical cord is tied either doubly with cord tapes or with special mechanical ties. Some prefer to delay tying the cord until it stops pulsating so that the baby can get an additional supply of blood. If this is done, then the baby must be held lower than the placenta so the blood reaches him.

The infant is then weighed and placed in its cot. The eyes are treated with silver nitrate or an antibiotic ointment to prevent ophthalmia neonatorum.

RESUSCITATION OF THE ASPHYXIATED NEWBORN

1. Oropharyngeal suction and oxygen delivered by mask and bag will initiate a gasp in 85 percent of cases.
2. When no gasp follows these measures are employed:
   a. Establishment of a clear airway is mandatory.
   b. Tracheal suction by direct laryngoscopy should precede intubation and insufflation.
   c. Ventilation with oxygen is given at 30 to 40 breaths per minute.
   d. When indicated, gentle cardiac massage, using two fingers on the lower sternum, is carried out at a rate of 120 to 140 per minute.
   e. Acidosis is prevented by the use of sodium bicarbonate, 0.9 mEq/ml, infused via an umbilical catheter or peripheral vein at a rate of 2 to 3 ml/minute.

Third Stage of Labor

BIRTH OF PLACENTA

Delivery of the placenta occurs in two stages: (1) separation of the placenta from the wall of the uterus and into the lower uterine segment and/or the vagina, and (2) actual expulsion of the placenta out of the birth canal.

Separation of Placenta Placental separation takes place, as a rule, within 5 minutes of the end of the second stage. Signs suggesting that detachment has taken place include:

1. Gush of blood from the vagina
2. Lengthening of the umbilical cord outside the vulva
3. Rising of the uterine fundus in the abdomen as the placenta passes from the uterus into the vagina
4. Uterus becoming firm and globular

Expulsion of Placenta   When these signs have appeared the placenta is ready for expression. If the patient is awake she is asked to bear down while gentle traction is exerted on the cord. If she is asleep or unable to bear down, pressure is made on the uterine fundus and the placenta is delivered in this way. It is wise to avoid rough manipulations of the uterus before placental separation has taken place, as such actions do not hasten delivery of the placenta and may lead to excessive bleeding.

The actual birth of the placenta takes place in one of two ways: (1) Duncan method (dirty Duncan), when the rough maternal edge comes first; or (2) Schultze mechanism (shiny Schultze), when the placenta comes out like an inverted umbrella with the glistening fetal membranes leading the way.

Examination of Delivered Placenta   Examination of the delivered placenta is performed to see that no parts are missing—i.e., left in the uterus. Torn blood vessels along the edge suggest that an accessory lobe may have remained in the uterus. Some obstetricians feel that examination of the placenta does not ensure that fragments have not been left behind, and they explore the uterine cavity manually after each delivery.

Delayed Separation and Delivery of Placenta   Delayed separation and delivery of the placenta may occur in several situations:

1. Placenta separated but trapped in the uterus by the cervix
2. Placenta separated incompletely
3. Placenta not separated at all
4. Placenta accreta, where the decidua is deficient and the chorionic villi have grown into the myometrium

Manual Removal of Placenta   At one time invasion of the postpartum uterus was believed to be so dangerous a procedure that a placenta that did not deliver spontaneously was left in situ even for days. Today we feel that prolonged retention of the afterbirth increases the danger of infection and hemorrhage. Current practice is to remove the placenta manually if it does not deliver within 30 minutes of the birth of the baby, provided bleeding is not excessive. If hemorrhage is profuse, the placenta must be removed immediately. The average blood loss during the third stage is 200 to 250 ml.

MANUAL EXPLORATION OF UTERUS
Manual exploration of the uterus is mandatory:

1. When examination of the placenta is inconclusive or there is suspicion that something has been left in the uterus

2. After a traumatic delivery to rule out lacerations of the uterus and cervix
3. When there is excessive postpartum bleeding
4. When a congenital anomaly of the uterus is suspected

The most common cause of excessive bleeding is mismanagement of the third stage. The most frequent fault is to try to hasten delivery of the placenta before it has separated. Kneading or massaging the uterus roughly when it is not ready to contract may cause partial separation of the placenta and result in postpartum hemorrhage.

OXYTOCICS

Oxytocics are drugs that stimulate the uterus to contract. Posterior pituitary extract causes clonic rhythmic contractions. The ergot alkaloids provoke a tonic type of contraction. The purpose of using these substances is to hasten placental delivery and so reduce uterine blood loss.

It is doubtful that the amount of blood lost during the delivery and the immediate postpartum period has any relationship to the rapidity of placental separation. In most cases detachment of the placenta from the wall of the uterus takes place within 5 minutes of the birth of the baby. After delivery of the placenta the uterine contractions decrease in strength and frequency; the normal puerperal uterus does not remain in a tonically contracted state, yet no excessive blood loss occurs. This suggests that the routine use of ecbolic drugs is unnecessary in normal deliveries and should be reserved for women who have conditions that increase the risk of postpartum hemorrhage, including: (1) over-distended uterus (multiple pregnancy, polyhydramnios), (2) high parity, (3) history of previous postpartum hemorrhage, (4) prolonged labor, especially when associated with ineffective uterine contractions, (5) deep general anesthesia, (6) difficult operative delivery, (7) induction or augmentation of labor by oxytocin.

Pitocin and Syntocinon Pitocin was originally the trade name for posterior pituitary extract that had been purified by removing the vasopressor substances almost completely. Today both Pitocin and Syntocinon are trade names for synthetic oxytocin. These substances may be given in several ways:

1. After birth of the baby, 10 units intramuscularly
2. After delivery of the placenta, 10 units intramuscularly
3. As an intravenous infusion using 5 to 10 units of oxytocin per liter of 5 percent glucose in water, given either before or after placental separation.

Ergometrine Ergometrine is given most commonly after the end of the third stage, either intramuscularly in the amount of 0.5 mg, or intravenously in a dose of 0.125 or 0.25 mg. A popular method of using ergometrine is to give 0.125 mg intravenously when the anterior shoulder has emerged from the symphysis pubis and the rest of the baby can be delivered at will. The birth of the rest of the baby is delayed 10 to 15 seconds. This gives the ergometrine time to reach the uterus and stimulate it to contract. The baby's buttocks are still in the uterine cervix and hold it open, so that the placenta is expelled from the uterus literally on the baby's heels. The aim of this technique is to speed expulsion of the placenta and reduce bleeding. Before employing this method the presence of twins must be ruled out. A rare complication is spasm of the cervix trapping the placenta. In such a case one must wait for the spasm to wear off.

REPAIR OF LACERATIONS

The cervix, vagina, and perineum must be examined carefully, lacerations repaired, and bleeding controlled.

Fourth Stage of Labor

The patient is kept in the delivery suite for 1 hour post partum under close observation. She is checked for bleeding, the blood pressure is measured, and the pulse is counted. The third stage and the hour after delivery are more dangerous to the mother than any other time.

Before the doctor leaves the patient he must do the following:

1. Feel the uterus through the abdomen to be sure it is firm and not filling with blood.
2. Look at the introitus to see that there is no hemorrhage.
3. See that the mother's vital signs are normal and that she is in good condition.
4. Examine the baby to be certain that it is breathing well and that the color and tone are normal.

ASEPSIS AND ANTISEPSIS

Anatomic Factors

The birth passage is divided into three parts:

1. The vulva and vaginal orifice, which are loaded with bacteria of all kinds.

2. The vagina, which contains some vaginal bacteria with their acidic secretion, a few fungi, and a number of leukocytes.
3. The uterine cavity, which is separated from the vagina by the mucous plug. There are no organisms here.

Natural Safeguards

1. During the first and second stages there is an increase in the vaginal secretion, which cleans the passage.
2. When the membranes rupture, the amniotic fluid flushes out the vagina.
3. As the baby passes through the vagina it distends the walls. Usually the birth of the baby is accompanied by another discharge of amniotic fluid, which helps wash out the vagina.
4. As the membranes and placenta pass through the vagina they also exert a cleaning, mop-like action.

Cleansing Procedures

The patient is given a bath; the vulva is washed, the rectum cleaned by an enema, and the bladder prevented from overfilling.

Personal Care by Attendants

All who come into contact with the woman in labor should:

1. Wash hands carefully
2. Wear gloves
3. Wear sterile masks to prevent passing bacteria from the nose and throat
4. Wear sterile gowns when delivering the woman
5. Avoid contact with infectious patients

BIBLIOGRAPHY

Atwood RJ: Parturitional posture and related birth behaviour. Acta Obstet Gynecol Scand Suppl 57, 1976
Flynn AM, Kelly J, Hollins G, Lynch PF: Ambulation in labour. Br Med J, 2:591, 1978
Friedman ML, McElin TW: Diagnosis of ruptured fetal membranes. Am J Obstet Gynecol 104:544, 1969

Fujikara T, Klionsky B: The significance of meconium staining. Am J Obstet Gynecol 121:45, 1975

Hendricks CH, Brenner WE, Kraus G: Normal cervical dilatation patterns in late pregnancy and labor. Am J Obstet Gynecol 106:1065, 1970

Liggins GC: Fetal influences on myometrial contractility. Clin Obstet Gynecol 16:148, 1973

Miller FC, Sachs DA, Yeh SY, et al: The significance of meconium during labor. Am J Obstet Gynecol 122:573, 1975

Wetrich DW: Effect of amniotomy upon labor. Obstet Gynecol 35:800, 1970

12.

Transverse Positions of the Occiput

LEFT OCCIPUT TRANSVERSE: LOT

Engagement is more frequent in the transverse diameter of the inlet than in the oblique, and left occiput transverse (LOT) is the most common position at the onset of labor (Fig. 1).

Diagnosis of Position: LOT

ABDOMINAL EXAMINATION

1. The lie is longitudinal.
2. The head is at or in the pelvis.
3. The back is on the left and toward the mother's flank.
4. The small parts are on the right and sometimes can be felt clearly.
5. The breech is in the fundus of the uterus.
6. The cephalic prominence (forehead) is on the right.

FETAL HEART
The fetal heart is heard loudest in the left lower quadrant of the mother's abdomen.

VAGINAL EXAMINATION

1. The sagittal suture is in the transverse diameter of the pelvis. If the head is in synclitism (Fig. 1B), the sagittal suture is midway between the symphysis pubis and the promontory of the sacrum. If there is anterior asynclitism (Fig. 1D) the sagittal suture is nearer the sacral promontory, while with posterior asynclitism (Fig. 1C) it is closer to the public symphysis.
2. The small posterior fontanelle is toward the mother's left, at 3 o'clock.

131

3. The bregma is on the right, at 9 o'clock.
4. If there is flexion the occiput is lower than the brow. If flexion is poor the occiput and brow are almost at the same level in the pelvis.

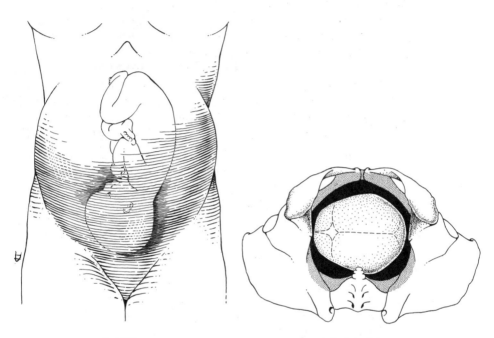

A. LOT.

B. Synclitism.

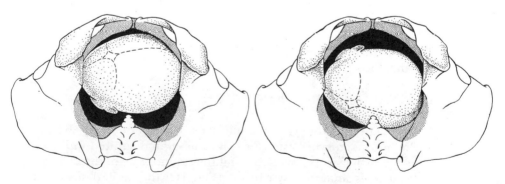

C. Posterior asynclitism.

D. Anterior asynclitism.

FIG. 1. Left occiput transverse.

Mechanism of Labor: LOT

DESCENT

Descent includes engagement, which may have taken place before labor (Figs. 2A and B). Descent continues throughout labor.

FLEXION

Resistance to descent causes the head to flex (Fig. 2B) so that the chin approaches the chest. This reduces the presenting diameter by 1.5 cm. The occipitofrontal diameter of 11.0 cm is replaced by the suboccipitobregmatic diameter of 9.5 cm.

INTERNAL ROTATION

The head enters the pelvis with the sagittal suture in the transverse diameter of the inlet and the occiput at 3 o'clock. The occiput then rotates 90° to arrive under the pubic symphysis. The sinciput comes to lie anterior to the sacrum. The sequence is LOT to LOA to OA (Figs. 2A and B). The shoulders lag behind 45° so that when the sagittal suture of the head is in the anteroposterior diameter of the pelvis the shoulders are in the left oblique. Thus the neck is twisted.

EXTENSION

Birth is by extension (Figs. 2E and F). The nape of the neck pivots under the pubis, while the vertex, bregma, forehead, face, and chin are born over the perineum.

RESTITUTION

When the head has made its exit, the neck untwists and the head turns back 45° to the left, resuming the normal relationship with the shoulders—OA to LOA (Fig. 2G).

EXTERNAL ROTATION

The shoulders now rotate 45° to the left to bring their bisacromial diameter into the anteroposterior diameter of the pelvis. The head follows the shoulder and rotates externally another 45° to the left—LOA to LOT (Fig. 2H).

TRANSVERSE POSITIONS OF THE OCCIPUT

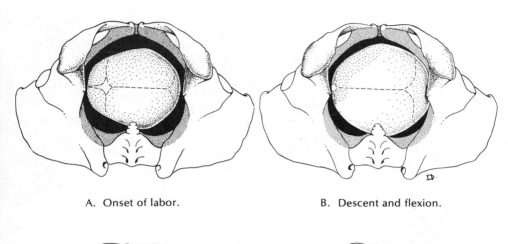

A. Onset of labor.   B. Descent and flexion.

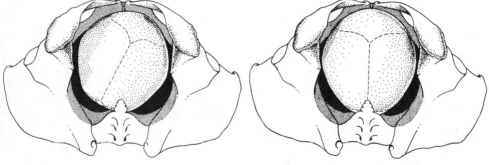

C. Internal rotation: LOT to LOA.   D. Internal rotation: LOA to OA.

FIG. 2. Mechanism of labor: LOT

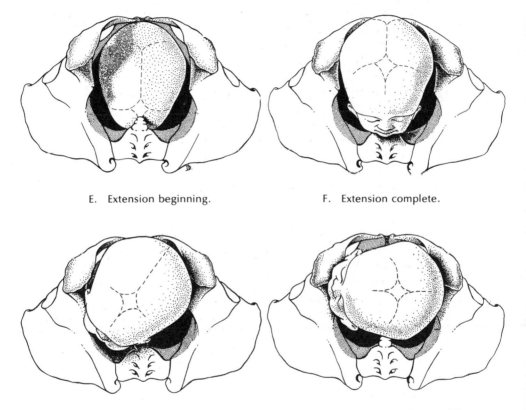

E. Extension beginning.   F. Extension complete.

G. Restitution: OA to LOA.   H. External rotation: LOA to LOT.

FIG. 2. (cont.) Mechanism of Labor: LOT.

Birth of Shoulders, Trunk, and Placenta

Birth of the shoulders, trunk, and placenta is the same as described in Chapter 10, "Anterior Positions of the Occiput and the Normal Mechanism of Labor." A summary of the mechanism of labor (LOT) is presented in Figure 3.

CLINICAL COURSE OF LABOR: LOT

Most fetuses that begin labor in the LOT position rotate the head 90° (LOT to LOA to OA) to bring the occiput under the pubic symphysis, from which position spontaneous delivery takes place.

Arrest of Progress

Arrest of progress can occur in any of these situations:

1. Anterior rotation of 90° to the OA position, but spontaneous delivery does not take place.
2. Anterior rotation of 45°, with cessation of progress in the LOA position.
3. No rotation. The head is arrested with the sagittal suture in the transverse diameter of the pelvis. This is known as transverse arrest.
4. In the rare case posterior rotation takes place, LOT to LOP. The mechanism of labor then becomes that of occipitoposterior positions.

Management of Arrested Cases

Providing the prerequisites for operative vaginal delivery are present, the following treatment is carried out:

1. Arrest in OA position: Forceps are applied to the sides of the fetal head, which is then extracted (see Chapter 25 for technical details).
2. Arrest as LOA: Forceps are applied to the fetal head, which is then rotated 45° to the OA position and extracted (see Chapter 25 for technical details).
3. Transverse arrest: LOT: Two operative technics are available.
   a. Manual rotation, 90°, LOT to LOA to OA, followed by forceps extraction (see Chapter 26 for technique).

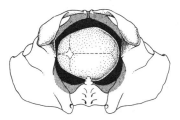

A. At onset of labor.

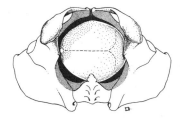

B. Descent and flexion.

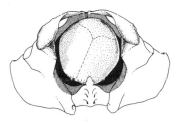

C. Internal rotation: LOT to LOA.

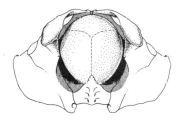

D. Internal rotation: LOA to OA.

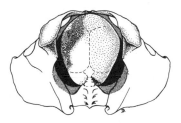

E. Extension beginning.

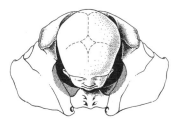

F. Extension complete.

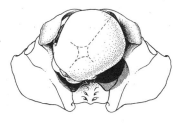

G. Restitution: OA to LOA.

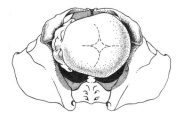

H. External rotation: LOA to LOT.

FIG. 3. Summary of the mechanism of labor: LOT.

b. Application of the forceps to the sides of the baby's head, rotation by the forceps of 90°, LOT to LOA to OA, and then extraction by the forceps (see Chapter 26 for technique).
4. Arrest as an occiput posterior is treated like other occiput posterior deliveries (see Chapter 13).

RIGHT OCCIPUT TRANSVERSE: ROT

ROT is similar to LOT. The difference is that the back and occiput are on the mother's right, and the limbs are on her left.

13.

Posterior Positions of the Occiput

GENERAL CONSIDERATIONS

Definition

The occiput and the small posterior fontanelle are in the rear segment of the maternal pelvis, and the brow and bregma are in the anterior segment.

Incidence

The incidence of this position is 15 to 30 percent. The exact incidence of posterior positions is difficult to ascertain, since most of them rotate anteriorly and are considered erroneously as being originally occipitoanterior. The posterior positions that rotate anteriorly with no difficulty are often not diagnosed, and only the persistent posteriors are regularly recognized. Right occiput posterior (ROP) is five times as common as left occiput posterior (LOP).

Etiology

The etiology of posterior positions of the occiput is the same as the etiology of other abnormal positions. Cephalopelvic disproportion is a frequent and serious complicating factor which must be considered at all times. The shape of the pelvic inlet influences the position of the occiput. Where the forepelvis is narrow there is a tendency for the back of the head with its long biparietal diameter to be pushed to the rear, so that the front of the head with its short bitemporal diameter can be accommodated by the small forepelvis. Hence posterior positions of the occiput are found often in android and anthropoid pelves.

139

RIGHT OCCIPUT POSTERIOR: ROP

Diagnosis of Position: ROP

ABDOMINAL EXAMINATION

1. The lie is vertical. The long axis of the fetus is parallel to the long axis of the mother (Fig. 1).
2. The head is at or in the pelvis.
3. The fetal back is in the right maternal flank. In most cases it cannot be outlined clearly.
4. The small parts are easily felt anteriorly on the left side. The maternal abdomen has been described as being alive with little hands and feet.
5. The breech is in the fundus of the uterus.
6. The cephalic prominence is on the left. It is not felt as easily as in anterior positions, because flexion is less marked.

FETAL HEART

Fetal heart tones are transmitted through the scapula and hence are heard in the right maternal flank, on the same side as the baby's back. Frequently the fetal heart sounds are indistinct. They can be transmitted through the baby's chest and in some cases are loudest in the left anterior lower quadrant of the abdomen. The location of the fetal heart sounds is not a reliable sign in determining how the baby is placed; hence a carefully made diagnosis of posterior position should not be changed because of the situation of the fetal heart. As the back rotates anteriorly, the fetal heart tones approach the midline of the abdomen.

VAGINAL EXAMINATION

1. The sagittal suture is in the right oblique diameter of the pelvis.
2. The small posterior fontanelle is in the right posterior segment of the pelvis.
3. The bregma is anterior and to the left of the symphysis pubis.
4. Since flexion is imperfect, the fontanelles may be close to the same level in the pelvis.
5. Where there is difficulty in diagnosis, the pinna (auricle) of the ear is found pointing to the occiput.

X-RAY EXAMINATION

Occasionally x-ray is helpful when diagnosis is in doubt.

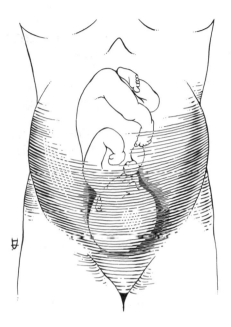

A. Abdominal view.

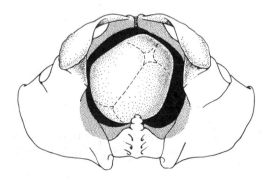

B. Vaginal view.

FIG. 1. Right occiput posterior.

Mechanism of Labor: ROP

Rotation of varying degree and direction can take place:

1. Anterior rotation
   a. Long arc rotation of 135°, ROP to ROT to ROA to OA. This occurs in 90 percent of occipitoposterior positions. The baby is born as an occipitoanterior.
   b. Rotation of 90°, ROP to ROT to ROA.
   c. Rotation of 45°, ROP to ROT. The result is deep transverse arrest.
2. No rotation. The position remains ROP.
3. Posterior rotation of 45°, ROP to OP, with the occiput turning into the hollow of the sacrum.

Spontaneous delivery can take place after:

1. Anterior rotation to OA with normal birth
2. Posterior rotation to OP with face to pubis delivery

Arrest can occur:

1. High in the pelvis, with failure to engage. These are often problems of disproportion.
2. In the midpelvis, with complete or partial failure of rotation.
   a. Deep transverse arrest, ROT
   b. Arrest with the sagittal suture in the right oblique diameter of the pelvis, ROP
   c. Arrest with the occiput in the hollow of the sacrum, OP
3. Arrest at the outlet.

LONG ARC ROTATION: 135° TO THE ANTERIOR

Descent The head enters the inlet with the sagittal suture in the right oblique diameter (Fig. 2A), and unless obstruction is encountered descent continues throughout labor. Engagement may be delayed, and the entire labor may take longer than in normal anterior positions.

Flexion Flexion (Fig. 2B) is imperfect and often is not complete until the head reaches the pelvic floor. The partial flexion and the resulting larger diameter of the presenting part contribute to the labor's being longer and harder for both mother and child.

Internal Rotation The occiput rotates 135° anteriorly under the symphysis pubis—ROP to ROT to ROA to OA (Figs. 2C-E).

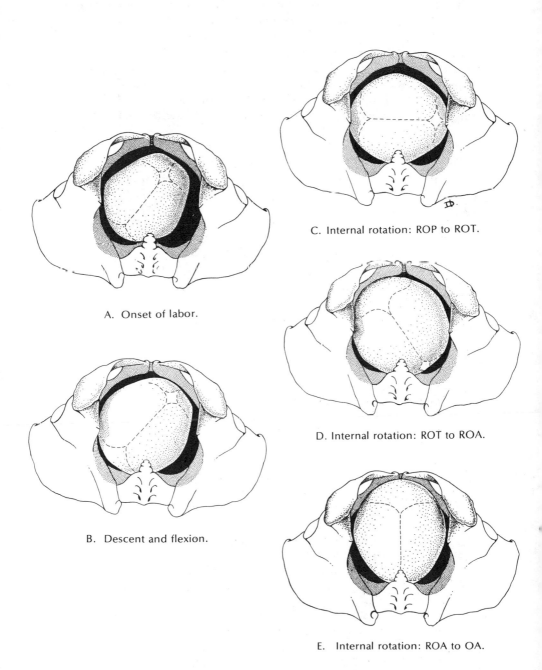

A. Onset of labor.

B. Descent and flexion.

C. Internal rotation: ROP to ROT.

D. Internal rotation: ROT to ROA.

E. Internal rotation: ROA to OA.

FIG. 2. ROP: long arc rotation.

Extension   The nape of the neck pivots in the subpubic angle, and the head is born by extension (Figs. 2F and G). The bregma, forehead, nose, mouth, and chin pass over the perineum in order.

Restitution   Restitution (OA to ROA) takes place to the right (Fig. 2H). The extent of restitution depends on how far the shoulders have followed the head during internal rotation. In most cases the shoulders turn with the head, lagging behind only 45°, and restitution is the usual 45°. Occasionally the shoulders may lag behind more or may swing back. The head then restitutes 90° or even 135°.

External Rotation   The anterior shoulder strikes the pelvic floor and rotates 45° toward the pubic symphysis so that the bisacromial diameter of the shoulders is in the anteroposterior diameter of the outlet. The head follows the shoulders, and the occiput rotates 45° to the right transverse position—ROA to ROT (Fig. 2I).

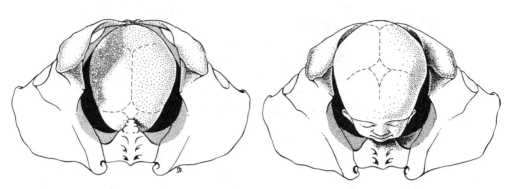

F. Extension beginning.

G. Extension complete.

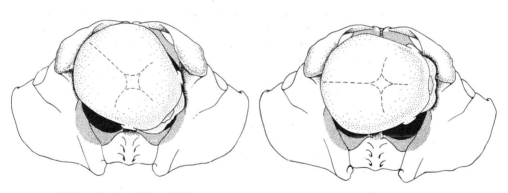

H. Restitution: OA to ROA.

I. External rotation: ROA to ROT.

FIG. 2. (cont.). ROP: long arc rotation.

SHORT ARC ROTATION: 45° TO THE POSTERIOR

Descent The head enters the inlet with the sagittal suture in the right oblique (Fig. 3A). Descent continues throughout labor.

Flexion Flexion (Fig. 3B) is imperfect, resulting in a longer presenting diameter.

Internal Rotation The occiput turns posteriorly 45° (ROP to OP) into the hollow of the sacrum (Fig. 3C). The sagittal suture is in the antero-posterior diameter of the pelvis. The bregma is behind the pubis.

RIGHT OCCIPUT POSTERIOR: ROP

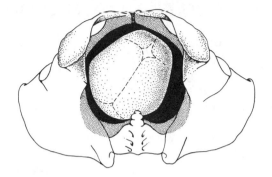

A. Onset of labor.

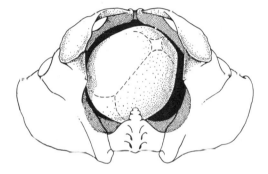

B. Descent and flexion.

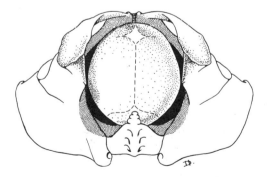

C. Internal rotation: ROP to OP.

FIG. 3. ROP: short arc rotation.

Birth of Head   Birth of the head is by a combination of flexion and extension (Fig. 3D–G).

There are two mechanisms of flexion:

1. Where there is good flexion the area anterior to the bregma pivots under the symphysis pubis. The presenting diameter is the suboccipitofrontal of 10.5 cm. The bregma, vertex, small fontanelle, and occiput are born by further flexion.
2. Where flexion is incomplete the root of the nose pivots under the symphysis. The presenting diameter is the larger occipitofrontal of 11.5 cm. This bigger diameter is more traumatic than the smaller one. By flexion, the forehead, bregma, vertex, and occiput are born over the perineum.

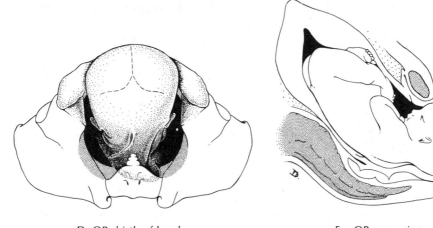

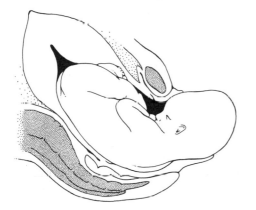

D. OP: birth of head.

E. OP: crowning.

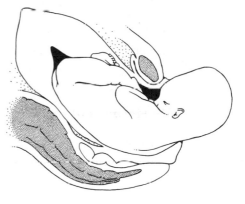

F. OP: flexion beginning.

G. OP: flexion complete.

FIG. 3. (cont.) ROP: short arc rotation.

Once the top and back of the head have been born by flexion, the occiput falls back toward the anus, and the nose, mouth, and chin are born under the symphysis pubis by extension (Figs. 3H and I).

Restitution of the occiput is 45° to the right oblique (OP to ROP) to resume the normal relationship of the head to the shoulders (Fig. 3J).

The anterior shoulder strikes the pelvic floor and rotates 45° toward the symphysis pubis, to bring the bisacromial diameter of the shoulders into the anteroposterior diameter of the pelvis (external rotation). The head follows, and the occiput rotates 45° to the right transverse position—ROP to ROT (Fig. 3K).

MOLDING

In persistent occipitoposterior positions the head is shortened in the occipitofrontal and lengthened in the suboccipitobregmatic and mentobregmatic diameters. The head rises steeply in front and in back. The caput succedaneum is located over the bregma. Molding (Fig. 4) and extensive edema of the scalp make accurate identification of the sutures and fontanelles difficult, thereby obscuring the diagnosis.

SUMMARIES

Summaries of both long arc and short arc rotations may be reviewed in Figures 5 and 6, respectively.

Management of the Progressing Case

1. Expectant observation is the best policy. Given sufficient time, most posterior positions of the occiput rotate anteriorly, and the baby is delivered spontaneously or by low forceps. Thus as long as the fetus and mother are in good condition and labor is progressing, there is no justification for hasty interference. The safe and wise rule is to leave occipitoposterior positions to nature, supplying only supportive measures until there is a definite indication for active intervention.

2. While it is believed that anterior rotation is helped by the mother's lying on the same side as the fetal limbs, most women remain in the position of greatest comfort.

3. Because the labor may be long and difficult for mother and child, care must be exercised to ensure adequate intake of fluids and nourishment. More judicious use of analgesia and sedation is required than in normal occipitoanterior positions.

4. When the head is delivered in the posterior position (face to pubis) the large back part of the head (biparietal diameter of

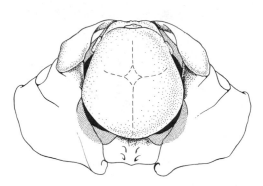

H. Extension: vaginal view.

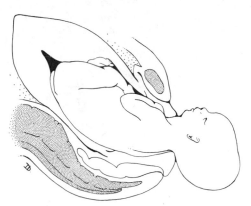

I. Extension: lateral view.

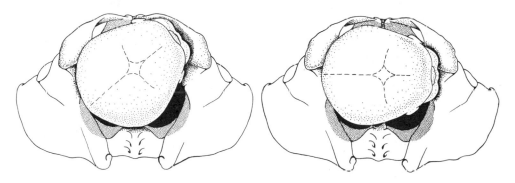

J. Restitution: OP to ROP.

K. External rotation: ROP to ROT.

FIG. 3. (cont.). ROP: Short arc rotation.

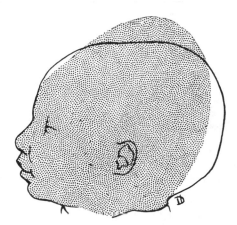

FIG. 4. Molding: ROP.

151

POSTERIOR POSITIONS OF THE OCCIPUT

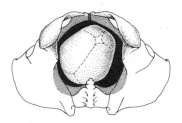

A. ROP: onset of labor.

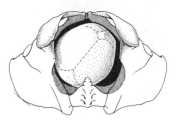

B. Descent and flexion.

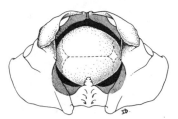

C. Internal rotation: ROP to ROT.

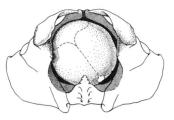

D. Internal rotation: ROT to ROA.

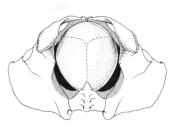

E. Internal rotation: ROA to OA.

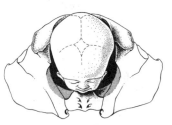

F. Extension.

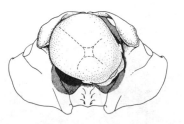

G. Restitution: OA to ROA.

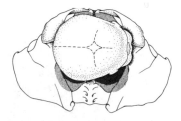

H. External rotation: ROA to ROT.

FIG. 5. Summary of long arc rotation: ROP to OA.

RIGHT OCCIPUT POSTERIOR: ROP

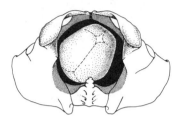

A. ROP: onset of labor.

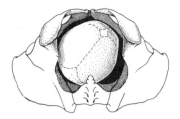

B. Descent and flexion.

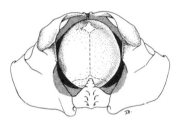

C. Internal rotation: ROP to OP.

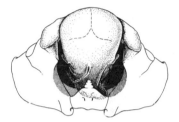

D. Birth by flexion.

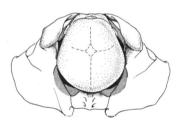

E. Head falls back in extension.

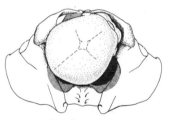

F. Restitution: OP to ROP.

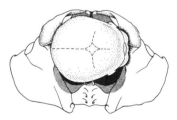

G. External rotation: ROP to ROT.

FIG. 6. Summary of short arc rotation: ROP to OP.

9.5 cm) causes greater stretching and more lacerations of the perineum than does the narrow anterior part of the head (bitemporal diameter of 8.0 cm). For this reason a large episiotomy is indicated. Frequently there is arrest at the perineum, and low forceps is the management of choice to save mother and child from the effects of a prolonged period of bearing down.

Indications for Interference

MATERNAL DISTRESS
Maternal distress is fatigue or exhaustion and is accompanied by the following signs:

1. Pulse above 100 beats/minute
2. Temperature above 100F
3. Dehydration, dry tongue, dry skin, concentrated urine
4. Loss of emotional stability

FETAL DISTRESS
Fetal distress is shown by:

1. Irregular fetal heart rate
2. Fetal heart rate below 100 or over 160 beats minute between uterine contractions
3. Passage of meconium in a vertex presentation

LACK OF PROGRESS
The cessation of descent and/or rotation indicates that labor is arrested and that interference is mandatory. Reasons for failure of descent and rotation include:

1. Cephalopelvic disproportion
2. Android midpelvis
3. Ineffective uterine contractions
4. Deflexion of the head
5. Uterine contraction ring preventing the shoulders from rotating anteriorly
6. Multiparity, pendulous abdomen, poor abdominal and uterine tone
7. A weak pelvic floor, failing to guide the occiput anteriorly

While the basic strategy of nonintervention is, up to a point, a wise one, it is not safe to wait too long; fine judgment is needed to decide the point at which further delay is undesirable or even harmful. Where the standard signs of fetal or maternal distress are present, the decision to interfere is based on clear-cut grounds. However, when the contractions are long, strong, and too frequent, the risk of intracranial damage is present and operative therapy must be instituted sooner, even though the fetal heart sounds are normal and no meconium has been passed.

In competent hands a wait of 2 hours during the second stage is sufficient. If, however, the attendant is not skilled in operative obstetrics, it may be safer to wait longer, but only if the baby and mother are in good condition.

Methods of Operative Vaginal Delivery in Arrested Occipitoposterior Position

Vaginal delivery by forceps is the procedure of choice, but only if the following prerequisites have been fulfilled:

1. The fetal head must be engaged—i.e., the biparietal diameter has passed through the pelvic inlet, and the bony presenting part has reached the level of the ischial spines.
2. There must be no cephalopelvic disproportion.
3. The cervix must be fully dilated.
4. The membranes have to be ruptured.
5. Accurate diagnosis of position and station is essential.

Under these conditions an arrest of progress in the second stage of labor of approximately 2 hours in a primigravida and 1 hour in a multipara is an indication for reevaluation and consideration of operative delivery. Fetal or maternal distress demands earlier interference. If the prerequisites are not present, vaginal delivery must not be attempted.

With forceps the fetal head can be delivered in the posterior position or it can be rotated to the anterior position before being extracted. The various maneuvers are described in Chapter 27. If an attempt at delivery with forceps fails, cesarean section is performed.

Management When Conditions for Immediate Vaginal Delivery Are Not Present

FETOPELVIC DISPROPORTION
If there has been no progress in the face of efficient uterine contractions and a diagnosis of fetopelvic disproportion has been made, cesarean section should be performed.

INTACT MEMBRANES

Intact membranes do not always help labor and often even seem to retard it. Therefore before the progress of labor can be considered halted, the membranes should be ruptured artificially and the patient given a further trial of labor. With these measures the patient frequently makes good progress in rotation and descent, and spontaneous delivery takes place.

INEFFECTIVE UTERINE CONTRACTIONS

Ineffective uterine contractions result in slow advance or none at all. There are two main groups of cases: (1) myometrial fatigue resulting from long labor and (2) inefficient uterine action, a condition frequently associated with posterior positions of the occiput, as well as with other malpresentations.

Two types of therapy are available: (1) the uterus can be rested or (2) it can be stimulated. Since in most cases the patient is weary, she should be helped to rest. Ten milligrams of morphine sulfate or 100 mg of Demerol gives the patient an hour or two of sleep, and an infusion of a liter (or more if needed) of 5 percent glucose in water improves her state of hydration. In many instances good labor starts soon after the patient awakens.

If effective labor does not begin, the uterus may be stimulated. The best method of doing this is to add 5 units of oxytocin to a liter of 5 percent glucose in water and to give this as an intravenous infusion. The drip is started slowly, at a rate of about 10 drops/minute, and the effect on the contractions and the fetal heart is observed. The subsequent speed is governed by the effect. The aim is to achieve good uterine contractions every 2 to 3 minutes, lasting 45 to 60 seconds (see Chapter 39).

UNDILATED CERVIX

The causes and management of failure of the cervix to dilate fully or to progress beyond 4 to 5 cm fall into several groups (see Chapter 38).

1. When the basic etiology is cephalopelvic disproportion, treatment by cesarean section is best for mother and child.
2. Artificial rupture of the bag of waters, by bringing the presenting part into closer apposition with the cervix, brings about more rapid dilatation in many instances.
3. When inefficient uterine action does not open the cervix, treatment is instituted to correct the defective contractions.
4. When some intrinsic disease of the cervix prevents it from dilating, cesarean section must be performed.
5. Dührssen's incisions can be made. Under direct vision the cervix is incised at 2, 6, and 10 o'clock. The baby is delivered with for-

ceps and the incisions repaired. These incision sites are chosen because their extension results in the least serious damage. It must be emphasized that deliveries through an incompletely dilated cervix or through Dührssen's incisions are done only when the cervix is thin and near full dilatation and never when the cervix is thick or less than half open. These procedures are performed rarely today. Better methods of therapy are available (see Chapter 34).

BIBLIOGRAPHY

Phillips RD, Freeman M: The management of the persistent occiput posterior position. Obstet Gynecol 43:171, 1974

14.

Malpresentations

GENERAL ETIOLOGIC FACTORS

Accidental Factors

This classification is used when there is no discovered cause for the malpresentation.

Maternal and Uterine Factors

1. Contracted pelvis. This is the most important factor.
2. Pendulous maternal abdomen. If the uterus and fetus are allowed to fall forward, there may be difficulty in engagement.
3. Neoplasms. Uterine fibromyomas or ovarian cysts can block the entry to the pelvis.
4. Uterine anomalies. In a bicornuate uterus the nonpregnant horn may obstruct labor in the pregnant one.
5. Abnormalities of placental size or location. Conditions such as placenta previa are associated with unfavorable positions of the fetus.

Fetal Factors

1. Large baby.
2. Errors in fetal polarity, such as breech presentation and transverse lie.
3. Abnormal internal rotation. The occiput rotates posteriorly or fails to rotate at all.
4. Fetal attitude: extension in place of normal flexion.
5. Multiple pregnancy.
6. Fetal anomalies, including hydrocephaly and anencephaly.

7. Polyhydramnios. An excessive amount of amniotic fluid allows the baby freedom of activity, and it may assume abnormal positions.

EFFECTS OF MALPRESENTATIONS

Effects on Labor

The less symmetrical adaptation of the presenting part to the cervix and to the pelvis plays a part in reducing the efficiency of labor.

1. The incidence of fetopelvic disproportion is higher.
2. Inefficient uterine action is common. The contractions tend to be weak and irregular.
3. Prolonged labor is seen frequently.
4. Pathologic retraction rings can develop, and rupture of the lower uterine segment may be the end result.
5. The cervix often dilates slowly and incompletely.
6. The presenting part stays high.
7. Premature rupture of the membranes occurs often.
8. The need for operative delivery is increased.

Effects on the Mother

1. Because greater uterine and intraabdominal muscular effort is required, and because labor is often prolonged with attendant lack of rest and inadequate nourishment, maternal exhaustion is common.
2. There is more stretching of the perineum and soft parts, and there are more lacerations.
3. Bleeding is more profuse, originating from:
   a. Tears of the uterus, cervix, and vagina
   b. The placental site, maternal exhaustion leading to uterine atony
4. There is a greater incidence of infection. This is caused by:
   a. Early rupture of the membranes
   b. Excessive blood loss
   c. Tissue damage
   d. Frequent rectal and vaginal examinations
5. The patient's discomfort seems out of proportion to the strength

of the uterine contractions. She complains bitterly of pain before the uterus is felt to harden, and continues to feel the pain after the uterus has relaxed.

6. Paresis of the bowel and bladder add to the patient's suffering.

Effects on the Fetus

1. The fetus fits the pelvis less perfectly, making its passage through the pelvis more difficult and leading to excessive molding.
2. The long labor is harder on the baby, with a greater incidence of anoxia, brain damage, asphyxia, and intrauterine death.
3. There is a higher incidence of operative delivery, increasing the danger of trauma to the baby.
4. Prolapse of the umbilical cord is more common than in normal positions.

15.

Face Presentation

GENERAL CONSIDERATIONS

Definition

The lie is longitudinal, the presentation is cephalic, the presenting part is the face, the attitude is one of complete extension, the chin (mentum, M) is the denominator and leading pole, and the presenting diameter is the submentobregmatic of 9.5 cm. In face presentations the part between the glabella and chin presents; in brow presentations it is the part between the glabella and bregma. However, positions intermediate to these are seen often.

Incidence

The incidence is less than 1 percent (one in 250) and is higher in multiparas than primigravidas. Primary face presentations are present before the onset of labor and are rare. Most face presentations are secondary, extension taking place during labor generally at the pelvic inlet. About 70 percent of face presentations are anterior or transverse, while 30 percent are posterior.

Etiology

Anything that delays engagement in flexion can contribute to the etiology of attitudes of extension. There is an association between attitudes of extension and cephalopelvic disproportion, and since this is a serious combination the presence of a small pelvis or a large head must be ruled out with certainty. Rare causes of extension include thyroid neoplasms, which act by pushing the head back; multiple coils of cord around the neck, which prevent flexion; and spasm or shortening of the extensor muscles of the neck. Anencephalic fetuses frequently present by the face. In many cases no cause can be found.

161

ANTERIOR FACE PRESENTATIONS

The following descriptions apply to the left mentum anterior (LMA) presentation. The mechanism for the right mentum anterior (RMA) presentation is similar to that for LMA except that the chin, small parts, and fetal heart are on the right side, while the back and cephalic prominence are on the left.

Diagnosis of Position: LMA

ABDOMINAL EXAMINATION

1. The long axes of the fetus and mother are parallel (Fig. 1A).
2. The head is at the pelvis. Early in labor the head is not engaged.
3. The back is on the right side of the mother's abdomen, but since it is posterior, it is often felt indistinctly. The small parts are on the left and anterior. Extension of the spine causes the chest to be thrown out and the back to be hollowed.
4. The breech is in the fundus.
5. The cephalic prominence (the occiput) is on the right. An important diagnostic sign of extension attitudes is that the back and the cephalic prominence are on the same side. When flexion is present, the cephalic prominence and the back are on opposite sides.
6. It must be kept in mind that in anterior face presentations the baby's back and occiput are posterior. When the chin is posterior, on the other hand, the back and occiput are anterior.

FETAL HEART
The fetal heart tones are transmitted through the anterior chest wall of the fetus and are heard loudest in the left lower quadrant of the maternal abdomen, on the same side as the small parts.

VAGINAL EXAMINATION

1. The clue to diagnosis is a negative finding—i.e., absence of the round, even, hard vertex. In place of the dome of the skull with its identifying suture lines and fontanelles, there is a softer and irregular presenting part. One suspects face or breech. Identification of the various parts of the face clinches the diagnosis. After prolonged labor marked edema may confuse the picture.
2. The long axis of the face is in the right oblique diameter of the pelvis (Fig. 1B).

3. The chin is in the left anterior quadrant of the maternal pelvis.
4. The forehead is in the right posterior quadrant of the pelvis.
5. Vaginal examination must be performed gently to avoid injury to the eyes.

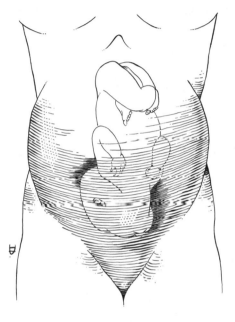

A. Abdominal view.

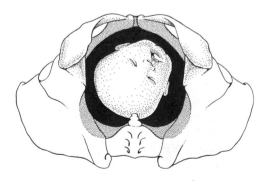

B. Vaginal view.

FIG. 1. Left mentum anterior.

X-RAY EXAMINATION

Occasionally radiologic examination is necessary in nonprogressing labors to diagnose the position and to estimate pelvic capacity.

LATE DIAGNOSIS

Because most face presentations make good progress, the diagnosis may not be made until the face has reached the floor of the pelvis or until advance has ceased.

Mechanism of Labor: LMA

EXTENSION

For some reason the head does not flex. Instead, it extends (Fig. 2), so that in place of an LOP or ROP there is an RMA or an LMA. The baby enters the pelvis chin first. The presenting diameter in face presentations (submentobregmatic) and in well flexed head presentations (suboccipitobregmatic) is 9.5 cm in each case. This is one of the reasons why most anterior face presentations come to spontaneous delivery.

DESCENT

With the chin as the leading part, engagement takes place in the right oblique diameter of the pelvis. Descent is slower than in flexed attitudes. The face is low in the pelvis before the biparietal diameter has passed the brim. When the forward leading edge of the presenting face is felt at the level of the ischial spines, the tracheobregmatic diameter is still above the inlet.

INTERNAL ROTATION

With descent and molding, the chin reaches the pelvic floor, where it is directed downward, forward, and medially. As it rotates 45° anteriorly toward the symphysis (LMA to MA), the long axis of the face comes into the anteroposterior diameter of the pelvis (Figs. 2C and D). With further descent the chin escapes under the symphysis. The shoulders have remained in the oblique diameter, so the neck is twisted 45°. An essential feature of internal rotation is that the chin must rotate anteriorly and under the symphysis, or spontaneous delivery is impossible. Anterior rotation does not take place until the face is well applied to the pelvic floor and may be delayed until late in labor. The attendant must not give up hope too soon.

ANTERIOR FACE PRESENTATIONS

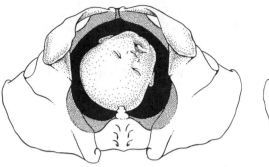 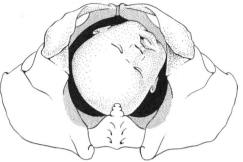

A. LMA: onset of labor.

B. Extension and descent.

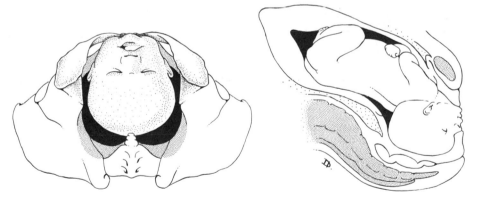

C. Vaginal view.

D. Lateral view.

C and D.   Internal rotation: LMA to MA.

FIG. 2. Mechanism of labor.

FLEXION

The head is born by flexion (Figs. 2E–G). The submental region at the neck impinges under the symphysis pubis. With the head pivoting around this point, the mouth, nose, orbits, forehead, vertex, and occiput are born over the perineum by flexion. The head then falls back (Figs. 2H and I).

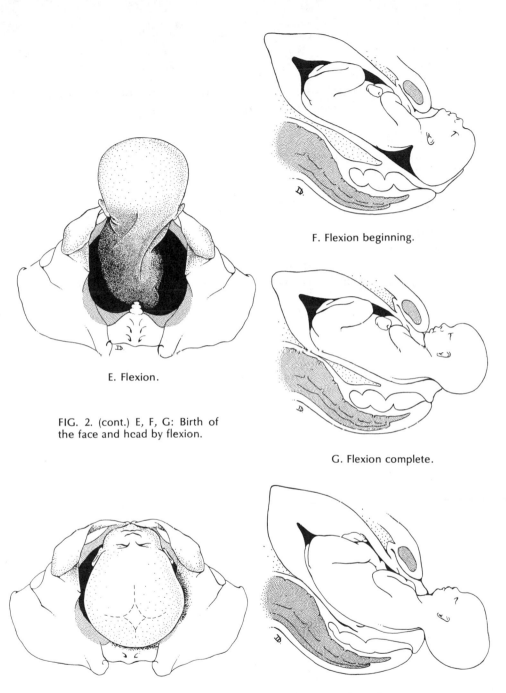

E. Flexion.

FIG. 2. (cont.) E, F, G: Birth of the face and head by flexion.

F. Flexion beginning.

G. Flexion complete.

H. Vaginal view.

I. Lateral view.

FIG. 2. (cont.) H, I: Head falls back in extension.

RESTITUTION

As the head is released from the vagina, the neck untwists and the chin turns 45° back toward the original side (Fig. 2J).

EXTERNAL ROTATION

The anterior shoulder reaches the pelvic floor and rotates toward the symphysis to bring the bisacromial diameter from the oblique to the anteroposterior diameter of the outlet. The chin rotates back another 45° to maintain the head in its correct relationship to the shoulders (Fig. 2K).

MOLDING

Molding (Fig. 3) leads to an elongation of the head in its antero-posterior diameter and flattening from above downward. The forehead and occiput protrude. The extension of the head on the trunk disappears after a few days.

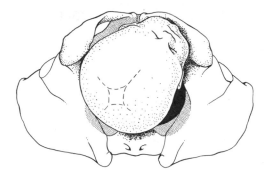

J. Restitution: MA to LMA.

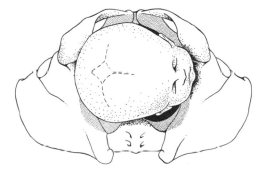

K. External rotation: LMA to LMT.
FIG. 2. (cont.) Head falls back in extension.

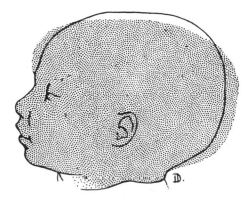

FIG. 3. Molding: face presentation.

Prognosis: Anterior Face Presentations

LABOR

Because the face is a poor dilator, and because attitudes of extension are less favorable, labor takes longer than in normal occipitoanterior positions. The labor is conducted with this in mind. Delay takes place at the inlet, but once the face presentation and the labor are well established steady progress is the rule. Over 90 percent of anterior face presentations deliver per vaginam without complications. Figure 4 summarizes the mechanism of labor with the LMA presentation.

MOTHER

The mother has more work to do, suffers more pain, and receives greater lacerations than in normal positions.

FETUS

The baby does well in most cases, but the prognosis is less favorable than in normal presentations. The outlook for the child can be improved by early diagnosis, carefully conducted first and second stages of labor, and the restriction of operative vaginal deliveries to easily performed procedures. Cesarean section is preferable to complicated, difficult, and traumatic vaginal operations.

The membranes rupture early in labor, and the face takes the brunt of the punishment so that it becomes badly swollen and misshapen. Its appearance is a great worry to the parents. The edema disappears gradually, and the infant takes on a more normal appearance. Edema of the larynx may result from prolonged pressure of the hyoid region of the neck against the pubic bone. For the first 24 hours the baby must be watched carefully to detect any difficulty in breathing.

Management of Anterior Face Presentations

1. DISPROPORTION   Disproportion is managed by cesarean section.
2. NORMAL PELVIS   In a normal pelvis anterior face presentations are left alone for these reasons:
   a. Most deliver spontaneously or with the aid of low forceps.
   b. Should conversion (flexion) be successful, the anterior face presentation is replaced by an occipitoposterior one (LMA to ROP or RMA to LOP). This does not improve the situation and may make it worse.
   c. If conversion is partially successful, the face is changed to a brow presentation. In this case a face presentation, which usually delivers spontaneously, is replaced by a brow, which cannot.

ANTERIOR FACE PRESENTATIONS

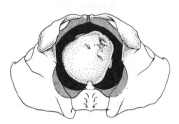

A. LMA: onset of labor.

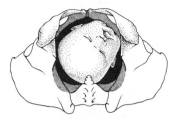

B. Extension and descent.

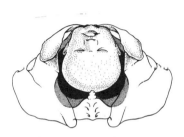

C. Internal rotation: LMA to MA.

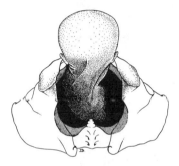

D. Flexion.

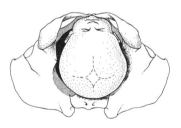

E. Extension.

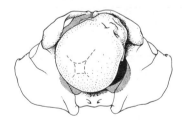

F. Restitution: MA to LMA.

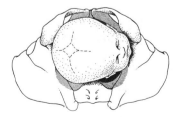

G. External rotation: LMA to LMT.

FIG. 4. Summary of mechanism of labor: LMA.

3. ARREST Arrest below the spines is treated best by extraction with low forceps. Arrest high in the pelvis is treated by cesarean section.

TRANSVERSE FACE PRESENTATIONS

The long axis of the face is in the transverse diameter of the pelvis, with the chin on one side and the forehead on the other (Fig. 5).

The following descriptions apply to the left mentum transverse (LMT) presentation. The mechanism of labor for the right mentum transverse (RMT) presentation is the same as that for LMT except that the chin, small parts, and fetal heart are on the right, while the back and cephalic prominence are on the left.

Diagnosis of Position: LMT

ABDOMINAL EXAMINATION

1. The long axis of the fetus is parallel to that of the mother.
2. The head is at the pelvis.
3. The back is on the right, toward the maternal flank. The small parts are on the left side.
4. The breech is in the fundus.
5. The cephalic prominence (the occiput) is on the right, the same side as the back.

FETAL HEART
The fetal heart is heard loudest in the left lower quadrant of the mother's abdomen.

VAGINAL EXAMINATION

1. The long axis of the face is in the transverse diameter of the pelvis.
2. The chin is to the left, at 3 o'clock.
3. The forehead is to the right, at 9 o'clock.

TRANSVERSE FACE PRESENTATIONS

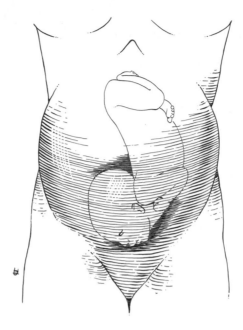

A. Abdominal view.

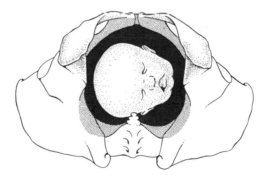

B. Vaginal view.

FIG. 5. Left mentum transverse.

Mechanism of Labor: LMT

A summary of the mechanism of labor for the LMT presentation is given in Figure 6.

EXTENSION
Extension to LMT occurs instead of flexion to ROT.

DESCENT
Engagement takes place in the transverse diameter of the pelvis. Descent is slow.

INTERNAL ROTATION
The chin rotates 90° anteriorly to the midline (LMT to LMA to MA). The chin comes under the symphysis.

FLEXION
The submental region of the neck impinges in the subpubic angle. Birth is by flexion, after which the head falls backward.

RESTITUTION
As the neck untwists, the head turns back 45°.

EXTERNAL ROTATION
The shoulders turn from the oblique into the anteroposterior diameter of the pelvis, and the head rotates back another 45°.

Clinical Course of Labor and Management: LMT

1. Anterior rotation takes place in the majority of cases, LMT to LMA to MA. The treatment is the same as LMA. Delivery is spontaneous or assisted by low forceps.
2. Arrest as LMT low in the pelvis is treated by rotation of the face (LMT to LMA to MA), either manually or by forceps. Once rotation has been achieved, the head is extracted with forceps.
3. Arrest as LMT high in the pelvis is treated by cesarean section.

TRANSVERSE FACE PRESENTATIONS

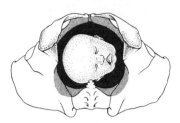

A. LMT: onset of labor.

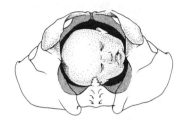

B. Descent.

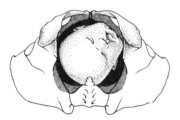

C. Internal rotation: LMT to LMA.

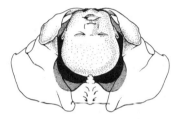

D. Internal rotation: LMA to MA.

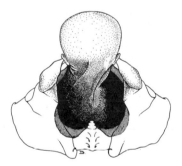

E. Birth by flexion.

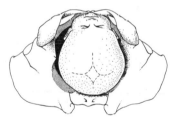

F. Extension.

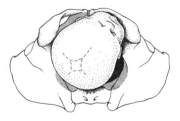

G. Restitution: MA to LMA.

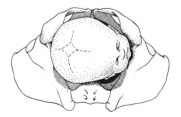

H. External rotation: LMA to LMT.

FIG. 6. Mechanism of labor: LMT.

POSTERIOR FACE PRESENTATIONS

Some 30 percent of face presentations are posterior. Most of these rotate anteriorly. The flexed counterpart of the posterior face is the anterior occiput; thus LMP flexes to ROA and RMP to LOA. Persistent posterior face presentations become arrested, as they cannot deliver spontaneously. The descriptions here are for the left mentum posterior (LMP) presentation.

Diagnosis of Position: LMP

ABDOMINAL EXAMINATION

1. The long axis of the fetus is parallel to the long axis of the mother (Fig. 7A).
2. The head is at the pelvis.
3. The back is anterior and to the right. The small parts are on the left and posterior.
4. The breech is in the fundus of the uterus.
5. The cephalic prominence (occiput) is to the right and anterior. It is on the same side as the back.

FETAL HEART
The fetal heart tones, transmitted through the anterior shoulder, are heard loudest in the left lower quadrant of the mother's abdomen.

VAGINAL EXAMINATION

1. The long diameter of the face is in the left oblique diameter of the pelvis.
2. The chin is in the left posterior quadrant of the pelvis (Fig. 8B).
3. The forehead is in the right anterior quadrant.

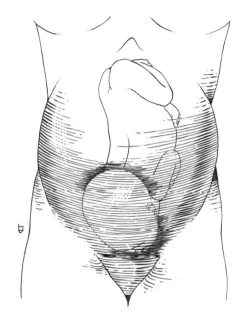

A. Abdominal view.

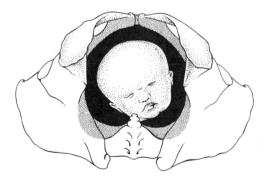

B. Vaginal view.

FIG. 7. Left mentum posterior.

Mechanism of Labor: LMP

There are two basic mechanisms:

1. Long arc rotation, with the chin rotating 135° to the anterior. About two-thirds of posterior face presentations do this and deliver spontaneously or with the aid of low forceps.
2. Short arc rotation of 45° to the posterior, with the chin ending up in the hollow of the sacrum. These cases become arrested as persistent posterior face presentations.

Long Arc Rotation: 135° to the Anterior

EXTENSION
Extension to LMP (Fig. 8) occurs instead of flexion to ROA.

DESCENT
Descent is slow. The presenting part remains high while the essential molding takes place. Without extreme molding the vertex cannot pass under the anterior part of the pelvic inlet.

INTERNAL ROTATION
The slow descent continues; the marked molding enables the chin to reach the pelvic floor, where it rotates 135° to the anterior and comes to lie under the symphysis. Since the original position was LMP, the sequence is LMP to LMT to LMA to MA in rotations of 45° between each step.

FLEXION
The submental area pivots under the symphysis, and the head is born by flexion. The head then falls backward.

RESTITUTION
The chin rotates back 45° as the neck untwists.

EXTERNAL ROTATION
With the rotation of the shoulders from the oblique into the antero-posterior diameter of the pelvis, the chin turns back another 45°.

POSTERIOR FACE PRESENTATIONS

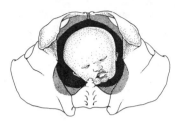

A. LMP: descent.

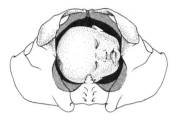

B. Internal rotation: LMP to LMT.

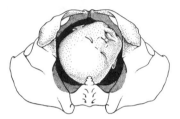

C. Internal rotation: LMT to LMA.

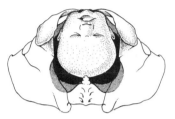

D. Internal rotation: LMA to MA.

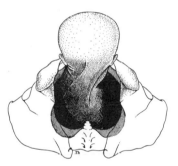

E. Birth by flexion.

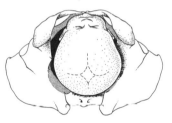

F. Head falls back in extension.

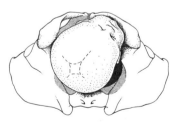

G. Restitution: MA to LMA.

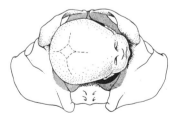

H. External rotation: LMA to LMT.

FIG. 8. LMP: long arc rotation.

Short Arc Rotation: 45° to the Posterior

EXTENSION
Extension to LMP takes place (Fig. 9).

DESCENT
Descent occurs with the help of extreme molding.

INTERNAL ROTATION
The chin rotates 45° posteriorly into the hollow of the sacrum (LMP to MP); impaction follows. The sacrum is 12 to 15 cm in length, while the fetal neck is only 5 cm. Flexion is impossible, and further advancement cannot take place unless the baby is so small that the shoulders and head can enter the pelvis together. This is rarely feasible, and arrest of progress results.

POSTERIOR FACE PRESENTATIONS

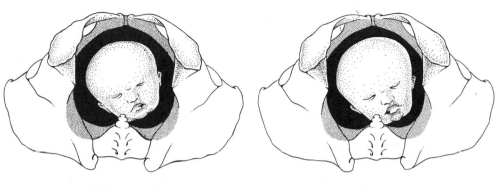

A. LMP: onset of labor.

B. Descent.

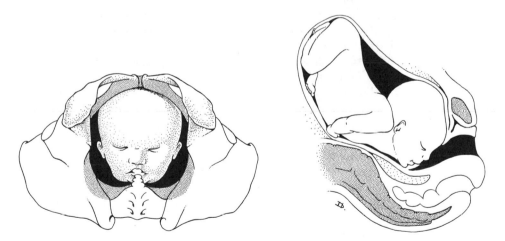

C. Vaginal view.

D. Lateral view.

C and D. Internal rotation: LMP to MP.

FIG. 9.   LMP: short arc rotation.

Prognosis: Posterior Face Presentations

The prolonged labor and difficult rotation are traumatic to both baby and mother. When the chin rotates posteriorly the prognosis is poor unless the situation is corrected. Maternal morbidity is directly proportional to the degree of difficulty of the birth. High forceps or version and extraction carry with them the most morbid postpartum courses.

Management of Posterior Face Presentations

1. DISPROPORTION Disproportion is managed by cesarean section.
2. NORMAL PELVIS Since two-thirds of posterior faces rotate anteriorly and deliver spontaneously, plenty of time should be given for this rotation to be accomplished. Internal rotation may not take place until late in labor when the face is distending the pelvic floor. Hence interference must not be rash.
3. PERSISTENT POSTERIOR FACE—MULTIPARA WITH NORMAL PELVIS Since persistent mentum posteriors cannot deliver spontaneously, operative interference is necessary. Several procedures are available.
    a. Flexion (conversion) from mentoposterior to occipitoanterior is the best treatment. One method of accomplishing this is by the *Thorn maneuver* (Fig. 10). The cervix must be fully dilated. With the vaginal hand the operator flexes the fetal head. Through the maternal abdomen he uses the other hand to flex the body by pushing on the breech. At the same time an assistant presses against the baby's thorax or abdomen to try and jackknife the infant's body. This procedure is performed under anesthesia and must be done soon after the membranes rupture. If the amniotic fluid has drained away, the dry uterine cavity and snug fit of the uterus around the baby make it difficult or impossible to carry out this treatment. Once flexion has been accomplished, the head is pushed into the pelvis and held in place.
    b. Rotation to a mentum anterior can sometimes be achieved by manual rotation, but in most cases forceps are required.
    c. Cesarean section is employed if the above maneuvers fail.
    d. Version and extraction, although once popular, have no place in the modern management of face presentations, except in the occasional case of a second twin.
    e. Destructive operation on the baby may be necessary if nothing else can be done and the baby is dead.

4. **PERSISTENT POSTERIOR FACE—PRIMIGRAVIDA WITH NORMAL PELVIS** Cesarean section gives the best results in most cases. Some authorities feel that flexion to occiput anterior or rotation to mentum anterior should be attempted before cesarean section is carried out.

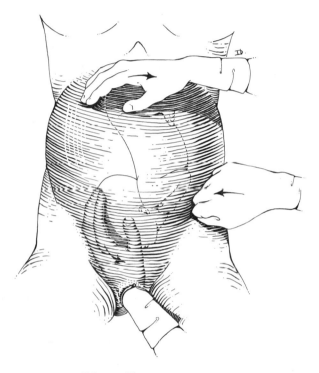

FIG. 10. Thorn maneuver.

16.

Brow Presentation

GENERAL CONSIDERATIONS

Definition

Brow presentation is an attitude of partial (halfway) extension, in contrast to face presentation in which extension is complete. The presenting part is the area between the orbital ridges and the bregma. The denominator is the forehead (frontum: Fr). The presenting diameter is the verticomental, which, at 13.5 cm, is the longest anteroposterior diameter of the fetal head.

Incidence

The incidence is under 1 percent, ranging from 1:3,000 to 1:1,000. Primary brow presentations—those that occur before labor has started—are rare. The majority are secondary—i.e., they occur after the onset of labor. Often the position is transitory, and the head either flexes to an occiput presentation or extends completely and becomes a face presentation.

Etiology

The causes are similar to those of face presentation and include anything that interferes with engagement in flexion.

1. Cephalopelvic disproportion is of great significance.
2. Some fetal conditions prevent flexion.
   a. Tumors of the neck, e.g., thyroid
   b. Coils of umbilical cord around the neck
   c. Fetal anomalies
3. Increased fetal mobility.
   a. Polyhydramnios
   b. Small or premature baby

184

4. Premature rupture of membranes when the head is not engaged. It is trapped in an attitude of extension.
5. Uterine abnormalities.
   a. Neoplasm of lower segment
   b. Bicornuate uterus
6. Abnormal placental implantation: placenta previa.
7. Iatrogenic: external version.
8. Idiopathic: nearly 30 percent are unexplained.

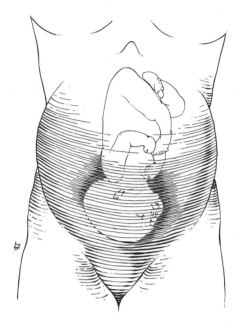

A. Abdominal view.

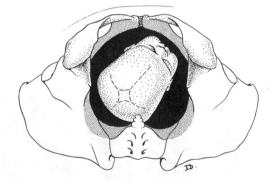

B. Vaginal view.

FIG. 1. Left frontum anterior.

LEFT FRONTUM ANTERIOR: LFrA

Diagnosis of Position: LFrA

ABDOMINAL EXAMINATION

1. The lie is longitudinal (Fig. 1A).
2. The head is at the pelvis but is not engaged.
3. The back is on the mother's right and posterior; it may be difficult to palpate. The small parts are on the left and anterior.
4. The breech is in the fundus of the uterus.
5. The cephalic prominence (occiput) and the back are on the same side (the right).

FETAL HEART

Fetal heart sounds are heard best in the left lower quadrant of the maternal abdomen.

VAGINAL EXAMINATION

1. The anteroposterior diameter of the head is in the right oblique diameter of the pelvis (Fig. 1B).
2. The brow, the area between the nasion and the bregma, presents and is felt in the left anterior quadrant of the pelvis.
3. The vertex is in the right posterior quadrant.
4. The bregma (anterior fontanelle) is palpated easily.
5. The frontal suture is felt, but the sagittal suture is usually out of reach.
6. Identification of the supraorbital ridges is a key to diagnosis.

X-RAY EXAMINATION

When labor has been prolonged and the landmarks on the fetal head are obscured by edema and molding, x-ray pelvimetry is helpful in making the diagnosis and assessing the pelvis.

LATE AND FAILED DIAGNOSIS

The difference, on vaginal examination, between the hard, smooth dome of the skull and the soft irregular face is great enough to diagnose the abnormal position or at least to suspect it. On the other hand, the feel of the vertex and that of the forehead may be similar, and molding and edema add to the difficulty of differentiation. Hence anything short of a most careful abdominal and vaginal examination with a high index of suspicion fails to identify the malposition. A good rule is that whenever there is failure of progress, one should examine the patient thoroughly, keeping brow presentation in mind.

Mechanism of Labor: LFrA

Presenting diameter is the verticomental, measuring 13.5 cm. It is the longest anterposterior diameter of the head. When engagement takes place it is accompanied by extensive molding, and when progress occurs it is slow.

Spontaneous labor and delivery can take place when there is the combination of (1) a large pelvis, (2) strong uterine contractions, and (3) a small baby. In these cases the following mechanism of labor (Fig. 2) occurs.

EXTENSION
The head extends and the verticomental diameter presents, with the forehead leading the way.

DESCENT
Descent is slow and late. Usually the head does not settle into the pelvis until the membranes have ruptured and the cervix has reached full dilatation.

INTERNAL ROTATION
The forehead rotates anteriorly 45° so that the face comes to lie behind the pubic symphysis (LFrA to FrA). A considerable amount of internal rotation may take place between the ischial spines and the tuberosities.

LEFT FRONTUM ANTERIOR: LFrA

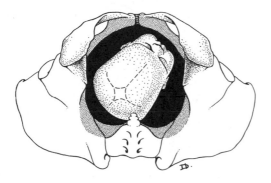

A. LFrA: Onset of labor.

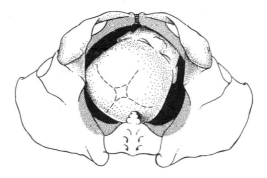

B. Descent.

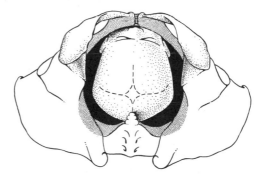

C. Internal rotation: LFrA to FrA.

FIG. 2. Labor: LFrA. Descent, internal rotation.

FLEXION
The face impinges under the pubis, and as the head pivots round this point the bregma, vertex, and occiput are born over the perineum (Figs. 3A-C).

EXTENSION
The head then falls back in extension (Figs. 4A and B), and the nose, mouth, and chin slip under the symphysis.

LEFT FRONTUM ANTERIOR: LFrA

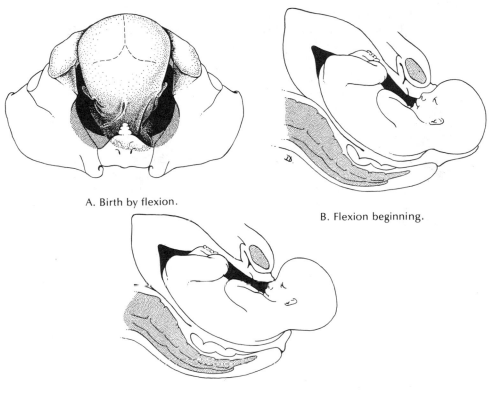

A. Birth by flexion.

B. Flexion beginning.

C. Flexion complete.

FIG. 3. Birth of brow and head by flexion.

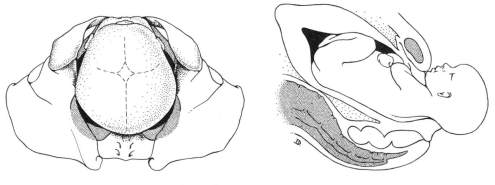

A. Vaginal view.

B. Lateral view.

FIG. 4. Head falls back in extension.

RESTITUTION
The neck untwists, and the head turns 45° back to the original side (Fig. 5A).

EXTERNAL ROTATION
As the shoulder rotates anteriorly from the oblique to the antero-posterior diameter of the pelvis, the head turns back another 45° (Fig. 5B).

MOLDING
Molding is extreme (Fig. 6). The verticomental diameter is compressed. The occipitofrontal diameter is elongated markedly, so that the forehead bulges greatly. The face is flattened, and the distance from the chin to the top of the head is long. This is exaggerated by the large caput succedaneum that forms on the forehead.

PROGNOSIS: BROW PRESENTATIONS

Labor

In most cases brow presentations do not deliver spontaneously. If the malposition is detected early in labor and if appropriate therapeutic measures are undertaken, the fetal and maternal results are good. Failure to recognize the problem leads to prolonged and traumatic labor.

Mother

Passage of a brow through the pelvis is slower, harder, and more traumatic to the mother than any other presentation. Perineal laceration is inevitable and may extend high into the vaginal fornices or into the rectum because of the large diameter offered to the outlet.

Fetus

Fetal mortality is high. The excessive molding may cause irreparable damage to the brain. Mistakes in diagnosis and treatment are the main causes of the poor fetal prognosis.

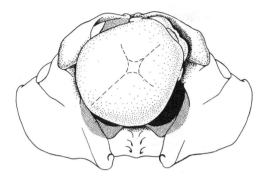

A. Restitution: FrA to LFrA.

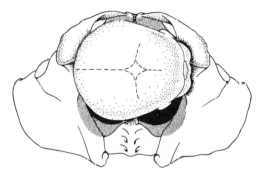

B. External rotation: LFrA to LFrT.

FIG. 5. Restitution, external rotation.

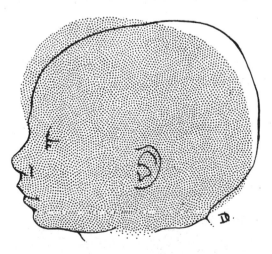

FIG. 6. Molding: brow presentation.

MANAGEMENT OF BROW PRESENTATIONS

X-ray pelvimetry helps in making the diagnosis and in assessing the pelvis.

1. NORMAL PELVIS: Since brow presentation may be transitory, and since spontaneous delivery is possible, a trial of labor is permissible in the hope that flexion to an occiput presentation, complete extension to a face presentation, or progress as a brow presentation will take place. If these steps fail within 12 hours, cesarean section should be performed.
2. DISPROPORTION AND ARREST HIGH IN THE PELVIS: These are managed by cesarean section.
3. PERSISTENT BROW PRESENTATION—MULTIPARA WITH NORMAL PELVIS: Since most brow presentations do not deliver spontaneously, operative interference is necessary. Once the head is fixed in the pelvis, the chance of spontaneous rectification is small.
   a. An attempt may be made to flex the head manually. This is done when the cervix is dilated sufficiently and as soon as possible after the membranes have ruptured.
   b. Sometimes the head can be flexed by forceps. The forceps are applied biparietally, and the head is pushed up just enough so that the brow can be rotated from one quadrant of the pelvis to the opposite one; flexion is attempted simultaneously.
   c. If the head cannot be flexed, an attempt is made to extend it to a face presentation.
   d. If gentle manipulations do not achieve correction, cesarean section should be carried out. Attempts at conversion are done best in the operating room, so that should cesarean be necessary it can be done without delay.
   e. Version and extraction are dangerous and are performed only in unusual situations, when other treatment is contraindicated.
4. PERSISTENT BROW PRESENTATION—PRIMIGRAVIDA WITH NORMAL PELVIS: Flexion or extension maneuvers may be attempted. Most authorities feel, however, that immediate cesarean section yields the best results and that no time should be wasted with other procedures.

BIBLIOGRAPHY

Kovacs SG: Brow presentation. Med J Aust 2:280, 1970

17.

Median Vertex Presentation: Military Attitude

DEFINITION

There is neither flexion nor extension; the occiput and the brow are at the same level in the pelvis. The presenting part is the vertex. The denominator is the occiput. The presenting diameter is the occipitofrontal, which at 11.0 cm is longer than the more favorable suboccipitobregmatic of 9.5 cm. Hence progress is slower and arrest a little more frequent. In many cases the military attitude is transitory, and the head flexes as it descends. Occasionally extension to a brow or face presentation takes place.

DIAGNOSIS OF POSITION: MEDIAN VERTEX PRESENTATION

ABDOMINAL EXAMINATION

1. The long axes of fetus and mother are parallel (Fig. 1A).
2. The head is at or in the pelvic inlet.
3. The back is in one flank, the small parts on the opposite side.
4. The breech is in the fundus.
5. Since there is neither flexion nor extension there is no marked cephalic prominence on one side or the other.

FETAL HEART
The feal heart tones are heard loudest in the lower quadrant of the mother's abdomen, on the same side as the fetal back.

MEDIAN VERTEX PRESENTATION: MILITARY ATTITUDE

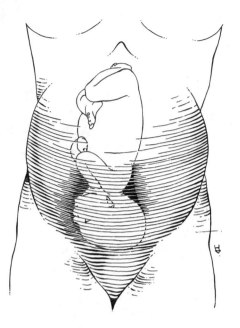

A. Abdominal view.

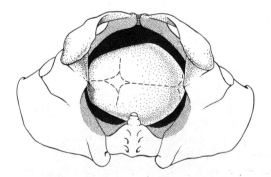

B. Vaginal view.

FIG. 1. Median vertex presentation: LOT.

VAGINAL EXAMINATION

1. The sagittal suture is felt commonly in the transverse diameter of the pelvis, as LOT or ROT (Fig. 1B).
2. The two fontanelles are equally easy to palpate and identify. They are at the same level in the pelvis.

X-RAY EXAMINATION
Occasionally radiologic examination is needed to diagnose the position and to assess the pelvis.

MECHANISM OF LABOR: MEDIAN VERTEX PRESENTATION

Engagement takes place most often in the transverse diameter of the inlet. The head descends slowly, with the occiput and the brow at the same level (there is neither flexion nor extension) and with the sagittal suture in the transverse diameter of the pelvis, until the median vertex reaches the pelvic floor. Now several terminations are possible:

1. Most often the head flexes, the occiput rotates to the anterior, and delivery takes place as an occipitoanterior position.
2. The head may become arrested in the transverse diameter of the pelvis. Operative assistance is necessary for deep transverse arrest.
3. The head may rotate posteriorly with or without flexion. The occiput turns into the hollow of the sacrum and the forehead to the pubis. The mechanism is that of persistent occipitoposterior positions. Delivery may be spontaneous or by operative methods.
4. In rare instances delivery can occur with the sagittal suture in the transverse diameter.
5. Occasionally the head extends, and the mechanism becomes a face or brow presentation.

PROGNOSIS: MEDIAN VERTEX PRESENTATION

While labor is a little longer and harder than normal on mother and child, the prognosis is reasonably good. Many cases flex and proceed to normal delivery.

MANAGEMENT OF MEDIAN VERTEX PRESENTATION

1. Since flexion occurs so frequently, there should be no interference as long as progress is being made.
2. When flexion takes place the management is that of occipito-anterior (see Chap. 10) or occipitoposterior (see Chap. 13) positions.
3. Cases in which the head extends are treated as face (see Chap. 15) or brow (see Chap. 16) presentations.
4. When arrest occurs in the normal pelvis with a persistent military attitude, vaginal delivery should be attempted by flexing the head, rotating the occiput to the anterior, and extracting the head by forceps (see Chap. 26).
5. Where disproportion is a complicating or etiologic factor, or where attempts at vaginal delivery fail, cesarean section should be performed.

18.

Breech Presentation

GENERAL CONSIDERATIONS

Definition

Breech presentation is a longitudinal lie with a variation in polarity. The fetal pelvis is the leading pole. The denominator is the sacrum. A right sacrum anterior (RSA) is a breech presentation where the fetal sacrum is in the right anterior quadrant of the mother's pelvis, and the bitrochanteric diameter of the fetus is in the right oblique diameter of the pelvis (Fig. 1).

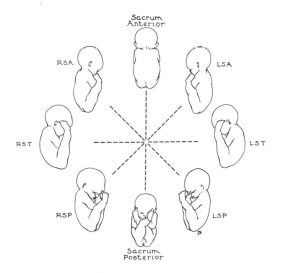

FIG. 1. Positions of breech presentation.

Incidence

Breech presentation at delivery occurs in 3 to 4 percent of pregnancies. The incidence is decreased as term is reached, and is increased in patients who go into labor before term. About 15 percent of babies presenting by the breech are preterm, three times the overall rate of preterm labor.

Etiology

Etiologic factors include prematurity, excess amniotic fluid, multiple pregnancy, placenta previa, contracted pelvis, fibromyomas, hydrocephalus, and large baby. Anything that interferes with engagement of the fetal head plays a part in the etiology of breech presentation. In many cases no reason can be found, and by exclusion the cause of the malposition is ascribed to pure chance. On the other hand, there is the habitual breech. Some women deliver all their children as breeches, suggesting that the pelvis is so shaped that the breech fits better than the head.

Notes and Comments

1. The patient feels fetal movements in the lower abdomen and may complain of painful kicking against the rectum.
2. Engagement before the onset of labor is uncommon. The patient rarely experiences lightening.
3. The uneven fit of breech to pelvis predisposes to early rupture of the membranes, with the danger of umbilical cord prolapse. The incidence of the latter, which is 4 to 5 percent, is higher with footling breeches. It is wise therefore when the bag of waters breaks to make a sterile vaginal examination to determine the exact state of the cervix and to make certain that the cord has not prolapsed.
4. In theory the breech is a poor dilator in comparison with the well flexed head, and labor, descent, and cervical dilatation are believed to take longer. While this is true in some cases, the mean duration of labor of 9.2 hours in primigravidas and 6.1 hours in multiparas suggests that in the majority of cases labor is not prolonged.
5. In frank breeches the baby's lower limbs, which are flexed at the hips and extended at the knees, lie anterior to and against the

baby's abdomen. This has the effect of a splint and by decreasing the maneuverability of the baby may result in delay or arrest of progress.

6. One of the dangers to the fetus in breech presentation is that the largest and least compressible diameter comes last.

7. There is an added risk in premature infants because the head is relatively larger in proportion to the rest of the body than in full-term babies. Thus while the small body slips through with no difficulty, it does not dilate the soft parts sufficiently to allow the head to pass easily.

8. On the one hand, the frank breech has the disadvantage of a large and less maneuverable presenting part and may have difficulty passing through the pelvis. On the other hand, it dilates the soft parts to the greatest degree and makes the most room for the head. The small footling breech slips through the pelvis easily but makes less provision for the aftercoming head.

9. Since the posterior segment of the pelvis is roomier than the anterior segment, the posterior parts of the baby are usually born first.

10. Because of the rapid passage of the head through the pelvis there is no time for molding to take place. The fetal head is round and symmetrical.

11. The baby which lay in utero as a frank breech lies with its hips flexed and the feet near its face for some time after birth.

12. The external genitalia are edematous.

13. The passage of meconium in a breech presentation does not have the same significance of fetal distress as in vertex presentation. The meconium is squeezed out of the intestine by the uterine contractions pressing the lower part of the baby's body against the pelvis.

CLASSIFICATION

There are four types of breech presentation:

COMPLETE Flexion at thighs and knees (Fig. 2A).

FRANK Flexion at thighs; extension at knees. This is the most common variety and includes almost two-thirds of breech presentations (Fig. 2B).

FOOTLING Single or double, with extension at thighs and knees. The foot is the presenting part (Fig. 2C).

KNEELING Single or double, with extension at thighs, flexion at knees. The knee is the presenting part (Fig. 2D).

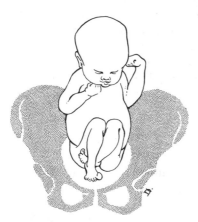

A. Complete breech.

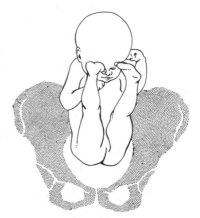

B. Frank breech.

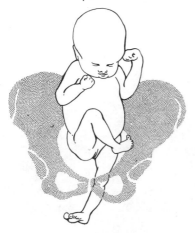

C. Footling breech.

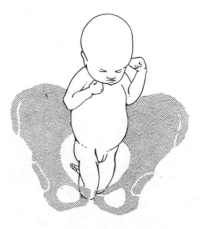

D. Kneeling breech.

FIG 2. Attitudes of breech presentation.

RIGHT SACRUM ANTERIOR: RSA

Diagnosis of Position

ABDOMINAL EXAMINATION

1. The lie is longitudinal (Fig. 3A).
2. A soft, irregular mass lies over the pelvis and does not feel like the head. One suspects breech. In a frank breech the muscles of the thighs are drawn taut over the underlying bones, giving an impression of hardness not unlike the head and leading to diagnostic errors.
3. The back is on the right near the midline. The small parts are on the left, away from the midline, and posterior.
4. The head is felt in the fundus of the uterus. If the head is under the liver or the ribs, it may be difficult to palpate. The head is harder and more globular than the breech, and sometimes it can be balloted. Whenever a ballotable mass is felt in the fundus, breech presentation should be suspected.
5. There is no cephalic prominence, and the breech is not ballotable.

FETAL HEART

The fetal heart tones are heard loudest at or above the umbilicus and on the same side as the back. In RSA the fetal heart is heard best in the right upper quadrant of the maternal abdomen. Sometimes the fetal heart is heard below the umbilicus; hence the diagnosis made by palpation should not be changed because of the location of the fetal heart.

VAGINAL EXAMINATION

1. The presenting part is high.
2. The smooth, regular, hard head with its suture lines and fontanelles is absent. This negative finding suggests a malpresentation.
3. The presenting part is soft and irregular. The anal orifice and the ischial tuberosities are in a straight line (Fig. 3B). The breech may be confused with a face.
4. Sometimes in frank breeches the sacrum is pulled down and is felt by the examining finger. It may be mistaken for the head because of its bony hardness.
5. The sacrum is in the right anterior quadrant of the pelvis, and the bitrochanteric diameter is in the right oblique.
6. Sometimes a foot is felt and must be distinguished from a hand.

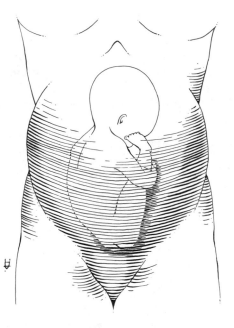

A. Abdominal view.

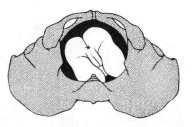

B. Vaginal view.

FIG. 3. Right sacrum anterior.

X-RAY EXAMINATION

Radiologic examination should be carried out in all patients with breech presentation. The position is confirmed, adequacy of the maternal pelvis is ascertained, and abnormalities such as hydrocephaly, anencephaly, and hyperextension of the fetal head are demonstrable.

MECHANISMS OF LABOR: BREECH PRESENTATIONS

Cephalic and breech presentations are like triangles. When the head presents, the base of the triangle leads the way: The largest and most unyielding part of the baby comes first, and the parts that follow are progressively smaller. When the breech presents, on the other hand, the apex of the triangle comes first and the succeeding parts are progressively bigger, with the relatively large head being last. In cases of cephalopelvic disproportion, by the time it is realized that the head is too big for this pelvis, the rest of the baby has been born and vaginal delivery must be carried on, with sad results for the baby.

In breech presentations there are three mechanisms of labor: (1) the buttocks and lower limbs, (2) the shoulders and arms, and (3) the head.

Mechanism of Labor: RSA

BUTTOCKS AND LOWER LIMBS

Descent Engagement has been achieved when the bitrochanteric diameter has passed through the inlet of the pelvis. In RSA the sacrum is in the right anterior quadrant of the maternal pelvis, and the bitrochanteric diameter is in the right oblique diameter of the pelvis (Figs. 4A and B). Since the breech is a less efficient dilator than the head, descent is slow and the breech may remain high until labor has been in progress for some time. In many instances the breech does not come down until the cervix is fully dilated and the membranes are ruptured.

Flexion In order to facilitate passage of the breech through the pelvis, lateral flexion takes place at the waist. The anterior hip becomes the leading part. Where the breech is frank, the baby's legs act as a splint along the body and, by reducing lateral flexion and maneuverability, may prevent descent into the pelvis.

Internal Rotation of Breech The anterior hip meets the resistance of the pelvic floor and rotates forward, downward, and toward the midline (Figs. 5A and B). The bitrochanteric diameter rotates 45° from the right oblique diameter of the pelvis to the anteroposterior. The sacrum turns away from the midline, from the right anterior quadrant to the right transverse (RSA to RST).

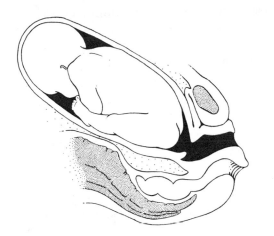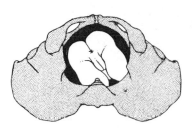

A. Lateral view.　　　　　　　　　　B. Vaginal view.

FIG. 4. RSA: onset of labor.

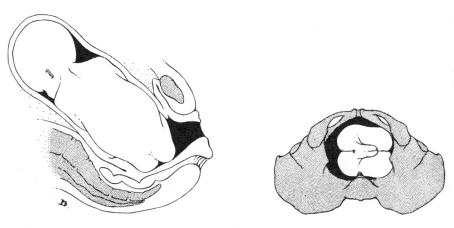

A. Lateral view.　　　　　　　　　　B. Vaginal view.

FIG. 5. Descent and internal rotation of buttocks.

Birth of Buttocks by Lateral Flexion   The anterior hip impinges under the pubic symphysis, lateral flexion occurs, and the posterior hip rises and is born over the perineum. The buttocks then fall toward the anus and the anterior hip slips out under the symphysis (Fig. 6).

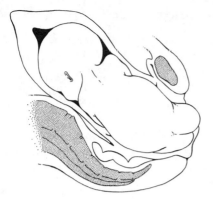

A. Breech crowning.

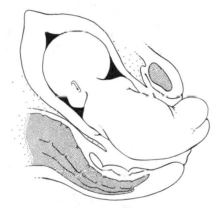

B. Birth of posterior buttock.

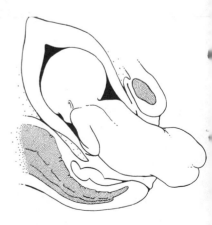

C. Birth of anterior buttock.

FIG. 6. Birth of the buttocks.

209

SHOULDERS AND ARMS

Engagement   Engagement of the shoulders takes place in the right oblique diameter of the pelvis, as the sacrum rotates RST to RSA (Fig. 7A).

Internal Rotation of Shoulders   The anterior shoulder rotates under the symphysis, and the bisacromial diameter turns 45° from the right oblique to the anteroposterior diameter of the outlet. The sacrum goes along, RSA to RST (Fig. 7B).

Birth of Shoulders by Lateral Flexion   The anterior shoulder impinges under the symphysis and the posterior shoulder and arm are born over the perineum as the baby's body is lifted upward (Fig. 7C). The baby is then lowered and the anterior shoulder and arms pass out under the symphysis.

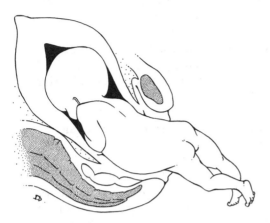

A. Feet born, shoulders engaging.

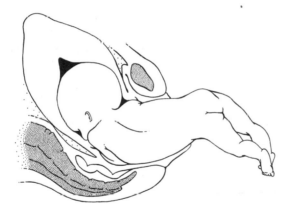

B. Descent and internal rotation of shoulders.

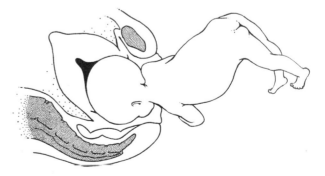

C. Posterior shoulder born: head has entered the pelvis.

FIG. 7. Birth of the shoulders.

HEAD

Descent and Engagement When the shoulders are at the outlet, the head is entering the pelvis (Fig. 8A). It enters the pelvis with the sagittal suture in the left oblique diameter. The occiput is in the right anterior quadrant of the pelvis.

Flexion Flexion of the head takes place just as in any other presentation. It is important that flexion is maintained.

Internal Rotation The head strikes the pelvic floor and rotates internally so that it comes to the outlet with the sagittal suture in the antero-posterior diameter, the brow in the hollow of the sacrum, and the occiput under the symphysis (Fig. 8B). The sacrum rotates toward the pubis, so that the back is anterior.

Birth of Head by Flexion The diameters are the same as in occipito-anterior positions but in reverse order. The nape of the neck pivots under the symphysis, and the chin, mouth, nose, forehead, bregma, and occiput are born over the perineum by a movement of flexion (Fig. 8C).

MECHANISMS OF LABOR: BREECH PRESENTATIONS

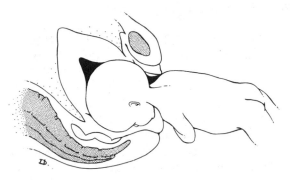

A. Anterior shoulder born; descent of head.

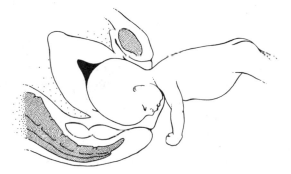

B. Internal rotation and beginning flexion of the head.

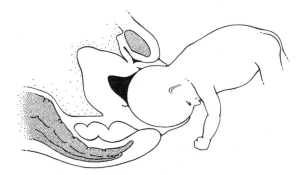

C. Flexion of the head complete.

FIG. 8. Birth of the head.

Mechanism of Labor: Sacrum Directly Anterior

Descent Engagement takes place with the bitrochanteric diameter in the transverse diameter of the inlet. The sacrum is directly anterior, behind the symphysis pubis (SA).

Flexion Flexion is the same as in RSA.

Internal Rotation The bitrochanteric diameter rotates 90° from the transverse diameter of the pelvis to the anteroposterior. The sacrum turns away from the midline to the transverse (SA to RST).

The rest of the mechanism of labor is the same as in RSA.

Mechanism of Labor: Sacrum Posterior

In the rare case, the sacrum and head rotate posteriorly so that the occiput is in the hollow of the sacrum and the face is behind the pubis. If the head is flexed (Fig. 9A), delivery occurs with the occiput posterior. The nasion pivots in the subpubic angle, and the nape of the neck, occiput, and vertex roll over the perineum. The face then emerges from behind the pubis. This method of delivery is helped by lifting up the child's body.

If the head is extended (Fig. 9B), the chin impinges behind the pubis and the submental area of the neck pivots in the subpubic angle. For delivery to take place the infant's body must be raised by the accoucheur so that the occiput, vertex, and forehead can pass over the perineum, in that order.

Delivery of the head from this position can be difficult. The best management of this complication lies in its prevention. Once the breech has been born, any tendency for the sacrum to rotate posteriorly must be restrained by the attendant and the breech encouraged to turn with the sacrum anteriorly toward the symphysis pubis.

Mechanism of Labor in Footling and Kneeling Breech

The mechanism of labor is the same as has been described in RSA with the difference being that in complete and frank breech presentations the buttocks form the leading part. In footling presentations it is one or both feet, and in kneeling breeches it is the knees.

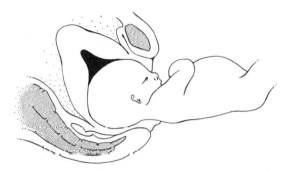

A. Head flexed.

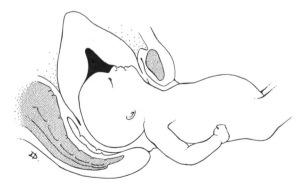

B. Head extended.

FIG. 9. Arrest of head: sacrum posterior.

PROGNOSIS: BREECH PRESENTATIONS

Mother

When spontaneous delivery takes place the maternal prognosis is good. Genital tract lacerations and hemorrhage may be caused by excessively rapid and forceful delivery of the baby through a pelvis that is too small or in which the soft parts have not been dilated sufficiently.

Fetus

The fetal mortality associated with vaginal delivery of full-term breech presentations is three times that of cephalic presentations. The worst prognosis is in premature breeches. The perinatal mortality is highest in double footling presentations and lowest when the breech is frank. Factors influencing the perinatal mortality include (1) prematurity, (2) congenital abnormalities, (3) prolapse of the umbilical cord, (4) fetal asphyxia from other causes, and (5) fetal injury.

The incidence of malformations, such as hydrocephaly, anencephaly, and dislocation of the hip, is higher than in cephalic presentation.

Prolapse of the umbilical cord is more common than in cephalic presentation, especially when the presentation is footling and when the mother is multiparous. Frank breech has the lowest incidence.

The danger of injury is as great in multiparas as in primigravidas. In difficult deliveries the risk of damage to the baby is 20 percent; in easy births it is 3.5 percent. The fetal outcome is worse when the diagnosis is not made before the onset of labor.

Intracranial hemorrhage, 10 times as common with breech as with cephalic presentations, is a major cause of fetal mortality. Sometimes the unmolded head has to pass rapidly and with difficulty through a borderline pelvis.

Significant long-term major abnormalities of the central nervous system are increased in breeches born per vaginam. These include (1) cerebral palsy, (2) epilepsy, (3) mental retardation, and (4) hemiplegia.

There is concern about "minimal brain damage," unrecognized at birth, among children born by breech in contrast to those in cephalic presentation. Problems such as difficulty in reading, writing, perception, and communication are twice as common in breech-born babies as in those delivered head first. It is not known whether the basic etiologic factor is anoxia or trauma.

Time of Death   About 15 percent of fetal deaths occur during labor. The remainder are divided more or less equally between fetal death in utero before the onset of labor, congenital anomalies incompatible with life, and neonatal death.

CAUSES OF DEATH OR DAMAGE TO THE BABY

1. Prematurity is the most common etiologic factor in the perinatal mortality of infants presenting by the breech.
2. Congenital malformation. The incidence of congenital malformation such as hydrocephalus in breech presentations is close to 8 percent, making prognosis less favorable.
3. Asphyxia.
   a. Prolonged compression of the umbilical cord between the pelvis and the aftercoming head.
   b. Actual prolapse of the cord.
   c. Aspiration of amniotic fluid and vaginal contents caused by active breathing before the head has been born.
   d. Prolonged and hard labor.
4. Injury to brain and skull.
   a. The aftercoming head passes through the pelvis rapidly. Instead of gradual molding taking place over several hours, there is rapid and sometimes excessive compression and decompression occurring within a few minutes. The ligaments of the brain are subjected to sudden and marked stretching, with the risk of laceration and intracranial hemorrhage. Injury to the brain may follow delivery through an incompletely dilated cervix or through a pelvis whose adequacy has been estimated incorrectly.
   b. Minute hemorrhages.
   c. Fractures of the skull.
5. Damage resulting from rough handling during the delivery.
   a. Fractures of the neck, humerus, clavicle, or femur.
   b. Cervical and brachial plexus paralyses.
   c. Rupture of the liver caused by grasping the baby too tightly around the abdomen while extracting it.
   d. Damage to fetal adrenal glands, which are relatively large.
   e. Injury to spinal cord.
   f. Traumatized pharynx caused by the obstetrician putting his finger in the baby's mouth to aid delivery.
   g. Damage to abdominal organs. Baby should be grasped by the hips and not the trunk.
6. Size of the baby.
   a. Large babies, over 8 pounds, may be too big for the pelvis.
   b. Premature babies have small bodies in relation to their heads. The little breech is not a good dilator and fails to make room for the head.

7. Rupture of membranes. It has been shown that the fetal mortality is significantly higher if the interval from rupture of the membranes to delivery is prolonged. The perinatal loss of mature infants was increased threefold if more than 24 hours elapsed from rupture of the bag of waters to delivery. If the latent period between rupture of membranes and onset of labor was over 12 hours, the fetal loss was increased three times in primigravidas and fivefold in multiparas. These findings do not hold for premature infants.

INVESTIGATION OF BREECH PRESENTATION AT TERM

Accessory Factors

These increase the risk and include (1) elderly primigravida, (2) precious baby, (3) history of infertility, (4) intrauterine growth retardation, (5) postterm pregnancy, (6) toxemia of pregnancy, (7) diabetes, and (8) uterine myoma.

Radiologic Examination

1. To assess the size and shape of the maternal pelvis. Bad prognostic features are:
   a. Interspinous diameter less than 9.0 cm.
   b. Foreward jutting of the sacrum.
   c. A narrow subpubic arch.
2. To confirm the presentation.
3. To diagnose the type of breech presentation—frank, complete, or footling.
4. To discover congenital anomalies such as anencephaly and hydrocephaly.
5. To rule out hyperextension of the fetal head.

Ultrasonic Examination

1. Confirm the presentation.
2. Discover fetal anomalies.
3. Measure the biparietal diameter of the fetal head and the abdominal and thoracic girth.
4. Compare the biparietal diameter of the fetal head and the measurements of the maternal pelvis.
5. Localize the placenta and rule out placenta previa.

Breech Score of Zatuchini and Andros

At the time of admittance to the labor ward of the patient with a breech presentation, a decision must be made whether a trial of labor is indicated or whether elective cesarean section is to be performed. The breech score is a numerical summary of several important parameters. While this index does not include all the factors which must be taken into consideration, and while it is not the final word, and although it is no substitute for clinical judgment, it is a valuable piece of information and is helpful in evaluating the situation.

	0 Points	1 Point	2 Points
Parity	Primigrav	Multip	
Gestational Age	39 weeks or more	38 weeks	37 weeks or less
Estimated Fetal Weight	>8 lb >3,630 g	7 to 8 lb 3,176–3,630 g	<7 lb <3,176 g
Previous Breech > 2,500 g	None	1	2 or more
Cervical Dilatation on Admission by Vaginal Examination	2 cm or less	3 cm	4 cm or more
Station on Admission	–3 or higher	–2	–1 or lower

There is statistical evidence to the effect that scores of 3 or less are associated with a high incidence of fetal morbidity, that prolonged labor is frequent, and that the rate of cesarean section is elevated. Thus, low scores are ominous and of great prognostic value. High scores, on the other hand, are less significant, are no guarantee of successful delivery, and are not a reason for complacency. It is suggested that a score of 3 or less is an indication for cesarean section.

MANAGEMENT OF BREECH PRESENTATION DURING LATE PREGNANCY

External Version

There is disagreement as to the advisability of external version during pregnancy. Since fetal mortality is higher in breech than in cephalic deliveries, many authorities believe that external version (turning the breech to a cephalic presentation) should be attempted in all cases (see Chap. 30 for technique). While the incidence of breech presentation decreases as term is neared, in most pregnancies the fetus has assumed its final position by the 34th week. The best time for external version is at 32 to 34 weeks' gestation. The procedure must be done gently and with no excessive force, since there is danger of placental separation or damage to the fetus. Version may succeed, be unsuccessful, or recur. Before attempting external version one must be certain of the position to avoid turning a cephalic presentation to a breech.

On the other hand, because (1) the fetal loss associated with external version is about the same as that with breech delivery, (2) at 32 to 34 weeks around 20 percent of fetuses present by the breech with all but 3 or 4 percent changing spontaneously to cephalic presentations, (3) experience in management of breech deliveries must be obtained so that proper care can be taken of those cases that persist as breeches (where external version fails or where the breech presentation recurs after successful version), and (4) the greater use of cesarean section has reduced the perinatal mortality greatly, many obstetricians believe that external version is unnecessary and inadvisable. External version is most difficult to perform in frank breeches (especially in the primigravida), and this is the commonest variety.

MANAGEMENT OF DELIVERY OF BREECH PRESENTATION

Classification of Breech Births

VAGINAL DELIVERY

1. SPONTANEOUS BREECH DELIVERY The entire infant is expelled by the natural forces of the mother, with no assistance other than support of the baby as it is being born.
2. ASSISTED BREECH (OR PARTIAL BREECH EXTRACTION) The infant is delivered by the natural forces as far as the umbilicus. The remainder of the baby is extracted by the attendant. In normal cases we believe this to be the best method.
3. TOTAL BREECH EXTRACTION The entire body of the infant is extracted by the attendant.

CESAREAN SECTION
The incidence is about 30 percent.

Elective Cesarean Section: Indicated or Considered In general, the following factors are unfavorable for vaginal delivery, and cesarean section may be safest for the fetus.

1. Presence of significant relative factors.

2. History of difficult delivery or damaged infant.
3. Chronic fetal distress, including intrauterine growth retardation, diabetes mellitus, and hypertensive disorders.
4. Breech score of 3 or less.
5. Abnormal pelvis, e.g., android.
6. Small pelvis.
7. Large baby.
   a. Over 3,600 g by clinical estimation.
   b. Biparietal diameter over 9.5 cm by ultrasound.
8. Hyperextension of the fetal head.
9. Footling breech. The limbs and pelvis of the footling breech deliver easily, but do not make room for the aftercoming head. Therefore, babies presenting in this way are delivered most safely by cesarean section, especially when they weigh between 1,000 and 2,000 g.
10. Premature but viable infant. Because infants presenting by the frank breech, weighing over 2,500 g, and delivering spontaneously per vaginam do well, routine elective cesarean section is not justified. The same cannot be said of babies weighing less than 2,500 g. Reasons for the bad results with premature breeches include the entrapment of the relatively large aftercoming head and the harmful effects, both physical and hypoxic, of labor and delivery on the preterm breech. Cesarean section may be a valid method of obviating these difficulties and improving results. The gestational age at which abdominal delivery is justified is a matter of individual judgment, varying between 28 and 32 weeks. These babies should be delivered in hospitals with high-risk units and specialized intensive care nurseries. The advances in pediatric care have reached the point where a baby weighing over 1,000 g is salvageable, providing there has been no intrauterine hypoxia. A point in opposition to routine cesarean section is the high incidence of congenital anomalies in babies presenting by the breech, even more so when the infant is premature. Therefore, cesarean section should be carried out only when serious anomalies have been ruled out by physical, radiological, and ultrasonic examination. The belief has evolved that strong consideration be given to delivering all breeches weighing between 1,000 and 2,000 g by cesarean section, unless there are reasons for not doing so.

Routine Cesarean Section   Because no clinical, radiologic, or ultrasonic assessment can guarantee a safe and easy birth of the aftercoming head, the suggestion has been made that all breeches be delivered by cesarean section. This idea has merit. However, until cesarean section becomes as safe for the mother, in the short and long term (including repeat cesarean section), as vaginal delivery, routine cesarean section will remain an unsatisfactory solution to the problems posed by breech presentation. As long as the indications for abdominal delivery are wide and include all questionable situations, of even the mildest degree, the majority of the remainder can be delivered safely per vaginam.

Trial of Labor   This is considered when the breech score is 4 or more, the breech is frank, and the indications for cesarean section are absent. The trial is carried on under the following conditions, with the understanding that any significant deviation from the normal is an indication for cesarean section.

1. The fetal heart rate is monitored continuously.
2. The progress of labor is observed meticulously.
3. Progressive cervical dilatation must take place.
4. Adequate descent of the breech must occur.
5. No heroic vaginal procedures are performed.
6. When progress is slow there is a strong probability that the baby is large, and cesarean section should be performed.
7. The association of a dysfunctional labor with a breech presentation is ominous. Stimulation by oxytocin is dangerous in such situations and cesarean section is the treatment of choice.

Management of Labor and Delivery in the Progressing Case

FIRST STAGE OF LABOR

1. Because most breech presentations progress to successful vaginal delivery, observant expectancy, supportive therapy, and absence of interference are the procedures of choice.
2. The patient is best in bed.
3. It is best to maintain intact membranes until the cervical dilatation is far advanced. Too frequent vaginal or rectal examinations, or any procedure that might contribute to premature rupture of the bag of waters, should be avoided.
4. When the membranes do rupture, vaginal examination is done to rule out prolapse of the umbilical cord and to determine the exact condition of the cervix.
5. Meconium is no cause for alarm as long as the fetal heart is normal.
6. An intravenous infusion of 5 percent glucose in water should be set up.

MANAGEMENT OF DELIVERY OF BREECH PRESENTATION

SECOND STAGE OF LABOR

Position for Delivery Once the cervix is fully dilated, the patient is placed on the delivery table. The firmness of the table and handbars that the patient uses to brace herself increases the effectiveness of the bearing down efforts and so expedites progress.

When the breech begins to distend the perineum, the patient is placed in the lithotomy position, with the legs in stirrups and the buttocks extending slightly past the end of the table. This is the best position in which to assist the birth and to handle complications.

During a contraction the pressure of the presenting part on the perineum stimulates the patient to move up the table and out of position. Shoulder braces are invaluable in preventing this.

An assistant should be scrubbed and gowned for every delivery.

The patient's bladder is catheterized.

Intravenous Infusion It is important for successful delivery of a breech presentation that good uterine contractions continue and that the patient retain the ability to bear down, and does so. Should the contractions become weak or irregular during the actual delivery, oxytocin can be added quickly to the infusion, to stimulate the uterus to more effective activity.

Assisted Breech The fetal heart is checked frequently. As long as the baby is in good condition, spontaneous delivery is awaited. Premature traction on the baby, especially between contractions, must be avoided, since it can lead to deflexion of the head and extension of the arms above or behind the head. It is important that the patient bear down with each contraction, and she must be encouraged to do so. Once the body has been born, the head is out of the upper contracting part of the uterus and in the lower segment, the cervix, or the upper vagina. Since these organs do not have the power to expel the head, its descent and delivery must be effected by the voluntary action of the abdominal muscles, with the attendant exerting suprapubic pressure. Fetal salvage is increased by calmness and slowness rather than by agitation and speed.

Our experience has been that in normally progressing cases the best results are obtained by a policy of:

1. No interference (except episiotomy) until the body is born to the umbilicus. This permits the cervix to become not only fully dilated but also paralyzed, an important factor in minimizing dystocia with the aftercoming head.
2. Hard bearing down by the mother during contractions.
3. The maintenance of suprapubic pressure during descent to aid delivery and to keep the head in flexion.

There are good reasons for using this technique:

1. It has proved successful.
2. It is safe. There is less trauma to the baby.
3. Flexion of the head is maintained.
4. The danger of extension of the arms above the head is reduced.
5. There is less chance of the cervix clamping down around the baby's head or neck.

Anesthesia   A combination of local and general anesthesia is employed. Pudendal block or perineal infiltration permits episiotomy without pain and facilitates delivery by relaxing the muscles. In addition, with each contraction the patient takes several breaths of an anesthetic vapor. This acts as an analgesic, eases the pain, and helps her to bear down more efficiently. Actual general anesthesia is not instituted until the baby is born to the umbilicus.

We have used epidural anesthesia with success. The drawback is that once the perineal dose takes effect, the reflex stimulation from pressure of the presenting part on the perineum may be reduced or removed and the patient's desire to bear down with each contraction lost. This unwanted effect can be obviated by omitting the perineal dose and using local anesthesia for the episiotomy. In this way the analgesic value of the epidural dose during labor is maintained without loss of the perineal reflex during the delivery.

Necessary Equipment   The procedure requires that certain equipment be at hand.

1. A warm, dry towel to be wrapped around the baby's body as soon as it is sufficiently born. The purposes of this are:
   a. To reduce the stimulating effect of cold air on the baby in the hope that respiration does not begin while the head is in the pelvis, resulting in aspiration of amniotic fluid or vaginal contents
   b. To make it easier to hold the slippery baby
2. Piper forceps for the aftercoming head, if it does not deliver easily with assistance
3. Equipment for resuscitation of the infant, ready for immediate use

Episiotomy   Since in many cases the breech dilates the perineum insufficiently to allow easy passage of the head, an adequate episiotomy is essential. It is safer to make a big episiotomy to avoid having to enlarge it while occupied with delivery of the head. A mediolateral incision is preferred. The perineotomy must be done at the optimum time—e.g., before the breech crowns or one is faced with the need for delivering the infant and making the incision simultaneously. On the other hand, if the incision is made too soon the blood loss can be excessive. Hence the episiotomy should be performed just before the buttocks crown or when the attendant feels that their birth will occur with the next one or two contractions.

Delivery of Breech

1. The patient is encouraged to bear down with the contractions but must rest between them.
2. When the buttocks are ready to crown, a wide mediolateral episiotomy is made and hemostasis secured.
3. As long as there is no fetal or maternal distress, spontaneous delivery to the umbilicus is awaited. Up to this point there is no urgency, and the operator should not interfere.
4. Once the umbilicus has been delivered, time becomes an important factor, and the remainder of the birth is expedited gently and skillfully. A free airway to the mouth should be available within 3 to 5 minutes to obviate anoxic brain damage.
5. The legs usually deliver spontaneously; if not they are easily extracted.
6. The baby is covered with a warm towel, and the body is supported.
7. A loop of umbilical cord is pulled down (Fig. 10) to minimize traction on it in case it is caught between the head and the pelvic wall. At the same time it is palpated for pulsations.
8. The anesthetist is asked to put the patient to sleep at this stage of the delivery.

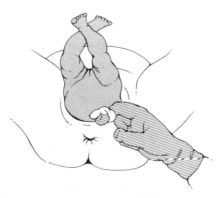

FIG. 10. Delivery of cord. Loop of umbilical cord being pulled down.

Delivery of Shoulders and Arms

1. The assistant exerts suprapubic pressure on the head to maintain its flexion.
2. The operator depresses the buttocks and delivers the body to the anterior scapula so that the anterior shoulder comes under the symphysis.
3. To deliver the anterior arm the accoucheur passes his hand up the baby's back, over the shoulder, and down the chest, thus sweeping the arm and hand out under the pubis with his finger (Fig. 11A).
4. The baby is raised so that the posterior scapula and then the posterior arm are born over the perineum by the same maneuver (Fig. 11B).
5. Some obstetricians deliver the posterior arm first.

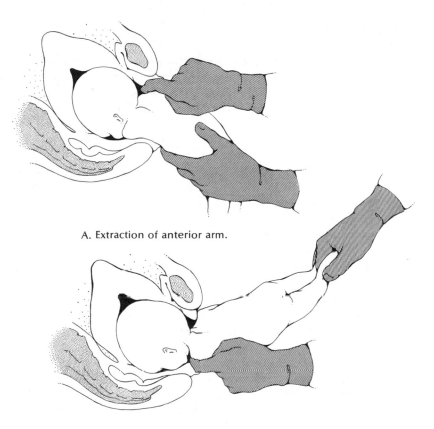

A. Extraction of anterior arm.

B. Extraction of posterior arm.

FIG. 11. Delivery of arms and shoulders.

Delivery of Head

1. In almost every case the back turns anteriorly spontaneously. This must be encouraged so that the head rotates the occiput to the pubis and the face toward the sacrum. Rarely, there is a tendency for the back to turn posteriorly. The obstetrician must counteract this and rotate the back anteriorly to prevent the head's rotating face to pubis, a serious and always avoidable complication.
2. Once the back has rotated anteriorly and the fetal head is in the anteroposterior diameter of the pelvis, the body is lowered so that the occiput appears under the symphysis and the nape of the neck pivots there (Fig. 12A).
3. At the same time the assistant maintains suprapubic pressure to guide the head through the pelvis and to keep it flexed.
4. The body is then raised gently so that there is slight extension at the neck.
5. Then by further suprapubic pressure (Kristellar maneuver) the head is delivered in flexion—the chin, mouth, nose, forehead, bregma, and vertex being born, in that order, over the perineum (Fig. 12B).
6. The speed of delivery of the aftercoming head must be considered. The rapid passage of the head through the pelvis causes sudden compression and decompression of the cranial contents. In the extreme, the ligaments of the brain tear, leading to hemorrhage, cerebral damage, and death. On the other hand, too slow delivery of the head results in asphyxia, which may also be fatal. Experience teaches the middle road: slow enough to prevent injury to the brain and sufficiently rapid to avoid asphyxia.

MANAGEMENT OF DELIVERY OF BREECH PRESENTATION

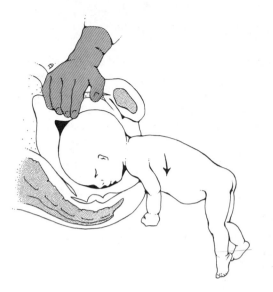

A. Body lowered so that nape of neck is in the subpubic angle. Assistant maintains flexion of the head.

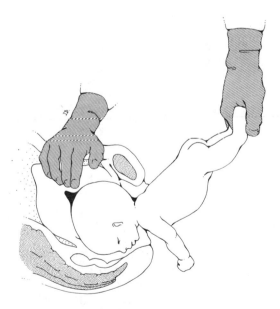

B. Kristellar maneuver: head born in flexion.

FIG. 12. Delivery of head.

ARREST IN BREECH PRESENTATION

Most babies who present by the breech are born spontaneously or with the help of but not interference from the attendant. The Kristellar maneuver (suprapubic pressure) is all that is needed to deliver the aftercoming head. However, progress may cease and active interference then becomes mandatory. Arrest may take place at the head, neck, shoulders and arms, or buttocks.

Arrest of the Head

Sometimes the body, shoulders, and arms are born, but the bearing-down efforts of the mother and the Kristellar maneuver are not successful in delivering the head. In cases where the head is arrested, several measures are available to extract it.

WIGAND-MARTIN MANEUVER
The body of the baby is placed on the arm of the operator, with the middle finger of the hand of that arm placed in the baby's mouth and the index and ring fingers on the malar bones (Fig. 13A). The purpose of the finger in the mouth is not for traction but to encourage and maintain flexion. With the other hand the obstetrician exerts suprapubic pressure on the head through the mother's abdomen.

MAURICEAU-SMELLIE-VEIT MANEUVER
The position is the same as the Wigand-Martin, with one finger in the baby's mouth and two on the malar bones. The difference is that the accoucheur places his other hand astride the baby's shoulders and produces traction in this way (Fig. 13B). The efficiency of this procedure is increased by an assistant's applying suprapubic pressure on the fetal head while the operator is performing the Mauriceau maneuver.

PIPER FORCEPS ON THE AFTERCOMING HEAD

1. The baby's feet are grasped by an assistant, and the body is raised (Fig. 13C). Care must be taken not to elevate the body too much for fear of damage to the sternomastoid muscles. A good way to keep the arms out of the way is to use a folded towel as described by Savage.
2. The right hand is placed in the vagina, and the left forceps blade is guided into place over the parietal bone. Should there be a rim of cervix still present, the blade must be inserted inside it.

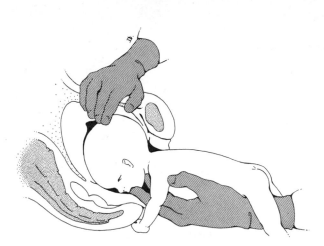

A. Wigand-Martin maneuver.

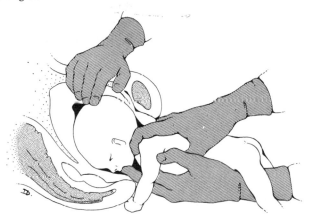

B. Mauriceau-Smellie-Veit maneuver.

C. Management of fetal arms (Savage) as Piper forceps are applied.

FIG. 13. Different maneuvers for arrest of head.

3. The right blade is then applied using the left hand as a guide.
4. The forceps are locked. The blades fit along the occipitomental diameter, one over each ear.
5. With the exception of simple suprapubic pressure, the best method of delivering the aftercoming head is by the use of the Piper forceps. In contrast to those maneuvers in which traction on the head is effected through the neck, the forceps exert traction directly on the head, thereby avoiding damage to structures in the baby's neck.
6. Traction is made and the head extracted slowly (see Chap. 29). This operation should be performed only when the head is in the pelvis. Any type of forceps can be used to deliver the aftercoming head. The Piper forceps have a double curve in the blades and in the shanks; the shanks are long, and the handles are depressed below the arch of the shanks. This instrument should be employed whenever possible, since it is easier to use and more efficient than regular forceps.

AIRWAY

When there is delay in delivery of the head and one is waiting for help or instruments, an ordinary vaginal retractor can be used temporarily to clear an airway in the vagina to the baby's mouth (Fig. 14). The retractor is placed in the vagina and pressure exerted posteriorly. The vaginal contents are sponged out so that air can get to the baby should it breathe.

CHIN TO PUBIS ROTATION

Anterior rotation of the chin is rare and occurs usually as part of posterior rotation of the back. The preferred management is as follows: (1) Institute deep anesthesia. (2) Cease all traction. (3) Dislodge the chin from behind the pubis. (4) Rotate the face posteriorly and the back anteriorly. (5) Flex the chin. (6) Effect engagement by suprapubic pressure. (7) Deliver the head with Piper forceps.

When this technique fails, the Prague maneuver (Fig. 15) may be used. Here the fingers are placed over the shoulders, and outward and upward traction is made. The legs are grasped with the other hand, and the body is swung over the mother's abdomen. By this procedure the occiput is born over the perineum. Since this method carries with it the danger of overstretching or breaking the neck of the infant, it is used rarely.

ARREST IN BREECH PRESENTATION

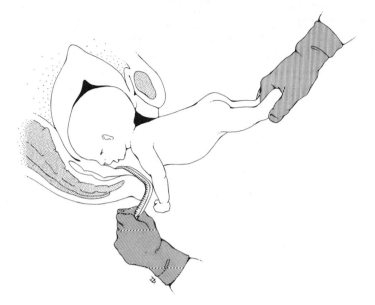

FIG. 14. Vaginal retractor providing airway to the baby's mouth and nose.

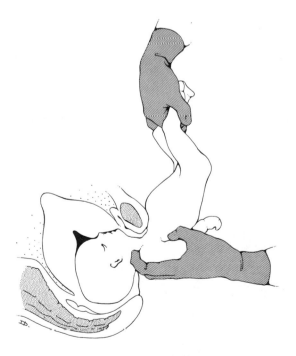

FIG. 15. Prague maneuver.

EMBRYOTOMY

When delivery of the head is not accomplished within reasonable time, the baby may die. If it does perish the mother's welfare alone should be considered. To save her from needless injury, reduction of the size of the child's head by perforation of the skull is preferable to its extraction by brute force.

Arrest of the Neck

Occasionally the cervix, which has opened sufficiently to allow the trunk and shoulders to be born, clamps down around the baby's neck, trapping the head in the uterus. The possibility of this happening is greater with the premature delivery, where the body has not yet developed its adipose tissue and is a poor dilating wedge. This dangerous situation calls for rapid action to break the spasm of the previously dilated cervix. This is accomplished by a single bold incision of the cervix with the scissors. The resultant relaxation of the spasm permits the head to be born.

Arrest of the Shoulders and Arms

Extended Arms   The arms are simply extended over the baby's head (Fig. 16A).

Nuchal Arms   There is extension at the shoulder and flexion at the elbow so that the forearm is trapped behind the fetal head (Fig. 16B). One or both arms may be affected.

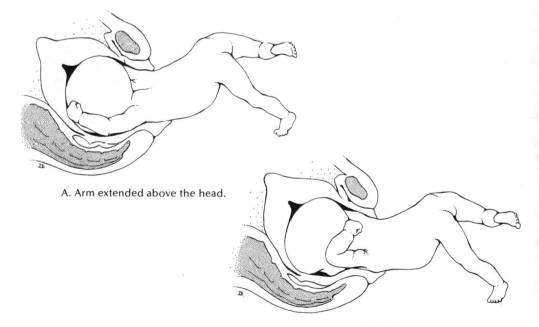

A. Arm extended above the head.

B. Nuchal arm.

FIG. 16. Extended and nuchal arms.

PROPHYLAXIS

One method of reducing the incidence of this complication is to resist the temptation of pulling on the baby's legs to speed delivery, especially when the uterus is in a relaxed state.

SIMPLE EXTRACTION

When this problem occurs an attempt should be made first to deliver the arms by sweeping them over the chest in the usual way. This succeeds in most cases of simple extension and in some instances of nuchal arms when the upper limb is not jammed tightly behind the head.

ROTATION OF BODY

If extraction fails in the case of a nuchal arm, the baby's body is rotated in the direction to which the hand is pointing (Fig. 16C). This dislodges the arm from behind the head and its delivery is then usually possible as described above (Fig. 16D). If both arms are nuchal, the body is rotated in one direction to free the first arm, which is then extracted, and then in the opposite direction to free the other arm.

FRACTURE

In the rare instance when rotation fails, the humerus or clavicle must be fractured. This can be done directly, or it can be effected by simply pulling on the arm until it breaks. Once this occurs delivery can be accomplished. Since the fracture usually heals rapidly and well, and since the choice may be between a dead baby and a broken arm, extreme measures are justified.

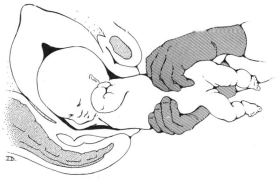

C. Nuchal arm: rotation of the trunk of the child 90° in the direction in which the hand is pointing.

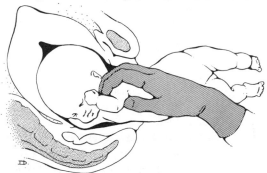

D. Nuchal arm: hand introduced into the uterus to flex and bring down the nuchal arm.

FIG. 16. (cont.) Extended and nuchal arms.

Failure of Descent of the Breech

ETIOLOGY
In any situation, the size of the passenger, the capacity of the pelvis, the dilatability of the maternal soft tissues, and the character of the uterine contractions all play a part in determining whether spontaneous delivery takes place. In frank breech presentation there is an added factor. The splinting effect of the baby's legs across its abdomen can reduce the maneuverability of the fetus to such an extent that progress is arrested.

DISPROPORTION
In the presence of good uterine contractions, nondescent of the breech is an indication, not for hasty interference, but for the most careful reassessment. Keeping in mind the fact that one of the causes of breech presentation is a large head that cannot engage easily, the accoucheur must be assured, not of the general capacity of the pelvis, but of its adequacy with respect to that particular baby. More and more evidence is appearing in the literature that when a breech fails to descend, in spite of good contractions, disproportion is present and cesarean section must be seriously considered.

DECOMPOSITION
If there is good evidence that vaginal delivery is feasible, progress and descent can be expedited by reducing the bulk of the breech, an operation known as decomposition. This is done by bringing down the legs, both whenever possible. When there is complete flexion at the hips and the knees, the feet can be reached easily. The hand is placed in the uterus, the membranes are ruptured, and a foot is grasped and brought down (Fig. 17A). Be sure it is not a hand. The same is done for the other foot. The position has been changed to a footling breech, and labor proceeds.

PINARD MANEUVER
If the breech is frank (flexion at the hips and extension at the knees), it may be impossible to reach the feet, as they are high in the uterus near the baby's face. In such situations the Pinard maneuver (Figs. 17B and C) is performed under anesthesia. With a hand in the uterus, pressure is made by the fingers against the popliteal fossa in a backward and outward direction. This brings about flexion of the knees to a sufficient extent that the foot can be grasped with the other fingers and delivered. When possible, both feet should be delivered. Unless there are urgent indications for immediate delivery, labor is allowed to carry on as with a footling breech.

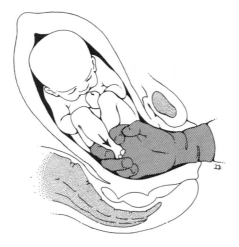

A. Decomposition of breech: bringing down a foot and leg.

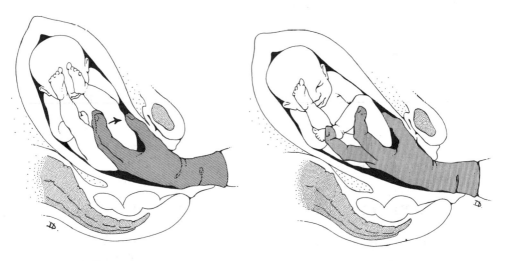

B. First step.

C. Second step.

B and C. Pinard maneuver.

FIG. 17 Breaking up the breech.

BREECH EXTRACTION

This operation is the immediate vaginal extraction of the baby when signs of fetal distress demand delivery without delay.

Prerequisites

There are certain conditions that must be present before this procedure may be performed. (1) The pelvis must be ample, with no disproportion. (2) The cervix must be fully dilated. (3) The bladder and rectum should be empty. (4) Expert and deep anesthesia is essential. (5) Good assistance is mandatory.

Procedure

The patient is placed in the lithotomy position, the bladder catheterized, and anesthesia administered. As described in a previous section, the breech is decomposed and the legs are brought down. The feet are pulled down if the breech is complete; the Pinard maneuver is used if the breech is frank. Instead of the patient going on to spontaneous delivery, the baby is extracted rapidly. Traction from below is substituted for uterine contractions from above, but the maneuvers for delivery of the shoulders, arms, and head are those already set forth in the management of arrested cases.

While expert and experienced obstetricians have reported good results with routine breech extraction as soon as the cervix is fully dilated, we believe that in the hands of the average doctor this operation is hazardous for both mother and child. We feel that it should be carried out only in urgent situations when cesarean section cannot be performed quickly and the baby must be delivered immediately.

HYPEREXTENSION OF THE FETAL HEAD

Hyperextension of the fetal head (Fig. 18) is seen most commonly in face presentation but also occurs with transverse lie and breech presentation. In the latter it is a serious problem.

Etiology

1. Spasm or congenital shortening of the extensor muscles of the neck.

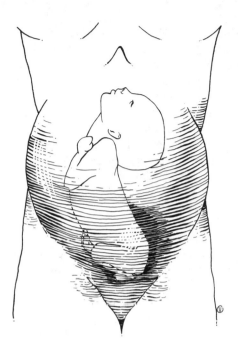

FIG. 18. Hyperextension of the fetal head.

2. Umbilical cord around the neck.
3. Congenital tumors of the fetal neck.
4. Fetal malformations.
5. Uterine anomalies.
6. Tumors in the placental site.

Diagnosis

The diagnosis is made by x-ray examination; the appearance is characteristic. When the head presents it is that of a face presentation. When the breech presents the appearance has been described as a "stargazing breech." In transverse lie the condition is seen as a "flying fetus."

Fetal Danger

There is a definite risk of damage to the lower cervical spinal cord of the fetus during vaginal delivery, greatest with breech presentation. The mechanisms by which the spinal injury is caused include (1) excessive longitudinal stretching of the spinal cord, (2) excessive flexion at the neck during delivery, (3) torsional forces. The resulting lesion is partial or complete laceration of the cervical spinal cord, occasional tears in the dura, and epidural hemorrhage. Dislocation or fracture of the cervical vertebrae is rare. Sudden extreme flexion, which is an integral part of vaginal breech delivery, is sufficient to damage the vulnerable spinal cord. Although the process of birth—more specifically the sudden flexion of the head as the fetus descends through the vagina—must be incriminated most of the time, there is evidence that occasionally the lesion occurs even before the onset of labor.

Fetal Prognosis

In a collected series of 73 cases the perinatal mortality rate was 13.7 percent in babies delivered vaginally in contrast to no deaths in those born by cesarean section. Medullary or vertebral injury occured in 20.6 percent of babies born per vaginam and in 5.7 percent delivered by cesarean section. Meningeal hemorrhage was found in 6.9 percent of children born vaginally, while none was noted following cesarean section.

Management

1. Radiography should be used whenever an abnormal presentation is suspected.
2. Breech presentation with hyperextension of the head should be delivered by cesarean section.
3. Transverse lie is treated by cesarean section.
4. Most face presentations will deliver safely per vaginam. If progress ceases or if the chin is posterior, cesarean section should be performed.

BREECH PRESENTATION IN AN ELDERLY PRIMIGRAVIDA

This is a special case. Unless there are overwhelming reasons for attempting vaginal delivery, cesarean section is the treatment of choice.

BIBLIOGRAPHY

Abroms IF, Bresnan MJ, Zuckerman JE, et al: Cervical cord injuries secondary to hyperextension of the head in breech presentation. Obstet Gynecol 41:369, 1973

Bird CC, McElin TW: A six year prospective study of term breech deliveries utilizing the Zatuchini-Andros prognostic scoring index. Am J Obstet Gynecol 121:551, 1975

Brenner WE, Bruce RD, Hendricks CW: The characteristics and perils of breech presentation. Am J Obstet Gynecol 118:700, 1974

Caterini H, Langer A, Sama JC et al: Fetal risk in hyperextension of the fetal head in breech presentation. Am J Obstet Gynecol 123:632, 1975

Daw E: Hyperextension of the fetal head—? the best mode of delivery. Practitioner 214:397, 1975

DeCrespigny LJC, Pepperell RJ: Perinatal mortality and morbidity in breech presentation. Obstet Gynecol 53:141, 1979

Fianu S: Fetal mortality and morbidity following breech delivery. Acta Obstet Gynaecol Scand Suppl 56, 1976

Karp LE, Doney JR, McCarthy T, Meis PJ, Hall M: The premature breech: trial of labor or cesarean section. Obstet Gynecol 53:88, 1979.

Kauppila O: The perinatal mortality in breech deliveries and observations on affecting factors. Acta Obstet Gynaecol Scand Supp 35, 1975

Rovinsky JJ, Miller JA, Kaplan S: Management of breech presentation at term. Am J Obstet Gynecol 115:497, 1973

19.

Transverse Lie

GENERAL CONSIDERATIONS

Definition

When the long axes of mother and fetus are at right angles to one another, a transverse lie is present. Because the shoulder is placed so frequently in the brim of the inlet, this malposition is often referred to as the shoulder presentation. The baby may lie directly across the maternal abdomen (Fig. 1), or it may lie obliquely with the head or breech in the iliac fossa (Figs. 2A and B). Usually the breech is at a higher level than the head. The denominator is the scapula (Sc); the situation of the head determines whether the position is left or right, and that of the back indicates whether it is anterior or posterior. Thus LScP means that the lie is transverse, the head is on the mother's left side, and the baby's back is posterior. The part which actually lies over the pelvic brim may be the shoulder, back, abdomen, ribs, or flank.

Incidence

The incidence of transverse lie is around 1:500. This is a serious malposition whose management must not be left to nature.

Etiology

Anything that prevents engagement of the head or the breech may predispose to transverse lie. This abnormality is more common in multiparas than primigravidas because of the laxness of the uterine and abdominal muscles. Included are such factors as placenta previa; obstructing neoplasm; multiple pregnancies; fetal anomalies; polyhydramnios; prematurity; fetopelvic disproportion; uterine abnormalities such as uterus subseptus, uterus arcuatus, and uterus bicornis; and contracted pelvis. In many instances no etiologic factor can be determined, and

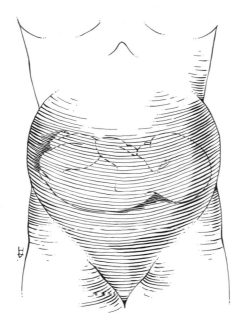

FIG. 1. Transverse lie: LScP.

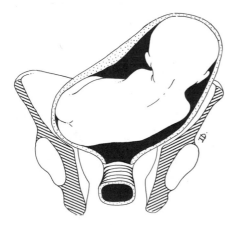

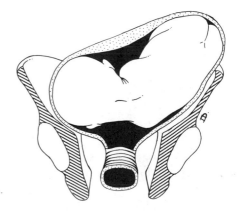

FIG. 2A. Oblique lie: breech in iliac fossa.   FIG. 2B. Oblique lie: head in iliac fossa.

we assume that the malposition is accidental. The head happens to be out of the lower uterine segment when labor starts, and the shoulder is pushed into the pelvic brim.

DIAGNOSIS OF POSITION: TRANSVERSE LIE

Abdominal Examination

1. The appearance of the abdomen is asymmetrical.
2. The long axis of the fetus is across the mother's abdomen.
3. The uterine fundus is lower than expected for the period of gestation. It has been described as a squat uterus. Its upper limit is near the umbilicus, and it is wider than usual.
4. Palpation of the upper and lower poles of the uterus reveals neither the head nor the breech.
5. The head can be felt in one maternal flank.
6. The buttocks are on the other side.

Fetal Heart

The fetal heart is heard best below the umbilicus and has no diagnostic significance regarding position.

Vaginal Examination

The most important finding is a negative one; neither the head nor the breech can be felt by the examining finger. The presenting part is high. In some cases one may actually feel the shoulder, a hand, the rib cage, or the back. Because of the poor fit of the presenting part to the pelvis the bag of waters may hang into the vagina.

X-Ray Examination

Radiologic examination will confirm the diagnosis and can detect certain abnormalities in the fetus or the pelvis.

MECHANISM OF LABOR: TRANSVERSE LIE

A persistent transverse lie cannot deliver spontaneously, and if uncorrected impaction takes place (Fig. 3A). The shoulder is jammed into the pelvis, the head and breech stay above the inlet, the neck becomes stretched, and progress is arrested. Transverse lies must never be left to nature.

Spontaneous Version

Spontaneous version takes place occasionally, more often with oblique than with transverse lies. Before or shortly after the onset of labor, the lie changes to a longitudinal one (cephalic or breech), and labor proceeds in the new position. Unfortunately, the chance of spontaneous version occurring is small, too small to warrant more than a very short delay in instituting corrective measures.

Neglected Transverse Lie

Neglected transverse lie results from misdiagnosis or improper treatment. At first the contractions are of poor quality and the cervix dilates slowly. Because of the irregularity of the presenting part, the membranes rupture early and the amniotic fluid escapes rapidly. As the labor pains become stronger the fetal shoulder is forced into the pelvis, the uterus molds itself around the baby, a state of impaction ensues, and progress is halted. From this impasse there is one of two outcomes:

1. Labor goes on; the upper part of the uterus becomes shorter and thicker, while the lower segment becomes progressively more stretched and thinner until it ruptures.
2. Uterine inertia sets in and the contractions cease. Intrauterine sepsis is followed by generalized sepsis.

In either event, fetal death is certain and maternal mortality possible. Transverse lies must not be neglected!

Complications

Because the presenting part does not fill the inlet, the membranes tend to rupture early and may be followed by prolapse of a fetal arm or the umbilical cord (Figs. 3B and C). Both are serious complications necessitating immediate action.

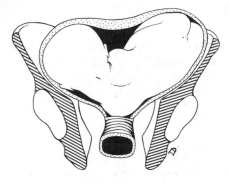

A. Impacted shoulder.

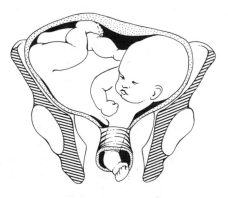

B. Prolapsed arm.

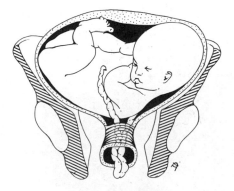

C. Prolapsed umbilical cord.

FIG. 3. Complications.

PROGNOSIS: TRANSVERSE LIE

Prognosis depends on the management. With early diagnosis and proper treatment the outcome is favorable. Neglect results in the death of all the infants and many mothers.

MANAGEMENT OF TRANSVERSE LIE

Management Before Labor

1. Careful abdominal, pelvic, and radiologic examinations are performed to rule out fetal and pelvic abnormalities.
2. External version to a breech or preferably a cephalic presentation should be attempted. This may have to be repeated as there is a tendency for the transverse lie to recur.
3. Elective cesarean section is indicated where conditions are incompatible with safe vaginal delivery. This includes such complications as placenta previa or fetopelvic disproportion.
4. In other cases the onset of labor is awaited, as there is a chance that the malposition will correct itself.

Management During Early Labor

In early labor external version should be attempted, and if successful the new presentation is maintained by a tight abdominal binder until it is fixed in the pelvis.

Management of Patient in Good Labor: Persistent Transverse Lie

Five points are considered:

1. Cause of the transverse lie
2. Parity of the patient
3. Cervical dilatation
4. State of the membranes
5. Condition of the child

CESAREAN SECTION
Cesarean section is the treatment of choice. It is safest for both mother and child. In some instances extraction of the infant through a

transverse lower segment incision may be difficult, and a vertical incision in the lower segment, which can be extended upward if necessary, is preferred by many obstetricians.

INTERNAL PODALIC VERSION AND EXTRACTION

This is a dangerous procedure for fetus and mother, especially if the membranes have been ruptured for some time and the amniotic fluid has drained away. The use of podalic version and extraction (turning the baby to a footling breech and delivering it as such*) is considered only in the following situations:

1. When the baby is premature, to the degree of nonviability, and the risk to the mother of cesarean section is not justified
2. Delivery of a second twin
3. When the patient is admitted to hospital with the membranes intact or ruptured a short time, the cervix fully or almost fully dilated, and prompt delivery is indicated and feasible.

Management of Neglected Transverse Lie

The following conditions are present:

1. There has been prolonged labor.
2. The membranes have been ruptured for a long time.
3. The lower uterine segment is stretched and thin.
4. Intrauterine infection is present.
5. Fetal impaction has taken place.
6. The cord, arm, or both have prolapsed.
7. The baby is dead.

Management under these circumstances is difficult.

1. Cesarean section, followed by hysterectomy if infection is present, is done in the interest of the mother even if the baby is dead.
2. Version and extraction may be considered. This carries a grave risk of rupturing the uterus and killing the mother.
3. In desperate situations a destructive operation on the child can be performed. Decapitation is carried out, the trunk is delivered, and then the head is extracted by forceps.

*See Chapter 30 for technique of internal podalic version.

CONCLUSION

Transverse lies at term, after failure of external version, are treated best by cesarean section. They must never be neglected or left to nature.

BIBLIOGRAPHY

Kawathekar P, Kasturilal MS, Srinivas P, Sudda G: Etiology and trends in the management of transverse lie. Am J Obstet Gynecol 117:39, 1973

20.

Compound Presentations

PROLAPSE OF HAND AND ARM OR FOOT AND LEG

Definition

A presentation is compound when there is prolapse of one or more of the limbs along with the head or the breech, both entering the pelvis at the same time. Footling breech or shoulder presentations are not included in this group. Associated prolapse of the umbilical cord occurs in 15 to 20 percent.

Incidence

Easily detectable compound presentations occur probably once in 500 to 1,000 confinements. It is impossible to establish the exact incidence because:

1. Spontaneous correction occurs frequently, and examination late in labor cannot provide the diagnosis.
2. Minor degrees of prolapse are detected only by early and careful vaginal examination.

Classification of Compound Presentation

1. Cephalic presentation with prolapse of:
   a. upper limb (arm-hand), one or both;
   b. lower limb (leg-foot), one or both;
   c. arm and leg together
2. Breech presentation with prolapse of the hand or arm

PROLAPSE OF HAND AND ARM OR FOOT AND LEG

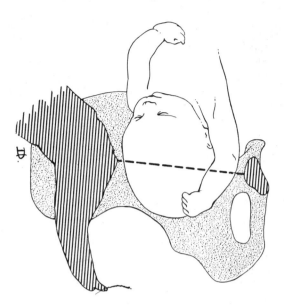

FIG. 1. Compound presentation: head and hand.

By far the most frequent combination is that of the head with the hand (Fig. 1) or arm. In contrast the head-foot and breech-arm groups are uncommon, about equally so. Prolapse of both hand and foot alongside the head is rare. All combinations may be complicated by prolapse of the umbilical cord, which then becomes the major problem.

Etiology

The etiology of compound presentation includes all conditions that prevent complete filling and occlusion of the pelvic inlet by the presenting part. The most common causal factor is prematurity. Others include high presenting part with ruptured membranes, multiparity, contracted pelvis, and twins.

Diagnosis

The condition is suspected when:

1. There is delay of progress in the active phase.

2. Engagement fails to occur.
3. The fetal head remains high and deviated from the midline during labor, especially after the membranes rupture.

Diagnosis is made by vaginal or rectal examination. In many cases the condition is not noted until labor is well advanced and the cervix fully dilated.

Prognosis

In the past authors suggested a poor prognosis for the child. However, the increased incidence of prematurity and associated prolapse of the cord make it difficult to evaluate accurately the danger to the fetus of uncomplicated prolapse of the hand or foot.

Because of the historically high fetal mortality associated with compound presentations, active therapy (repositioning of the prolapsed part or version and extraction) was the most popular method of management. Recent studies have shown that the high fetal and maternal death rates resulted from overzealous treatment and not from the compound presentation itself. With conservative management the results should be no worse than with other presentations.

Mechanism of Labor

The mechanism of labor is that of the main presenting part. Because the diameter is increased, the chance of arrested progress is greater. In many cases labor is not obstructed, and the leading part is brought down to the outlet. If dystocia occurs, the baby remains high and operative treatment is needed.

MANAGEMENT OF COMPOUND PRESENTATIONS

In choosing the therapeutic procedure, these factors are considered:

1. Presentation
2. Presence or absence of cord prolapse
3. State of the cervix
4. Condition of the membranes
5. Condition and size of the baby
6. Presence of twins

Progressing Case

The best treatment for compound presentations (in the absence of complications such as prolapse of the cord) is masterful inactivity. In most cases, as the cervix becomes fully dilated and the presenting part descends, the prolapsed arm or leg rises out of the pelvis, allowing labor to proceed normally. Hence as long as progress is being made there should be no interference.

Arrest of Progress

1. REPOSITION OF THE PROLAPSED PART: In a normal pelvis if progress is arrested the arm or leg should be replaced, under anesthesia, and the head pushed into the pelvis. If the head is low in the pelvis and the cervix fully dilated, the head is extracted with forceps. High forceps must never be used.
2. CESAREAN SECTION: If there is cephalopelvic disproportion, if reposition is not feasible or is unsuccessful, or if there is some other condition that militates against vaginal delivery, cesarean section should be performed.
3. INTERNAL PODALIC VERSION AND EXTRACTION: This procedure carries with it the danger of uterine rupture and fetal death. Hence it should not be used in the management of uncomplicated compound presentations. An exception is made in the case of a second twin.

Prolapse of the Cord

In 13 to 23 percent the compound presentation is complicated by prolapse of the umbilical cord. This then becomes the major and urgent problem, and treatment is directed primarily to it (see Chap. 21).

BIBLIOGRAPHY

Weissberg SM, O'Leary JA: Compound presentation of the fetus. Obstet Gynecol 41:60, 1973

21.

The Umbilical Cord

THE NORMAL UMBILICAL CORD

The umbilical cord links the fetus to the placenta and is the fetal lifeline. The cord is between 30 and 60 cm in length, the average being 50 cm. It is covered on the outside by the amnion, which blends with the fetal skin at the umbilicus. On the inside of the cord is the thick myxomatous Wharton's jelly. Through the jelly, and protected by it, run the umbilical vessels, one vein and two arteries, in a spiral arrangement. The circulation is the reverse of the adult in that the vein carries oxygenated blood to the fetus, while the arteries bring venous blood back to the placenta.

The fetal surface of the placenta is covered by amniotic membrane, under which course the large blood vessels, branches of the umbilical vein and arteries. Normally the cord inserts into the center of the placenta.

ABNORMALITIES OF THE UMBILICAL CORD

Length

On record are cords as short as 0 cm and as long as 104 cm.

1. A short cord may result in delay in descent of the fetus, fetal distress, separation of the placenta from the wall of the uterus, inversion of the uterus, and rupture leading to hemorrhage and possible fetal exsanguination.
2. A long cord is subject to entanglement, knotting, encirclement of the fetus, and prolapse.
3. When the cord is absent the fetus is attached directly to the placenta at the umbilicus. Omphalocele is always present.

Single Umbilical Artery

This occurs in 1 percent of single births and in 7 to 14 percent of multiple pregnancies. The condition is associated with a high rate of congenital fetal anomalies.

Battledore Placenta

Instead of being at the center, the cord is inserted at the margin of the placental disc. This condition has no known clinical significance.

Velamentous Insertion

In this case the vessels of the cord break up into branches before reaching the placenta, so that the cord inserts into the membranes rather than the placental disc. The result is that large vessels course under the membrane and are unprotected by Wharton's jelly.

Vasa Previa

In this situation the velamentous vessels lie over the cervix, in front of the presenting part. Rupture leads to fetal bleeding, which may be fatal. The clinical picture is similar to placenta previa.

CORD ENTANGLEMENTS

The most common variety of cord entanglement is the umbilical cord around the fetal neck. Four coils have been seen from time to time and as many as nine have been reported. The cord may be looped around the trunk, shoulders, and upper or lower limbs. This condition is associated with excessive amounts of amniotic fluid, long cords, and small infants.

During pregnancy trouble is unusual. Sometimes as the fetus descends during labor the coils tighten sufficiently to reduce the flow of blood through the cord, thus causing fetal anoxia.

Only rarely are cord entanglements responsible for fetal or neonatal death. However, abnormalities of the fetal heart, meconium-stained amniotic fluid, and babies requiring resuscitation are seen more often when there is an entanglement of the cord. Significantly lower Apgar scores have been reported. Radical or hasty delivery is almost never indicated for cord abnormalities other than prolapse.

KNOTS OF THE CORD

True Knot

Occasionally a true knot of the umbilical cord is noted after delivery. This complication can occur when there is a long cord, large amounts of amniotic fluid, a small infant, monoamniotic twins, or an overactive fetus or as a result of external version. In many instances the knot is formed when a loop of cord is slipped over the infant's head or shoulders during delivery.

Rarely is the knot pulled tightly enough to cause the death of the fetus from restriction of the circulation in the cord. The umbilical vessels, protected by the thick myxomatous Wharton's jelly, are rarely occluded completely. The fetal mortality associated with true knots of the umbilical cord is low. In these cases there is flattening or dissipation of Wharton's jelly and venous congestion distal to the knot, as well as partially or completely occlusive vascular thrombi.

False Knots

The blood vessels are longer than the cord. Often they are folded on themselves and produce nodulations on the surface of the cord. These have been termed false knots.

PROLAPSE OF THE UMBILICAL CORD

In this situation the umbilical cord lies beside or below the presenting part. Although an infrequent complication—less than 1 percent (0.3 to 0.6 percent)—its significance is disproportionately great because of the high fetal mortality rate and the increased maternal hazard from the operative procedures used in treatment.

Compression of the umbilical cord between the presenting part and the maternal pelvis reduces or cuts off the blood supply to the fetus, and if uncorrected leads to death of the baby.

Classification of Prolapsed Cord

UMBILICAL CORD PRESENTATION   The membranes are intact.
UMBILICAL CORD PROLAPSE   The membranes are ruptured. The cord may occupy three positions (Fig. 1):

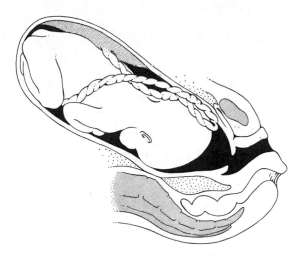

A. Cord prolapsed at the inlet.

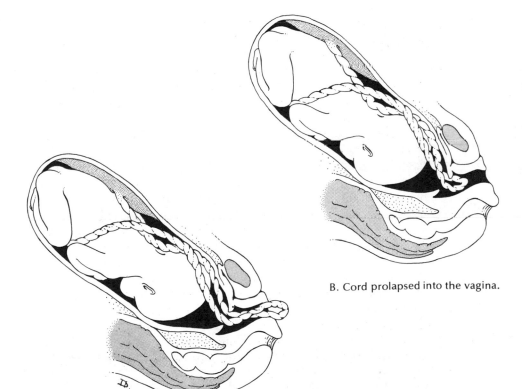

B. Cord prolapsed into the vagina.

C. Cord prolapsed through the introitus.

FIG. 1. Prolapsed umbilical cord.

1. It may lie beside the presenting part at the inlet. Such an occult prolapse may be more common than is generally accepted. It could kill a baby during labor without leaving a trace of evidence at vaginal delivery.
2. It may descend into the vagina.
3. It may pass through the introitus and out the vagina.

Etiology

Whenever the presenting part does not fit closely and fails to fill the inlet of the pelvis, danger of prolapse of the umbilical cord exists. Compound presentation and rupture of the bag of waters increases the risk.

FETAL ETIOLOGY

1. ABNORMAL PRESENTATION Abnormal presentation occurs in almost half the cases of prolapse of the cord. Since 95 percent of all presentations are cephalic, the greatest number of prolapsed cords occur when the head leads the way. The highest relative incidence, however, is in the following order: (1) transverse lie; (2) breech presentation, especially the footling variety; and (3) cephalic presentation.
2. PREMATURITY Two factors play a part in the failure to fill the inlet: (1) the smallness of the presenting part, and (2) the frequency of abnormal positions in premature labors. The fetal mortality is high. One reason for this is that small babies withstand trauma and anoxia badly. The second is the reluctance to submit the mother to a major operation when the chance of saving the baby is almost nil.
3. MULTIPLE PREGNANCY The factors involved here include interference with good adaptation, greater frequency of abnormal presentation, high incidence of polyhydramnios, and rupture of the membranes of the second twin while it is still high.
4. POLYHYDRAMNIOS When the membranes rupture, the large amount of fluid pours out and the cord may be washed down.

MATERNAL AND OBSTETRIC ETIOLOGY

1. CEPHALOPELVIC DISPROPORTION Disproportion between pelvis and baby causes failure of engagement, and rupture of the membranes may be attended by prolapse of the cord.
2. HIGH PRESENTING PART Temporary delay of engagement may

occur even in the normal pelvis, especially in multiparas. Should the membranes rupture during this period, the cord may come down.

CORD AND PLACENTAL ETIOLOGY

1. LONG CORD The longer the umbilical cord the easier it is for it to prolapse.
2. LOW-LYING PLACENTA When the placenta is located near the cervix it hinders engagement. In addition, insertion of the cord is nearer the cervix.

IATROGENIC ETIOLOGY
One-third of prolapses of the cord are produced during obstetric procedures.

1. Artificial rupture of the membranes. When the head is high, or when there is an abnormal presentation, rupture of the membranes may be attended by prolapse of the cord.
2. Disengaging the head. Elevation of the head out of the pelvis to facilitate rotation.
3. Flexion of an extended head.
4. Version and extraction.
5. Insertion of a bag (rarely used today).

Diagnosis: Prolapse of the Cord

The diagnosis of prolapse of the cord is made in two ways: (1) seeing the cord outside the vulva, and (2) feeling the cord on vaginal examination. Since the fetal mortality is high once the cord has protruded through the introitus, means of earlier diagnosis must be sought.

VAGINAL EXAMINATION
Vaginal examination should be performed:

1. When there is unexplained fetal distress, and especially if the presenting part is not well engaged. Unfortunately fetal distress may be a late sign.
2. When the membranes rupture with a high presenting part.
3. In all cases of malpresentation when the membranes rupture.
4. When the baby is markedly premature.
5. In cases of twins.

Prognosis: Prolapse of the Cord

LABOR
Labor is not affected by the prolapsed cord.

MOTHER
Maternal danger is caused only by traumatic attempts to save the child.

FETUS
The uncorrected perinatal mortality is around 35 percent. The baby's chances depend on the degree and duration of the compression of the cord and the interval between diagnosis and delivery. The fetal results depend upon the following factors:

1. The better the condition of the baby at the time of diagnosis, the greater its chance of survival. A strongly pulsating cord is a sign of hope, while a cord with a weak pulse is an ill omen.
2. The sooner the baby is delivered after the cord comes down, the better are the results. Delay of over 30 minutes increases the fetal mortality four times.
3. The more mature the fetus, the greater is its ability to withstand traumatic processes.
4. The less traumatic the actual delivery of the child, the better is the prognosis for mother and baby.
5. Cervical dilatation is probably the most important point. If the cervix is fully dilated when the diagnosis is made, many babies can be saved. The less the dilatation, the worse the prognosis. The exception to this situation is when rapid cesarean section can be done, in which case the prognosis is equally good or better when the cervix is dilated only a small degree.
6. The fetal mortality increases as the interval between rupture of the membranes and delivery increases.

Management of Prolapsed Cord

NO INTERFERENCE
The prolapsed cord is ignored and labor allowed to proceed under the following conditions:

1. When the baby is dead.
2. When the baby is known to be abnormal (e.g., anencephaly).

3. When the fetus is so premature that it has no chance of survival. There is no point in subjecting the mother to needless risk.

TEMPORARY MEASURES

Measures to lessen cord compression and improve the condition of the infant include the following:

1. The attendant places a hand in the vagina and pushes the presenting part up and away from the cord. At the same time preparations are made for delivery.
2. The patient is placed in the knee-chest or Trendelenburg position, with the hips elevated and the head low.
3. The woman is given oxygen by mask.
4. The fetal heart is checked carefully and often.
5. Vaginal examination is made to ascertain presentation, cervical dilatation, station of the presenting part, and condition of the cord.

CERVIX FULLY DILATED

When the cervix is fully dilated these measures are carried out with these presentations:

1. Cephalic presentation, head low in the pelvis: Extraction by forceps.
2. In other situations cesarean section is the best treatment if it can be performed without delay.
3. If cesarean section cannot be carried out immediately the following procedures are indicated:
   a. Cephalic presentation, head high: Internal podalic version and extraction as a breech. There is the danger of rupturing the uterus, but since this is a desperate attempt to save the child, the chance is taken.
   b. Breech presentation: Extraction as a footling breech.
   c. Transverse lie: Internal podalic version to a footling breech and immediate extraction.

CERVIX INCOMPLETELY DILATED

When the cervix is incompletely dilated, these measures are carried out:

1. Cesarean section is the treatment of choice as long as the child is mature and in good condition. The fetal results with cesarean section are far superior to other methods of delivery. The danger

to the mother is considerably less than forceful delivery through an undilated cervix. While preparations for surgery are being made, the measures previously described for reducing compression of the cord are carried out.

2. Reposition of the cord may be attempted if cesarean section cannot be performed. The cord is carried up into the uterus, and the presenting part is pushed down into the pelvis and held there. Reposition of the cord is successful occasionally, but in most cases valuable time is lost in attempting it.
3. These measures failing, the mother is kept in the Trendelenburg position in the hope that pressure is kept off the cord so that the child survives until the cervix is dilated enough to enable delivery.
4. Manual dilatation of the cervix, cervical incisions, and other forceful methods of opening the cervix are almost never justified. Their success is small, and the risk to the mother is great.

Prophylaxis

Obstetric manipulations that encourage premature rupture of the membranes (such as artificial rupture of the membranes when the leading part is unengaged or when there is a malpresentation) and that increase the incidence of prolapse of the umbilical cord should be avoided. Patients whose membranes rupture at home, either before or during labor, should be admitted to hospital.

BIBLIOGRAPHY

Savage EW, Kohl SG, Wynn RW: Prolapse of the umbilical cord. Obstet Gynecol 36:502, 1970
Tipton RH, Chang AM: Nuchal encirclement by the umbilical cord. J Obstet Gynecol Br Commonw 78:901, 1971

22.

Shoulder Dystocia

GENERAL CONSIDERATIONS

Definition

True shoulder dystocia refers to the following situation: The presentation is cephalic; the head has been born, but the shoulders cannot be delivered by the usual methods. There is no other cause for the difficulty.

Incidence

The general incidence is less than 1 percent (0.15 to 0.2 percent). In babies weighing over 4,000 g the incidence is 1.6 percent.

Etiology

Shoulder dystocia is associated with maternal obesity, excessive weight gain, oversized infants, history of large siblings, and maternal diabetes.

MECHANISM OF THE SHOULDERS

Normal Mechanism

In most cases the shoulders enter the pelvis in an oblique diameter. As labor progresses the shoulders descend and, under the rifling effect of the birth canal, rotate the bisacromial diameter toward the anteroposterior diameter of the pelvis. By this mechanism the anterior shoulder comes under the pubic symphysis a little to the side of the midline and is then delivered.

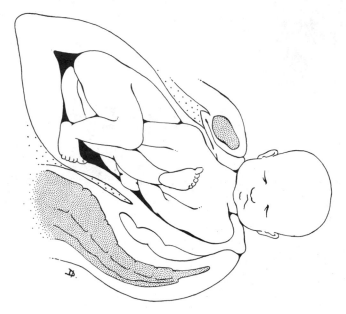

FIG. 1. Shoulder dystocia: bisacromial diameter in the anteroposterior diameter of the pelvis.

Mechanism in Shoulder Dystocia

Impaction of the shoulders is favored when they attempt to enter the pelvis with the bisacromial diameter in the anteroposterior diameter of the inlet (Fig. 1), instead of utilizing one of the oblique diameters. Rarely do both shoulders impact above the pelvic brim. Usually the posterior shoulder can negotiate its way past the sacral promontory, but the anterior one becomes arrested against the pubic symphysis. Some authors restrict the definition of shoulder dystocia to cases where the shoulders try to enter the pelvis with their bisacromial diameter in the anteroposterior diameter of the inlet.

Causes of Dystocia after Birth of the Head

1. Short umbilical cord
2. Abdominal or thoracic enlargement of the infant (anasarca, monsters, neoplasms)
3. Locked or conjoined twins
4. Uterine constriction ring
5. True shoulder dystocia

EFFECTS OF SHOULDER DYSTOCIA

Effects on the Fetus

With each uterine contraction large amounts of blood are transferred from the baby's trunk to its head. The angulation of the neck and the compression of the chest, which interfere with cardiac function, impair the venous return. The intracranial vascular system of the fetus cannot compensate for the excessive intravascular pressure. Under these conditions anoxia develops and may be accompanied by hemorrhagic effusions. If this condition persists too long the baby suffers irreparable brain damage. It may die during the attempts at delivery or in the neonatal period.

Complications

1. Fetal
   a. Death, intrapartum or neonatal.
   b. Immediate birth injuries, such as brachial plexus palsy and fractured clavicle, occur in 20 percent.
   c. Late neuropsychiatric abnormalities are seen in 30 percent of survivors.
2. Maternal: Lacerations of the birth canal.

CLINICAL PICTURE

The clinical picture has been described by Morris:

> The delivery of the head with or without forceps may have been quite easy, but more commonly there has been a little difficulty in completing the extension of the head. The hairy scalp slides out with reluctance. When the forehead has appeared it is necessary to press back the perineum to deliver the face. Fat cheeks eventually emerge. A double chin has to be hooked over the posterior vulval commissure, to which it remains tightly opposed. Restitution seldom occurs spontaneously, for the head seems incapable of movement as a result of friction with the girdle of contact of the vulva. On the other hand, gentle manipulation of the head sometimes results in a sudden 90 degree restitution as the head adjusts itself without descent to the anteroposterior position of the shoulders.
> Time passes. The child's head becomes suffused. It endeavors unsuccessfully to breathe. Abdominal efforts by the mother or by her attendants produce no advance; gentle head traction is equally unavailing.

Usually equanimity forsakes the attendants. They push, they pull. Alarm increases. Eventually

By greater strength of muscle
Or by some infernal juggle

the difficulty appears to be overcome, and the shoulders and trunk of a goodly child are delivered. The pallor of its body contrasts with the plum-colored cyanosis of the face, and the small quantity of freshly expelled meconium about the buttocks. It dawns upon the attendants that their anxiety was not ill-founded, the baby lies limp and voiceless, and too often remains so despite all efforts at resuscitation.

DIAGNOSIS

Diagnosis can be made only after the head has been delivered. Certain signs then appear:

1. There is a definite recoil of the head back against the perineum.
2. Restitution rarely takes place spontaneously. Because of the friction with the vulva, the head seems incapable of movement.
3. The problem is usually recognized when traction from below and pressure from above fail to deliver the child.
4. Vaginal examination is made to rule out other causes of difficulty, as listed above under "Causes of Dystocia after Birth of the Head."

MANAGEMENT OF SHOULDER DYSTOCIA

Prophylaxis

While this complication cannot be prevented, the results can be improved by recognizing the situations in which it occurs and by insisting on expert obstetric care for these patients. It has been suggested that a prolonged second stage of labor is a warning sign.

Accessory Measures

1. Anesthesia is administered, or if already in progress it should be deepened; complete muscle relaxation is of great value. Time is precious, and while the anesthesia is being given the operator must act.
2. The respiratory tract is cleared of mucus and debris to provide a clear airway.

3. Vaginal examination of the infant and the pelvis is made to rule out the other complications that prevent descent of the body: short umbilical cord, locked or conjoined twins, enlargement of abdomen or thorax, and uterine constriction ring.
4. An episiotomy, preferably mediolateral and large, is made to make room and to prevent tears into the rectum.

Basic Method of Delivery of Shoulders

Gentle backward traction is made on the delivered head, without forced rotation and without excessive angulation (Fig. 2A). At the same time the patient is told to bear down, if she is awake; if she is asleep, pressure on the fundus is made by an assistant at the same time that traction is being exerted on the head. The traction must be smooth and continuous, and sudden jerks avoided. The duration of these efforts should rarely exceed 4 to 5 seconds. If the cause of the difficulty is merely the friction of large shoulders in the oblique or transverse diameters, these simple measures almost always produce advancement. One or two efforts, however, are sufficient. If they fail, this method of delivery should be abandoned.

OPERATIVE METHODS OF TREATING SHOULDER DYSTOCIA

Delivery of Anterior Shoulder

1. The hand is placed deeply in the vagina behind the anterior shoulder.
2. With the next contraction the axis of the shoulders is rotated into an oblique diameter of the pelvis (Fig. 2B).
3. Firm traction is made on the head, deflecting it toward the floor.
4. Suprapubic pressure is exerted; this usually succeeds in bringing the anterior shoulder into and through the pelvis.
5. Sometimes the extraction may be furthered by the operator's hooking a forefinger under the axilla.

Extraction of Posterior Shoulder and Arm

1. The hand is placed deeply into the vagina behind the posterior shoulder (Fig. 3A).

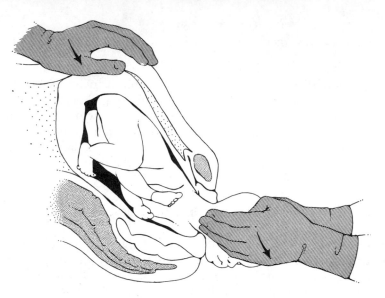

A. Basic method of delivering shoulders.

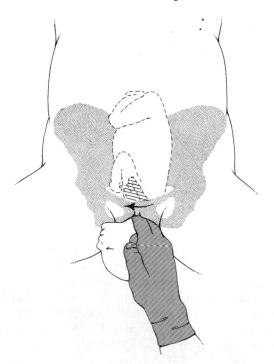

B. Shoulder dystocia: rotation of bisacromial diameter from anteroposterior diameter pelvis into the oblique.

FIG. 2. Delivery of anterior shoulder.

OPERATIVE METHODS OF TREATING SHOULDER DYSTOCIA

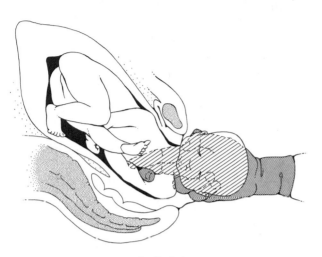

A. First step.

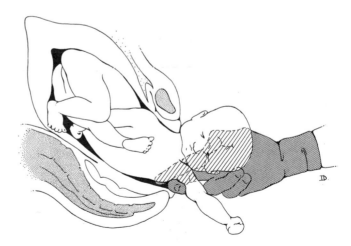

B. Second step.

FIG. 3. Extraction of posterior shoulder and arm.

2. The arm is grasped and carried up over the front of the baby's abdomen. The hand is then seized and extracted with the arm (Fig. 3B).
3. Once this is accomplished the anterior shoulder delivers. If it does not, the body is rotated 180° so that the anterior shoulder is now posterior. It is then delivered in the same way as the first one.

Screw Principle of Woods

1. The position of the head is LOT. This technic is not possible until the posterior shoulder has passed the spines.
2. Downward pressure is made on the baby's buttocks through the mother's abdomen by the operator's hand (Fig. 4A).
3. Two fingers of the left hand are placed on the anterior aspect of the posterior shoulder. Pressure is made against the shoulder so that is moves counterclockwise, the posterior aspect leading the way (Fig. 4B). It is turned 180°, past 12 o'clock. In this way the posterior shoulder is delivered under the pubic arc. The head has turned from LOT to ROT.
4. The posterior shoulder has been delivered, and the anterior shoulder is now posterior.

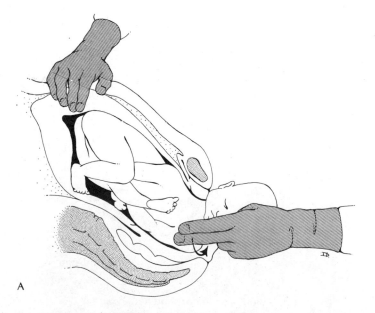

A

FIG. 4. Screw principle of Woods. A through D represent steps one through four in this maneuver.

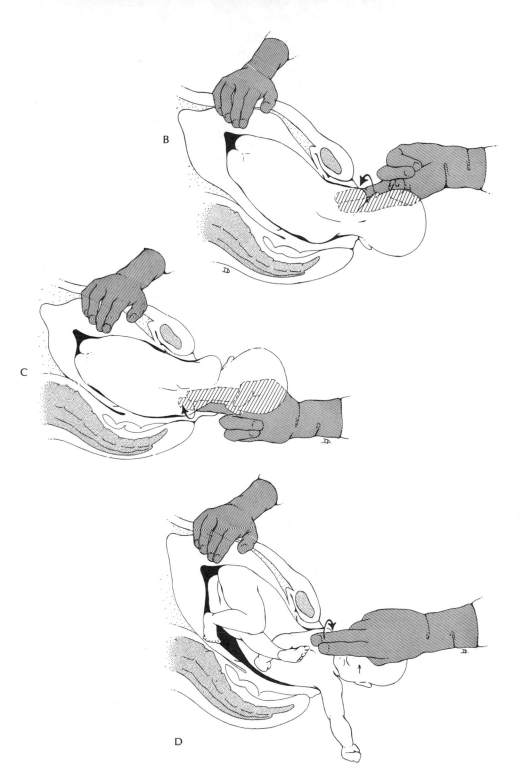

B

C

D

5. Pressure is again made on the baby's buttocks in a downward direction.

6. At the same time two fingers are placed against the anterior aspect of the newly posterior shoulder. By pressure against the shoulder, it is moved in a clockwise direction, the posterior aspect leading the way (Fig. 4C). It is turned 180°, past 12 o'clock, and the posterior shoulder is again delivered (Fig. 4D). The head rotates from ROT to LOT.

BIBLIOGRAPHY

Benedetti TJ, Gabbe SG: Shoulder Dystocia. Obstet Gynecol 52:526, 1978
Morris WIC: Shoulder dystocia. J Obstet Gynaecol Br Emp 62:302, 1955

23.

Multiple Pregnancy

INCIDENCE

Hellin's law propounds the following rates of multiple pregnancy:

Twins	1:89
Triplets	$1:89^2$
Quadruplets	$1:89^3$
Quintuplets	$1:89^4$

Another way of expressing the approximate incidence is:

Twins	1:100
Triplets	1:10,000
Quadruplets	1:750,000

The etiology of multiple pregnancy has not been proved. Genetic factors have been implicated in monozygous replication, excessive gonadotropic stimulation in dizygous twins. A tendency to plural births runs in families, more often on the maternal side. The incidence is higher in multiparas and in colored races.

An American survey noted that the mean birthweight and duration of pregnancy for the single fetus was 3,377 g and 280.5 days, for twins 2,395 g each and 261.6 days, and for triplets 1,818 g each and 246.8 days. For a comparable period of gestation the mean weight of a singleton is 200 to 800 g greater than that of a twin.

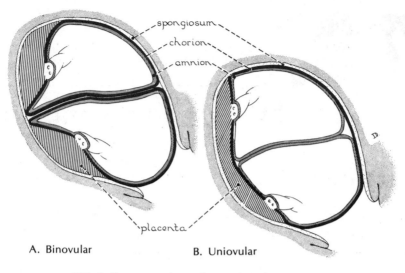

FIG. 1. Placenta and membranes in twin pregnancy.

TWIN PREGNANCY

Dizygous: Double Ovum

About 75 percent of twins are binovular (Fig. 1A). Two fetuses develop from the fertilization of two ova liberated during the same menstrual cycle. The incidence of double ovum twins is influenced by heredity, race, maternal age, and parity. Each twin has its own placenta, chorion, and amniotic sac. When the ova are implanted near each other, the two placentas may seem to fuse. The circulations, however, remain completely separate. These children are fraternal twins. They resemble each other only to the extent that siblings of the same age would. They may be of different sex and sometimes look entirely dissimilar. Weinberg's rule states that the number of dizygous twins in any population is twice the number of twins of different sex; the remainder are monozygous. Dizygous twinning is the result of multiple ovulation, which may be caused by high levels of gonadotropic hormones overstimulating the ovary. The artificial induction of ovulation by clomiphene or gonadotropins may increase the incidence of multiple pregnancy.

Monozygous: Single Ovum

Some 25 percent of twins are uniovular (Fig. 1B); these are identical or true, twins. They represent complete cleavage of the blastodermic vesicle. There is one egg fertilized by a single sperm, and therefore the offspring arise from the same germ plasm. The frequency of single ovum twinning is independent of heredity, race, maternal age, and parity. These children are always of the same sex and look alike. Incomplete division results in anything from conjoined twins to double monsters. There is one placenta, one chorion, and two amniotic sacs. The blood circulations of the twins intercommunicate in the common placenta. In some cases a stronger twin monopolizes the circulation, which results in poor development of the other fetus. The undersized member tends to remain inferior into adult life. The smaller twin does not catch up to the larger in weight, length, head circumference, or the scores of intelligence tests. It is possible that the inability of the placenta to transmit adequate amounts of nutrition to the smaller twin leads to a cellular deficit that may restrict the final growth potential.

Placentas of Twins

The only time that twins can be proved to be fraternal is when they are of different sexes. Identical twins may have one or two chorionic sacs, but only when there is a single chorionic sac can identicity be proved. Thus twins with one chorion are always identical. Twins of the same sex with two chorionic sacs may be identical or fraternal, and no examination of the placenta or membranes can establish the true status.

Monoamniotic Twins

Monoamniotic twins—with both babies lying in one amniotic cavity—are rare. The exact incidence is not known. There are two etiologic theories:

1. At first there are two amnions. Early in the pregnancy the partition between them breaks down, and a single amniotic sac results.
2. A single ovum gives rise to two blastodermic vesicles, which split after formation of the amnion. Thus there is only one original sac.

Because the fetuses are not separated by membrane there is a great likelihood of knotting, tangling, and strangulation of the cords, resulting in fetal death. Therefore the prognosis for monoamniotic twins is poor. If after the birth of the first baby the umbilical cord is observed to be twisted or knotted, or if there is no second bag of waters, the other twin should be delivered immediately.

Twin Transfusion Syndrome

This occurs in monozygous twins with a single placenta in which arteriovenous fistulization leads to a parabiotic relationship. The donor twin is anemic (as low as 8 g of hemoglobin), while the recipient is plethoric (hemoglobin as high as 27 g) and is in danger of developing neonatal cardiac failure. The difference in weight is as much as 1,000 g. The smaller twin may be associated with oligohydramnios; polyhydramnios is more common in the larger infant. The placenta of the donor twin is pale and swollen or atrophied; that of the recipient is large and congested.

Management includes (1) exchange transfusion, (2) venesection of the recipient, (3) treatment of hypoglycemia. Neonatal mortality has been reported to be as high as 70 percent.

Superfetation

Superfetation is the fertilization of a second ovum at a later ovulation. There is doubt that superfetation takes place because (1) pregnancy suppresses ovulation, (2) the cervical canal is occluded by a plug of mucus, which acts as a barrier to the ascent of sperm, and (3) after the 14th week the uterine cavity is sealed off by the enlarging fetal sac. However, a few cases have been reported in which the possibility of superfetation exists.

Superfecundation

Superfecundation is the fertilization of two ova expelled at the same ovulation but fertilized at different copulations. This can be proved only if the resulting children are of identifiably different races.

DIAGNOSIS OF MULTIPLE PREGNANCY

1. Suggestive findings:
   a. Familial history is positive.
   b. The uterus and abdomen seem larger than expected for the period of amenorrhea.
   c. Uterine growth is more rapid than normal.
   d. There is unexplainably excessive weight gain.
2. Positive signs:
   a. Palpation of two heads or two breeches.

DIAGNOSIS OF MULTIPLE PREGNANCY

b. Two fetal hearts auscultated at the same time by two observers and differing in rate by at least 10 beats per minute.

c. X-ray of the abdomen shows two skeletons. These may appear by the 18th week or sooner, but a second skeleton cannot be ruled out until the 25th week.

d. Ultrasonography demonstrates the presence of two or more fetal skulls.

3. The diagnosis of twins is not easy unless there is a high index of suspicion. The frequency of premature labor makes the diagnosis even more difficult.

EFFECTS OF MULTIPLE PREGNANCY

Maternal Effects

1. Because the volume of the intrauterine contents is large, symptoms ranging from discomfort to actual abdominal pain are frequent. Pressure against the diaphragm leads to dyspnea.
2. The mechanical and metabolic loads increase with the multiplicity of the pregnancy.
3. Polyhydramnios, an excessive amount of amniotic fluid, is more common than in single pregnancies.
4. The incidence of preeclampsia is increased.
5. Anemia is prevalent.
6. Excessive weight gain occurs for several reasons, including overeating, water retention, the presence of more than one fetus, and polyhydramnios.
7. Complaints of fetal overactivity are frequent.

Fetal Effects

1. While the individual child is smaller than average, the combined weight of the babies is larger than that of a single child. One twin may be 50 to 1,000 g heavier than the other. In half the cases the children are of term size. In one-eighth of pregnancies both babies are under 1,500 g. The remaining three-eighths are between 1,500 and 2,500 g.
2. The combination of small babies and large amounts of amniotic fluid leads to an increased incidence of malpresentation.
3. Fetal mortality is increased in twin pregnancy to four times that of singletons. The gross mortality varies from 9 to 14 percent. While malpresentations and congenital abnormalities play a part, the major cause of death is prematurity. Birth weight is an important factor; 2,000 g seems to be a critical point. The survival rate of twins born after 36 weeks' gestation is several times higher than that of twins born before this period.
4. The risk to the second twin is greater than to the first. Reasons for this include:
   a. Greater incidence of operative deliveries.
   b. Too long an interval between the birth of the first and second twins.
   c. Reduction of the uterine capacity after the birth of the first baby: This may alter the placental hemodynamics and result in fetal anoxia.

    d. The second twin occupies a less favorable position in the actively contracting upper uterine segment.

    e. There is an increased incidence of malpresentation in the second twin.

5. The least possible delay should be permitted between delivery of the children. After the first is born it may be wise to give the mother oxygen to breathe in an effort to prevent anoxia of the second twin. The greater loss of the second twin is the result of death in the neonatal period rather than before or during labor.

6. Congenital malformations are more common in twins than in singletons.

7. Kurtz found that in no set of triplets did the combined weights reach 7,500 g, indicating that triplets average under 2,500 g. The second and third babies have a higher mortality than the first.

Effects on Labor

1. Overstretching of the uterus by the large combined weights of the babies, two placentas, and copious amniotic fluid, leads to the following:

    a. Premature labor occurs, on the average, 3 weeks before term.

    b. Early rupture of the membranes is frequent and is one cause of premature labor.

    c. Most twin labors are satisfactory. Sometimes the overlengthened uterine muscles produce weak and inefficient contractions, resulting in slow progress.

    d. The increased incidence and danger of postpartum hemorrhage must be kept in mind.

    e. Malpresentations are common.

    f. Umbilical cord prolapse is caused by rupture of the membranes with the gushing out of large amounts of fluid, especially with the second twin.

    g. Multiple pregnancy accelerates the problem of cervical incompetence and can result in effacement and dilatation as early as the first trimester.

2. In 80 percent of cases the second twin is born within 30 minutes of the first.

3. The two babies are born first and then the two placentas.

4. The combinations of presentations (Fig. 2) are, in descending order of frequency:

    a. Two vertices (most common and most favorable presentation)

    b. Vertex and breech

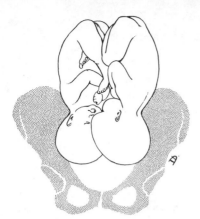

A. Two vertexes.

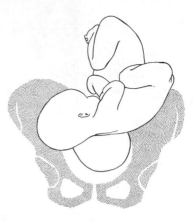

D. Vertex and transverse lie.

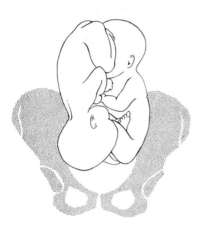

B. Vertex and breech.

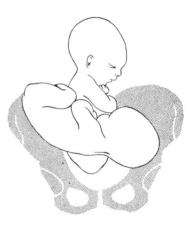

E. Breech and transverse lie.

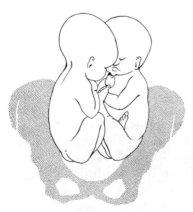

C. Two breeches.

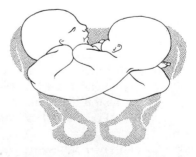

F. Two transverse lies.

FIG. 2. Twin presentations.

   c. Two breeches
   d. Vertex and transverse lie
   e. Breech and transverse lie
   f. Both in the transverse lie

MANAGEMENT OF MULTIPLE PREGNANCY

Management During Pregnancy

Early diagnosis enables the parents to make preparations for more than one child and alerts the doctor to the problems of multiple pregnancy. The two main complications, premature labor and preeclampsia, call for special care during the prenatal period.

1. The patient should cease outside work by 24 weeks. She needs frequent rest periods.
2. Travel is restricted, since the probability of early labor is strong.
3. Coitus is forbidden during the last 3 months.
4. It is believed that one reason for premature labor is the inability of the cervix to contain the enlarging products of conception. If at any time the cervix becomes effaced and open, the patient should be put to bed.
5. Prenatal visits are made more often so that the presence of toxemia can be noted as soon as possible.
6. Since the greatest cause of fetal mortality is preterm labor, the maintenance of the pregnancy to 36 to 37 weeks is desirable. Many obstetricians believe that bed rest, at home or in hospital, helps to achieve this goal. Rest in bed during pregnancy has two important effects: it delays the onset of labor, and it promotes intrauterine fetal growth; multiple gestation may represent a form of intrauterine growth retardation. The period of bed rest, with rising for meals and use of the bathroom, is from the 28th to the 36th week. Once the babies have attained a good size, the patient may resume her usual activities. It is important that the diagnosis of multiple pregnancy be made as early as possible, and routine ultrasonic screening of all pregnant women at 20 weeks has been suggested.

Management During Labor

1. Accurate diagnosis of the presentations is essential. X-ray examination is used when needed.

2. Sedatives and analgesics are administered with care, since small babies are quite susceptible to drugs that depress the vital centers.

3. The higher incidence of postpartum hemorrhage calls for precautionary measures, even to the extent of having crossmatched blood available, especially if the mother is anemic.

4. Watchful expectancy is the procedure of choice during labor. The best results are obtained when the least interference is employed.

5. When delivery is near, the patient is placed on the delivery table and an intravenous infusion of 5 percent glucose in water is started. This precautionary measure has two uses: (a) Should uterine atony occur, either before or after the birth of the baby, oxytocin can be added to the solution to stimulate the myometrium. (b) If postpartum hemorrhage does take place, the route for the administration of fluids or blood is available immediately.

6. The first baby is delivered in the usual way, as if it were a single pregnancy.

7. The umbilical cord must be clamped doubly. This is to prevent the second baby from bleeding through the cord of the first in uniovular twins, in whom the placental circulations communicate.

8. Intravenous egometrine should not be given before birth of the second twin is complete. The strong contraction that results may be dangerous to the baby still in utero, especially if it is placed badly.

9. Careful examination is made to determine the position and station of the second baby. If the vertex or breech is in or over the inlet and the uterus is contracting, the membranes should be ruptured artificially, care being taken that the cord does not prolapse. If uterine inertia has set in, an oxytocin drip may be given to reestablish uterine contractions; when this has been achieved, amniotomy is performed. The presenting part is guided into the pelvis by the vaginal hand. If necessary, pressure is made on the fundus with the other hand. Since the first baby has already dilated the birth canal, the second one descends rapidly to the pelvic floor.

10. Once the presenting part is on the perineum it is delivered spontaneously or by simple operative measures.

11. If the presentation is abnormal, if fetal or maternal distress supervenes, or if spontaneous delivery of the second twin has not taken place within 15 minutes, operative interference is considered, since the risk to the second baby increases with time.

The second baby should be extracted as a breech if it so presents, and by version and extraction if it is a cephalic presentation or transverse lie. We do not believe in routine version and extraction for normal positions.

12. The sudden reduction of the intrauterine contents by delivery of the first twin may lead to premature separation of the placenta, endangering the second baby.

13. The placentas are delivered after both twins have been born.

14. Cesarean section is never performed when the presence of twins is the sole indication. The reason for operative delivery is some accompanying complication, such as toxemia of pregnancy, antepartum hemorrhage (placenta previa and abruptio placentae), transverse lie, or prolapse of the umbilical cord. Twin pregnancy does not impose a special threat to the integrity of a preexisting low transverse cesarean scar. It is not necessary to schedule a repeat cesarean any earlier for a twin pregnancy than for a singleton.

15. On rare occasions the second twin has been delivered by cesarean section following vaginal delivery of the first. In most cases the indication was transverse lie. Other situations include premature separation of the placenta, uterine inertia, fetal distress, prolapsed cord, and breech presentation. The incidence of fetal loss has been reported to be as high as 23 percent of second twins delivered by cesarean section.

TRIPLET PREGNANCY

Daw analyzed a series of 14 triplet pregnancies. He noted a poor rate of growth, a finding that fits the theory of "uterine crowding." There was a high incidence of females. Most of the first infants presented by the head, with an equal distribution of cephalic and breech presentation among the second and third triplets. The fetal mortality rate was 31 percent.

The prognosis for fetal survival was associated with several factors:

1. It was higher in older mothers.
2. Female infants did better than males.
3. The second and third infants fared worse than the first.
4. Fetuses presenting by the breech had a higher perinatal mortality rate, independent of birth order.
5. Parity did not have much effect on fetal survival.
6. The maturity of the infants at birth had more importance than the weight.

The poor prognosis for triplets delivered as breeches suggests that cesarean section might be the better way to deliver triplets. It may also be safer for the mother because it eliminates the risks of manipulations in the overdistended uterus.

LOCKING OF TWINS

Locking of twins is the situation in which one baby impedes the descent and delivery of the other. The problem is more common in primigravidas. Small babies are more likely to lock than large ones. This complication is so rare that most obstetricians never see a case. There are four varieties:

1. COLLISION The contact of any fetal parts of one twin with those of its co-twin, preventing the engagement of either (Fig. 3A).
2. IMPACTION The indentation of any fetal parts of one twin onto the surface of its co-twin, permitting partial engagement of both simultaneously (Fig. 3B).
3. COMPACTION The simultaneous full engagement of the leading fetal poles of both twins, thus filling the true pelvic cavity and thereby preventing further descent or disengagement of either twin.
4. INTERLOCKING The intimate adhesion of the inferior surface of a twin's chin with that of its co-twin above or below the pelvic inlet (Fig. 3C). If this occurs within the true pelvis, compaction results.

There are four main categories of locked twins:

1. Breech-vertex (most common)
2. Vertex-vertex
3. Vertex-transverse lie
4. Breech-breech

Interlocking is a rare condition. The incidence is 1 per 1,000 twin gestations. However, in the situation in which both twins occupy longitudinal lies, when the fetal poles are opposite to each other, and when the first presents as a breech, the incidence is 1 per 100 cases.

In interlocking the first infant presents as a breech and the second is cephalic. Interlocking takes place between the chins. The first child delivers uneventfully until the scapula is born. The interlocking makes further descent impossible. Unless the condition is corrected rapidly, the first child will die of asphyxia.

LOCKING OF TWINS

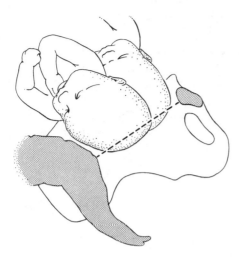

A. Collision.

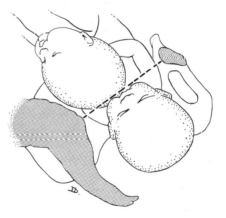

B. Impaction.

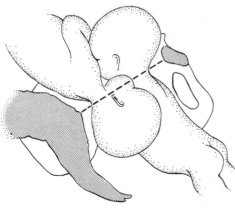

C. Interlocking.

FIG. 3. Locking of twins.

Diagnosis and Prevention

Early diagnosis is rare. True locking occurs only in the second stage of labor and treatment must be instituted before the condition progresses to the point of irreversibility. The following are recommended:

1. An x-ray is taken for every twin gestation during labor.
2. If twin A is presenting as a breech and twin B by the head, the x-ray is repeated after 2 hours of active labor.
3. If there is collision of the twins or suspicion of interlocking, cesarean section should be performed.

Management

MANAGEMENT OF COLLISION, IMPACTION, COMPACTION

1. Strong traction and fundal pressure must be avoided.
2. In general, an attempt is made under deep anesthesia to push the second twin out of the way and out of the pelvis before traction is applied to the first twin and its delivery effected.
3. The second twin is delivered in the usual way.
4. If this method fails and the babies are alive, cesarean section is performed.
5. Embryotomy is a last resort.

MANAGEMENT OF CHIN TO CHIN INTERLOCKING

1. Under anesthesia an attempt is made to unlock the chins, so that the second twin can be pushed out of the way, enabling the first to be born. Traction on the first twin must be avoided as this aggravates the problem.
2. If this does not succeed within a short time, the first baby dies from asphyxia and trauma in the attempted delivery. The following treatment is carried out:

   a. The first twin is decapitated.
   b. The second is delivered.
   c. The head of the first is extracted by forceps.
   d. A couple of strong sutures should be placed in the head of the first twin above the line of decapitation. Later, by traction on these sutures, the head can be fixed, making it easier to apply the forceps.

3. Cesarean section is contraindicated. It would entail pulling the body of the first twin, which is outside of the vulva, back through the vagina, uterus, and peritoneal cavity. This would carry with it grave danger to the mother of peritonitis and general sepsis when there is nothing to gain by this procedure.

Prognosis

The maternal prognosis is good, but fetal prognosis is bad. The perinatal mortality is between 40 and 50 percent. As many as 60 to 70 percent of the deaths are in the first twin, and half of these result from embryotomy.

CONJOINED TWINS

Conjoined twins are uniovular twins in whom the embryonic area failed to split completely and the two individuals remain attached. Siamese twins are one variety.

INCIDENCE
The incidence is from 1:100,000 to 1:50,000 births. In twin gestation the incidence is from 1:900 to 1:650. Most are female.

ETIOLOGY
Because these fetuses originate from a single ovum they are monovular, monozygotic, and monoamniotic, with the same sex and chromosomal pattern. The basic defect is thought to be an incomplete, delayed fission of the inner cell mass, which takes place after the fourteenth day following fertilization. The cause of this event is not known; it is not a new dominant mutation.

DIAGNOSIS
Antepartum diagnosis of multiple gestation is made in only 50 percent to 70 percent of cases. Certain steps are advised:

1. Ultrasonography is performed whenever twins are suspected. The presence of conjoined twins is suggested by the inability to separate the images of the two fetuses, which implies a union at that point.
2. X-ray. Criteria for the diagnosis of conjoined twins include:
   (a) The heads are at the same level and in the same body plane.
   (b) The spines are in unusually close proximity. (c) The spines

are unusually extended. (d) The fetuses do not change position relative to each other after movement, manipulation, or the passage of time.

3. Amniography (the injection of a dye into the amniotic fluid followed by radiologic examination) is carried out when conjoined twinning is suspected on ultrasonic or x-ray examination. This may demonstrate the presence or absence of a union between the two infants, and if present, its location.

4. During labor, when a twin pregnancy is associated with dystocia, one should consider the possibilities of conjoined twins, locked twins, or congenital anomalies.

CLASSIFICATION

1. Thoracopagus—joined at the chest: 40 percent.
2. Xiphopagus or omphalopagus—joined at the anterior abdominal wall from the xiphisternum to the level of the umbilicus: 34 percent.
3. Pyopagus—joined at the buttocks: 18 percent.
4. Ischiopagus—joined at the ischium: 6 percent.
5. Craniopagus—joined at the head: 2 percent.

MANAGEMENT

The decision as to whether delivery should be per vaginam or by cesarean section is based on the possibility of survival of the infants, their size, where they are joined, and the attitudes of the parents.

1. At term, cesarean sections offers the best chance for the fetuses and obviates damage to the mother from a difficult delivery.
2. If the gestation is well before term, the babies are small, and, especially, if they are dead, vaginal delivery can be effected, although dystocia is common.
3. The only group of conjoined twins who do not seem to be affected by dystocia is the craniopagus type. Because of their site of union they can be delivered one after the other.
4. In the case of fetal death with term-sized infants, cesarean section is preferable to protect the mother.

FETUS PAPYRACEUS

This is a rare condition, the reported incidence being 1:12,000 live births and 1:184 twin pregnancies.

FETUS PAPYRACEUS

The mechanism of papyraceus formation involves the death and compression of one twin resulting in a small, underdeveloped, and wafer-thin body that resembles old parchment. Most of the fetal deaths occur in the second trimester, rarely in the third. The etiology is unknown.

The diagnosis is usually made during labor or after delivery of the papyraceus. Antepartum diagnosis is rare. When there is suspicion that a twin pregnancy is not progressing properly, the diagnosis can be made by serial ultrasonic examinations that show evidence of fetal death.

The presence of the papyraceus has little effect on the mother or the viable baby. In rare instances the dead fetus may obstruct labor. At times the undiagnosed papyraceus is retained in utero, and this may lead to post partum hemorrhage or infection.

BIBLIOGRAPHY

Allen MS, Turner UG: Twin birth—identical or fraternal twins? Obstet Gynecol 37:358, 1971

Babson SG, Phillips DS: Growth and development of twins dissimilar in size at birth. New Engl J Med 289:937, 1973

Compton HL: Conjoined twins. Obstet Gynecol 37:27, 1971

Daw, E: Triplet pregnancy. Br J Obstet Gynaecol 85:505, 1978

Farooqui MO, Grossman JH, Shannon RA: A review of twin pregnancy and perinatal mortality. Obstet Gynecol Surv 28:144, 1973

Fox RL, Nathanson HG, Tejani N: Interlocking twins. Obstet Gynecol 46:53, 1975

Jeffrey RL, Bowes WA, Delaney JJ: Role of bed rest in twin gestation. Obstet Gynecol 43:822, 1974

Khunda S: Locked twins. Obstet Gynecol 39:453, 1972

Kohl SG, Casey G: Twin gestation. Mt Sinai J Med 42:523, 1975

Livinat EJ, Burd L, Cadkin A, et al: Fetus papyraceus in twin pregnancy. Obstet Gynecol 51:415, 1978

Nissen ED: Collision, impaction, compaction, and interlocking. Obstet Gynecol 11:514, 1958

Quigley JK: Monoamniotic twin pregnancy. Am J Obstet Gynecol 29:354, 1935

Vaughn TC, Powell LC: The obstetrical management of conjoined twins. Obstet Gynecol 53:67S, 1979

24.

Obstetric Forceps

The obstetric forceps, invented by Peter Chamberlen at the beginning of the 17th century, is an instrument designed for extraction of the fetal head. While many varieties of forceps have been described, the basic design and purpose remain unchanged.

PARTS OF THE FORCEPS

1. There are handles by which to grip the forceps.
2. The lock holds the forceps together. It is so constructed that the right one fits on over the left. For this reason, unless the particular situation necessitates doing otherwise, the left blade should be applied first. The main types of lock are:
   a. The English lock (e.g., Simpson forceps) has a shoulder and flange in each shank which fit into each other (Fig. 1A). Articulation is fixed at a given point.
   b. The French lock (e.g., Tarnier and De Wees) has a pinion and screw (Fig. 1B). The left shank bears a pivot fitting into a notch on the right shank. After articulation the pivot is tightened by screwing it home.
   c. The sliding lock (e.g., Kjelland) is built into the left blade only (Fig. 1C). The right blade fits into the lock, but articulation is not fixed. This type of lock is useful when application is not perfect, as when the head is asynclitic.
3. The shank connects the handle and the blade. A short-shanked instrument is satisfactory when the fetal head is low in the pelvis. When the head has not reached the perineum a longer shank is needed.
4. The blades, which enclose the head, may be solid or fenestrated. They are designed to grasp the head firmly but without excessive compression. The solid blades may cause less trauma, but the fenestrated blades are lighter, grip the fetal head better, and are less likely to slip. The edges are smooth to reduce damage to the soft tissues.

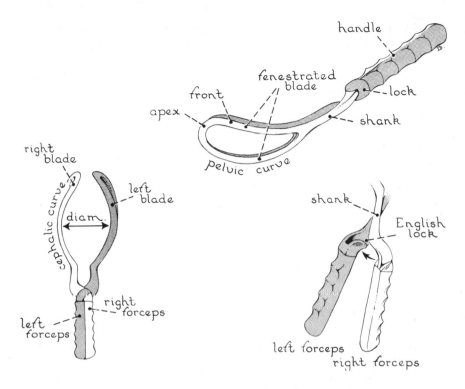

A. Simpson forceps showing the various parts.

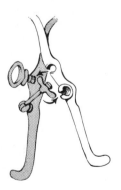

B. French lock.

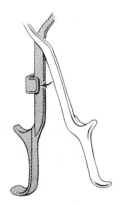

C. Sliding lock.

FIG. 1. Obstetric forceps.

5. Forceps are right or left depending on the side of the maternal pelvis to which they are applied. Since most forceps cross at the lock, the handle of the right forceps is held in the operator's right hand and fits the right side of the pelvis. The left blade fits the left side of the maternal pelvis, and its handle is held in the left hand of the operator.
6. The front of the forceps is the concave side.
7. The apex is the tips of the blades.
8. The diameter is the widest distance between the blades. It measures about 7.5 cm.
9. The forceps have two curves:
   a. The cephalic curve fits the shape of the baby's head and reduces the danger of compression.
   b. The pelvic curve follows the direction of the birth canal. It makes application and extraction easier, and decreases damage to the maternal tissues.

TYPES OF FORCEPS

There are many general-duty forceps and several with specialized functions (Figs. 2 and 3). We believe that the new obstetrician should learn to use one instrument well, so that he becomes thoroughly at home with it. Once he has achieved this experience he must try other instruments, so that he has several familiar types at his command.

1. SIMPSON FORCEPS This is the common parent forceps. It has a cephalic and a pelvic curve. The shank is straight. The lock is of the English variety. This is a good general-duty forceps and is used widely and successfully for all obstetric forceps operations.
2. DELEE FORCEPS This is the Simpson forceps with a few minor modifications. The shank is a little longer to keep the handle away from the anus. The handle is changed to secure lightness, a better grip, and ease of cleaning.
3. TUCKER-MCLANE FORCEPS The blades are solid.
4. KJELLAND FORCEPS The pelvic curve is almost nonexistent, making the instrument ideal for rotating the fetal head. Rotation can be accomplished simply by twisting the closed handles instead of sweeping them through a wide arc, as is necessary when using forceps with a deep pelvic curve. The sliding lock makes the locking of the blades easier. Delivery can be accomplished with the same instrument; no reapplication is needed.
5. BARTON FORCEPS The construction is such that an exact cephalic application can be made without disturbing the relation-

ship of the head to the pelvis. The blades are joined to the shank at an angle of 135°. The posterior blade is attached to the shank in a fixed manner. The anterior blade is hinged at its junction to the shank, allowing movement through 45°. This feature, plus the sliding lock, allows the blades to be locked even when there is marked asynclitism. This is a good forceps for rotation of a head in transverse arrest.

6. PIPER FORCEPS The blade of this forceps is similar to that of the Simpson forceps. The shank has been lengthened and curved downward so that the handles are lower than the blades. Thus the forceps has a double pelvic curve, which facilitates application to the aftercoming head in breech presentations.

7. DEWEES FORCEPS The blades are standard. The handles are modified so that an axis-traction bar can be attached.

8. AXIS-TRACTION FORCEPS These are forceps specially designed so that a traction apparatus can be attached either to the blades at the bases of the fenestra (Tarnier and Milne-Murray) or to the handles (DeWees). The traction bar is attached to the forceps by a series of joints, which has the effect of a universal joint. The forceps are applied to the head in the usual way, and the traction apparatus is attached. The baby's head is then extracted by pulling only on the traction bar. The advantages of this technic are:

a. The line of traction is in the axis of the birth canal.

b. The universal joint permits the blades to rotate with the head and thus to follow the natural rotation of the head as it accommodates itself to the maternal pelvis in its descent.

c. Axis traction was of value in difficult high and midforceps deliveries. Since in modern obstetrics we try to eliminate these traumatic operations, axis traction is needed rarely today.

OBSTETRIC FORCEPS

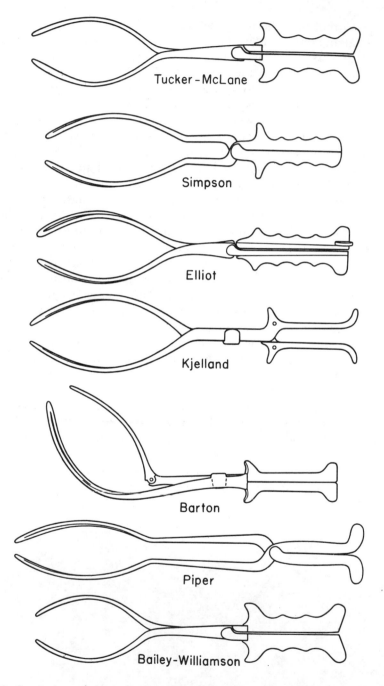

FIG. 2. Front view of some commonly used forceps. (From Douglas and Stromme. *Operative Obstetrics*, 2nd ed, 1965. Courtesy of Appleton-Century-Crofts.)

TYPES OF FORCEPS

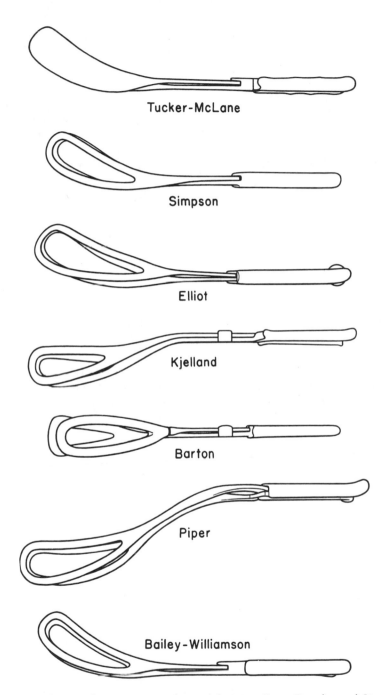

Tucker-McLane

Simpson

Elliot

Kjelland

Barton

Piper

Bailey-Williamson

FIG. 3. Lateral view of some commonly used forceps. (From Douglas and Stromme. *Operative Obstetrics,* 2nd ed, 1965. Courtesy of Appleton-Century-Crofts.)

APPLICATION OF FORCEPS

Cephalic Application

A cephalic application is made to fit the baby's head (Fig. 4A). An ideal cephalic application in occipitoanterior positions is biparietal, along the occipitomental diameter, with the fenestra including the parietal bosses and the tips lying over the cheeks. The concave edges should point to the denominator and the convex edges toward the face.

With this application, pressure on the head causes the least damage. If the forceps are applied so that one blade lies over the face and the other over the occiput, a relatively small degree of compression may cause tentorial tears and intracranial hemorrhage.

Pelvic Application

A pelvic application is made to fit the maternal pelvis (Fig. 4B), regardless of how the forceps grip the fetal head. The best pelvic application is achieved when:

1. The left blade is next to the left side of the pelvis.
2. The right blade is on the right side of the pelvis.
3. The concave margin is near the symphysis pubis.
4. The convex margin is in the hollow of the sacrum.
5. The diameter of the forceps is in the transverse diameter of the pelvis.

Perfect Application

A perfect application (Fig. 4C) is achieved when both the cephalic and pelvic requirements have been fulfilled. When the occiput has rotated under the symphysis pubis and the sagittal suture is in the anteroposterior diameter, an ideal application is possible.

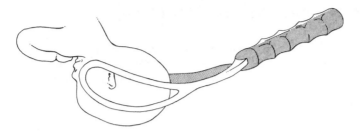

A. Cephalic application.

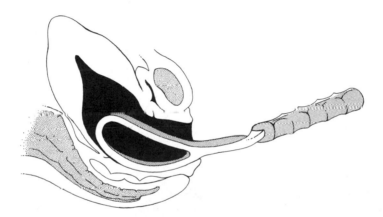

B. Pelvic application.

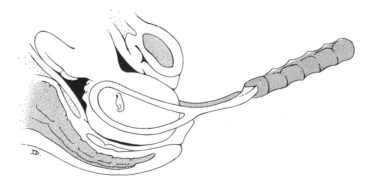

C. Perfect application.

FIG. 4. Application of forceps.

FUNCTIONS OF OBSTETRIC FORCEPS

Of the six original uses of forceps—traction, rotation, compression, dilation, leverage, irritation—only traction and rotation are acceptable today. Compression of the head may be an unavoidable accompaniment but is never a function of forceps.

Traction

In other than expert hands the use of forceps should be restricted to that of traction (Fig. 5A). The direction of traction must be along the pelvic curvature, and as the station changes during descent so does the line of traction. The direction of pull should be perpendicular to the plane of the level at which it is being applied. The higher the level, the more posterior the line of traction.

Rotation of Head from Posterior or Transverse Positions

An important principle must be remembered when using the forceps for rotation. The handles should be swung through a wide arc in order to reduce the arc of the blades (Figs. 5B and C). This lowers the incidence and extent of vaginal lacerations and at the same time makes the operation easier. Rotation is carried out best in the midpelvis.

FUNCTIONS OF OBSTETRIC FORCEPS

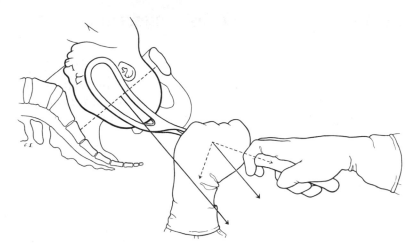

A. Traction with forceps.

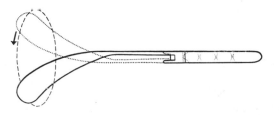

B. Rotation with forceps, incorrect technique.

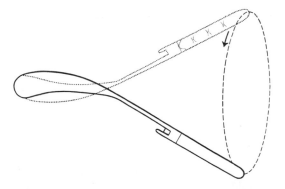

C. Rotation with forceps, correct technique.

FIG. 5. Traction and rotation with forceps. (From Douglas and Stromme. *Operative Obstetrics,* 2nd ed, 1965. Courtesy of Appleton-Century-Crofts.)

CLASSIFICATION OF FORCEPS OPERATIONS

Low Forceps

Low forceps is the application of forceps after the head has become visible, the skull (not the caput) has reached the perineal floor, and the sagittal suture is in or near the anteroposterior diameter of the pelvis. The station is +3.

Midforceps

Midforceps is the application of forceps before the criteria of low forceps have been met but after engagement has taken place. The biparietal diameter has passed through the inlet and the lowest part of the skull has reached the level of the ischial spines. The station is 0 to +2. Frequently rotation is not complete. This can be a difficult operation, even for the experienced obstetrician.

High Forceps

The head has entered the pelvis but is not engaged. The widest diameter has not passed through the inlet, and the bony presenting part has not reached the level of the ischial spines. The danger of damage to both baby and mother is great, and this operation is rarely carried out.

Floating Forceps

The whole fetal head is above the pelvic brim. This procedure is not performed today, having been superseded by cesarean section.

Summary

The average case fits nicely into these categories. However, when there is extreme molding, marked asynclitism, large caput succedaneum, attitude of extension, or abnormal pelvis, errors are often made in thinking that the station is lower than it really is. The operator believes he is about the perform a midforceps operation and finds himself doing a high forceps.

ACOG Classification

In 1964 the Executive Board of the American College of Obstetricians and Gynecologists adopted the following classification of forceps deliveries.

OUTLET FORCEPS The application of forceps when the scalp is or has been visible at the introitus without separating the labia, the skull has reached the pelvic floor, and the sagittal suture is in the anteroposterior diameter of the pelvis.

MIDFORCEPS The application of forceps when the head is engaged but the conditions for outlet forceps have not been met. In the context of this term, any forceps delivery requiring artificial rotation, regardless of the station from which extraction is begun, shall be designated a midforceps delivery. The term low midforceps is disapproved. A record shall be made of the position and station of the head when the delivery is begun. In addition, a description of the various maneuvers and of any difficulties encountered in the application of the forceps and in the extraction of the infant shall be recorded.

HIGH FORCEPS The application of forceps at any time prior to full engagement of the head. High forceps delivery is almost never justified.

CONDITIONS AND PREREQUISITES

Before obstetric forceps may be used safely certain conditions, requirements, or prerequisites must be present.

1. An adequate pelvis with no disproportion is an absolute condition. Failure to observe this rule may lead to disaster for fetus and mother.
2. There must be no serious bony or soft tissue obstruction, such as presenting ovarian cysts or uterine fibromyomas.
3. The fetal head must be engaged so that the bony skull (not the caput succedaneum) is at least at the level of the ischial spines. In modern times forceps are not employed unless the station is +1, +2, or lower.
4. The cervix must be completely dilated and retracted. Disregard for this rule leads to tears of the cervix, hemorrhage, and possible "failed forceps."
5. Accurate diagnosis of position and station (Fig. 6) is essential.
6. The membranes should be ruptured. If they are not there is increased chance of the blades slipping, and there is danger of pulling the placenta away from the uterine wall. If the bag of waters is intact is should be broken. Frequently this results in better labor and progress, so that the need for forceps is obviated.
7. The patient is placed on a good delivery table, with her legs in

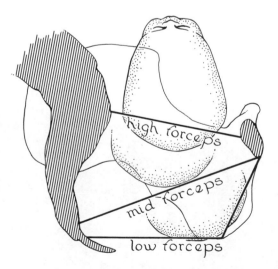

FIG. 6. Classification of forceps operations according to station.

stirrups and her buttocks well down and a little past the end of the table.

8. Some form of anesthesia—general, conduction, or local—should be used. This achieves both relaxation and relief of pain.
9. The bladder must be emptied by using a rubber catheter before the forceps are applied. An empty bladder occupies less space than a full one and is less liable to injury.
10. The rectum should be empty. This is usually already accomplished by an enema earlier in labor.
11. The operation is performed under strictly aseptic conditions.

INDICATIONS FOR USE OF FORCEPS

Fetal Distress

Signs that suggest the baby is suffering from lack of oxygen include:

1. Irregular fetal heart beat
2. Bradycardia, under 100 beats per minute, between uterine contractions
3. Late decelerations of the fetal heart rate
4. Rapid fetal heart—more than 160 beats per minute
5. Passage of meconium in cephalic presentations

Once fetal distress has developed the baby must be delivered immediately, providing the prerequisites have been met.

The more serious signs are irregularity and slowness of the fetal heart. Prolapse of the umbilical cord may be in the background. Occasionally a loop of cord around the baby's neck tightens as the fetus descends; the flow of blood through the cord is reduced, and hypoxia or anoxia results, with bradycardia as a clinical sign. Often babies who demonstrate intrauterine bradycardia or pass meconium are born in good condition and remain so. Thus when signs of distress are present and delivery can be expedited by an easy low forceps delivery, this should be done immediately. On the other hand, in the panicky attempt to save a baby with possible anoxia one should beware of damaging it or even killing it by a difficult, traumatic, and sometimes needless forceps extraction.

Maternal Conditions

An extraction of the baby for maternal reasons is justified if the risk to mother and child is less than that of waiting for spontaneous delivery.

Maternal distress or exhaustion is shown by dehydration, concentrated urine, and pulse and temperature above 100. These patients are not in shock, they are simply becoming exhausted.

When there is maternal disease—cardiac disease, tuberculosis, toxemia, or any debilitating condition—forceps can be used to shorten the second stage and obviate the need for prolonged bearing-down efforts by the patient.

It is essential in these situations that the forceps delivery be easy. The patient is not helped by a difficult forceps extraction with attendant lacerations and hemorrhage.

Failure of Progress in the Second Stage

1. Failure of descent
2. Failure of internal rotation

Providing the conditions for the use of forceps have been met, lack of advancement in the presence of good uterine contractions for 1 hour in a multipara or 2 hours in a primigravida is an indication for assessment of the situation and probable delivery of the baby by forceps. A delay of only 2 hours in the second stage is permitted, because experience has shown that the incidence of fetal and maternal damage definitely rises after this period.

Situations that predispose to arrest of progress include: *2nd stage*

1. Poor uterine contractions
2. Minor degrees of relative disproportion caused by such conditions as a large baby or prominent ischial spines
3. Abnormal fetal position such as posterior position of the occiput or attitudes of extension.
4. A rigid perineum, which the advancing head cannot thin out
5. Diastasis of the rectus abdominis muscle, which reduces the efficiency of the bearing-down effects of the patient
6. A lax pelvic floor, which inhibits proper rotation of the head

Elective Outlet Forceps: Prophylactic Forceps

This procedure is prophylactic in that it is designed to prevent fetal asphyxia and death and to reduce injury and needless suffering of the mother. It is done in conjunction with early episiotomy. The reasoning is:

1. It is better to do the episiotomy before the tissues are over-

stretched. This may reduce the incidence of relaxation of the perineum and pelvic floor and of prolapse of the uterus in later life.

2. It saves the mother a period of bearing down and may prevent painful hemorrhoids.
3. The extraction of the baby with outlet forceps is less damaging than prolonged pounding of the head on the perineum.

In a study by the Collaborative Perinatal Project the offspring of 30,000 gravidas, delivered spontaneously or by low forceps, were followed to 4 years of age. The data showed that, when compared with infants born spontaneously, the incidence of neonatal death or subsequent neurologic impairment was no higher in those born by low forceps. These findings suggest that the procedure is safe. Whether the operation is "protective" to the infant is less certain.

Optimum Time to Use Forceps

The indications, conditions, and time limits, as detailed previously, cannot be considered rigid and unchangeable. The attendant must at all times exercise his prerogative to modify the indications to suit the situation at hand. Sometimes interference is carried out sooner than usual, while in other instances more time is allowed before operative measures are instituted.

Once fetal distress is present, interference is mandatory. However, rather than waiting for marked bradycardia with subsequent desperate activity by the obstetrician, it is better to extract the infant while it is still in good condition and better able to stand the trauma of the operation and anesthesia. In cases of prolonged labor with slow advance, for example, the possibility of fetal distress should be anticipated.

Maternal distress is a definite indication for operative delivery. One should not permit the patient to become completely exhausted before offering assistance. Once the second stage has been reached the patient must be observed carefully for signs of fatigue. When they appear, extraction should be carried out without waiting for the usual time limit to expire.

The rule to wait until progress in the second stage has ceased for 1 hour in a multipara and 2 hours in a primipara is not absolute. Often the attendant can decide much sooner whether there is hope for advancement. For instance, when the head is on the perineum there is no justification in running out the clock when an episiotomy or low forceps would be of assistance to the fetus, the mother, and the perineum.

The best time to use forceps is a matter of judgment. One should not resort to operative delivery needlessly or too quickly. On the other hand, one must not wait so long that the life of the baby and the health of the mother are jeopardized.

CONTRAINDICATIONS TO USE OF FORCEPS

1. Absence of a proper indication
2. Incompletely dilated cervix
3. Marked cephalopelvic disproportion
4. Unengaged fetal head
5. Lack of experience on the part of the operator

DANGERS OF FORCEPS

Maternal Dangers

1. Lacerations of vulva, vagina, cervix, and extension of episiotomy
2. Rupture of the uterus
3. Hemorrhage from lacerations and uterine atony
4. Injury to bladder and/or rectum
5. Infection of genital tract
6. Atony of bladder leading to urinary infection
7. Fracture of coccyx

Fetal Dangers

1. Cephalhematoma
2. Brain damage and intracranial hemorrhage
3. General depression and asphyxia
4. Late neurologic sequelae
5. Fracture of skull
6. Facial paralysis
7. Brachial palsy
8. Bruising
9. Cord compression
10. Death

Serious injuries to the fetus delivered by forceps consist mainly of damage to the falx cerebri, the tentorium cerebelli, and the associated venous sinuses and other vessels. Lacerations are caused by excessive force and excessive compression. These injuries are associated mainly with deliveries from the midpelvis or higher. The dangers are especially great when (1) the forceps are applied in other than the biparietal diameter, (2) the fetal head is drawn through the least favorable diameters of the pelvis, (3) forceful rotation is made at the wrong level of the pelvis, (4) excessive force is used in other than the correct line of the axis of the pelvis.

MIDPELVIC ARREST: FORCEPS OR CESAREAN SECTION

Midpelvic arrest is one of the chief problems in the labor room. When the fetal head is floating the obvious solution is cesarean section. Once engagement has or appears to have taken place, however, a difficult decision must be made—i.e., whether to allow a further trial of labor, to effect delivery by midforceps, or to perform cesarean section. We resist the urge to do an abdominal operation which may be unnecessary, but at the same time we fear the dangers to mother and child of an ill-advised, difficult, and traumatic vaginal extraction by forceps.

Should midforceps ever be used? Some maintain that the danger of obvious and hidden damage is too great, and that this procedure must be replaced by cesarean section. In opposition to this extreme view is the belief that the easy midforceps is safer and has fewer long-term effects than cesarean section. However, the heavy traction of the past is no longer acceptable, and abdominal delivery is preferable to a difficult vaginal forceps delivery.

Providing there is no cephalopelvic disproportion, midforceps when performed properly by competent hands and on correct indications need not be mutilating to the mother nor impose undue hazard on the fetus. When the head is engaged deeply, with the biparietal diameter at the level of the ischial spines and the station at +2, midforceps is the procedure of choice, especially when uterine inertia or maternal fatigue results in arrest in the second stage. The midforceps operation is an important part of obstetrics.

MIDFORCEPS DELIVERY

Advantages

1. The procedure is safe as long as there is no disproportion.
2. The operation is often surprisingly easy, with excellent results in selected cases.
3. Frequently all that is needed is rotation of the head to a more favorable position.

4. Soft tissue dystocia can be overcome.
5. It is effective in getting the head past a localized area of minor disproportion.
6. It is helpful when the patient can no longer push.
7. Subsequent births are often easy.

Disadvantages

1. There is danger of fetal damage.
2. Maternal lacerations are possible.
3. Fear of another difficult delivery leads to the avoidance of pregnancy.
4. Fear of another pregnancy leads to loss of libido.

CESAREAN SECTION

Advantages

1. The modern operation, especially the low transverse variety, is safe.
2. When done in time, before the baby is injured by prolonged obstructed labor, the fetal results are good.
3. You may be sorry for the cesarean section you failed to do, never for those you did.

Disadvantages

1. It is a major surgical procedure and leads to increased morbidity.
2. Future pregnancies, in most cases, are managed by repeat cesarean section. This limits the size of the family.
3. Cesarean section is not the answer to every obstetric problem.

FAILED FORCEPS OR CATASTROPHIC SUCCESS

An attempt to deliver the child by forceps may fail completely; or it may produce a damaged or dead baby and leave the mother with a lacerated pelvis. Pitfalls that contribute to making a wrong decision include the following:

1. Misunderstanding the significance and the relationship of station and the level of the biparietal diameter. Station zero means that the presenting part has reached the level of the ischial spines. In most women when the station is zero the biparietal diameter is at or just through the pelvic inlet. Thus when forceps are applied at station zero, the essence of the procedure lies, not in extracting the presenting part from the midpelvis, but in dragging the biparietal diameter all the way from the inlet, through the midpelvis and the outlet. This is a difficult and potentially dangerous procedure. On the other hand, when the station is +2 and the biparietal diameter is at or below the spines, a midforceps operation is often easy and safe. Hence we must always consider both the station of the presenting part and the level of the biparietal diameter.

2. Unrecognized disproportion, caused by:
   a. Small or abnormal pelvis.
   b. Large baby. This is the most treacherous of all situations, especially in a multipara who had a normal delivery previously. An anticipated easy birth turns into the nightmare of a difficult forceps extraction, vaginal and cervical lacerations, postpartum hemorrhage, and too often a damaged or dead infant. Whenever progress has ceased, the size of the baby must be reassessed before any action is taken.

3. Misdiagnosis of station.
   a. Rectal examination may be adequate for the management of normal labor, but it is inaccurate and unreliable and leads to serious errors when a problem exists. In such cases careful, sterile vaginal examination on a table is mandatory before a decision is made.
   b. Caput succedaneum (edema of the scalp). In prolonged labor the caput may be 1 to 2 cm thick, and hence the bony skull is at a correspondingly higher level in the pelvis. It is important to ascertain the station of the skull and not the edematous scalp. A large caput indicates strong contractions, great resistance, or both. A small or absent caput suggests that the contractions and/or the resistance of the pelvic tissues are weak.
   c. Molding. Excessive molding makes the head pointed by lengthening its long axis: therefore the biparietal diameter is at a greater distance from the leading part of the skull. In such situations engagement may not have taken place when the station is zero. Not only is the forceps operation difficult, but the pressure of the instrument on a brain already under stress increases the risk of permanent damage. Extreme molding is a sign of trouble.

4. Misdiagnosis of position. In descending order of importance, the steps in the use of forceps are diagnosis of position, application, and traction. It is obvious that if the exact position of the fetal head is not known the forceps cannot be applied correctly. Difficulty in applying forceps demands a complete reevaluation of the situation and not forceful delivery. Whenever labor ceases to advance, the possibility of an abnormal position or a malpresentation (such as brow) must be kept in mind.

5. Incorrect diagnosis of cervical dilatation. Often the patient thought to be ready for delivery is found during the final vaginal examination to have an incompletely dilated cervix. Except in the rarest situation, forceps must not be applied through a cervix that is not open fully. This may be a sign of disproportion, and forceful vaginal delivery leads to catastrophe. If there is no disproportion and the mother and fetus are in good condition, labor should proceed until sufficient advancement has been made. If there is disproportion or fetal and maternal distress, cesarean section is indicated.

6. Misdiagnosis of inefficient uterine action. The erroneous assumption that the lack of progress is the result of poor contractions leads to trouble in two ways: (1) Forceps are applied too soon. (2) An oxytocin infusion may dilate the cervix and jam the fetal head into the pelvis just far enough to encourage the performance of a misguided forceps extraction.

7. A constriction ring is a localized area of myometrial spasm that grips the fetus tightly and prevents descent, either spontaneously or by forceps.

8. Premature interference. This involves the use of forceps either before the patient is ready and the prerequisites are fulfilled, or when there are no valid indications. The factors here are:
   a. An impatient doctor
   b. Pressure from the patient and her family to do something
   c. Anesthesia administered too soon because of (1) error in deciding how far advanced in labor the patient is, (2) fear of precipitate delivery, and (3) a rambunctious patient

9. Indecision and stubbornness.
   a. The doctor does not make up his mind and waits too long; by the time he decides to act, the baby and mother are already in bad shape.
   b. Stubbornness is of two kinds. In the first place is the doctor who simply cannot admit to an error in judgment and proceeds to compound it. In the second situation is the doctor who refuses to obtain consultation.

c. A treacherous problem occurs when small advancement does take place. This encourages the accoucheur to go on when cesarean section would be preferable.

TRIAL FORCEPS AND FAILED FORCEPS

Once a decision has been made to attempt delivery by means of forceps, one of several outcomes is possible.

1. Final vaginal examination reveals an unfavorable situation or the presence of unexpected disproportion, and vaginal delivery is abandoned in favor of cesarean section or a further trial of labor.
2. An easy, atraumatic operation produces a healthy child.
3. An excessively forceful, difficult, and ill-advised procedure is carried out, and a damaged or dead infant is born.
4. Failed forceps fall into two categories.
   a. Failure of application. The forceps cannot be applied properly to the fetal head.
   b. Failure of extraction. The forceps are applied, but despite an all-out effort delivery cannot be accomplished. By the time the attempt is stopped the baby may be injured.
   Causes of failed forceps include: (1) disproportion, (2) malposition, (3) cervix not fully dilated, (4) constriction ring, and (5) premature interference.
5. Trial forceps. The principle of trial forceps postulates that after successful application has been achieved gentle traction is made. Should the head come down easily, the operation is continued and the baby delivered. If, on the other hand, the operator feels that an undue amount of force would be required to extract the head, the forceps are removed and cesarean section is carried out. In order to avoid delay, all preparations for cesarean should be made before the vaginal delivery is attempted. To a degree, every forceps delivery is a trial. Of course if there is obvious disproportion a trial of forceps is contraindicated.

VACUUM EXTRACTOR

In 1964 James Yonge had described the use of a cupping glass on the fetal scalp to assist the delivery of the fetal head. Saemann and Arnott each reported the use of vacuum instruments in 1829. James Y. Simpson demonstrated the use of a vacuum extractor in 1848. The modern apparatus was made by Malmstrom in 1954, and the modified instrument, now in general use, was developed in 1957.

The modern instrument consists of an all metal cup of four sizes— 30, 40, 50, and 60 mm in diameter. The largest diameter is in the interior of the cup. A rubber tube extends from the cup to a pump, which creates the suction. Attached to the cup and inside the tubing is a chain by which traction on the cup is effected. The scalp is drawn into the cup (Fig. 7), and an artificial caput succedaneum is formed. A dusky ring remains after the cup is removed; this is gone by the time the baby leaves the hospital.

Indications

The indications are much the same as those for forceps. The vacuum extractor cannot be used for face presentations, nor on the after-coming head in breeches.

1. Second stage of labor
   a. Maternal exhaustion or disease (e.g., heart)
   b. Fetal distress
   c. Failure of descent or rotation
   d. Elective outlet application
2. First stage of labor

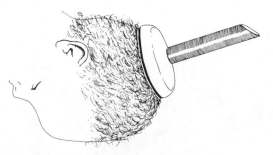

FIG. 7. Vacuum extractor in place.

    a. Inertic labor
    b. Fetal distress

Contraindications

1. Absolute
    a. Cephalopelvic disproportion
    b. Face presentation
    c. Aftercoming head in a breech
2. Relative
    a. Partially dilated cervix. While it is preferable for the cervix to be fully dilated, the vacuum extractor can be used when the cervix is incompletely dilated with little or no injury to fetus or mother. In properly selected cases cesarean section can be avoided.
    b. Unengaged head. Under ideal conditions the extractor should not be used when the head is high. However, in some cases of fetal distress the delivery can be effected more quickly by the vacuum extractor than by cesarean section.
    c. Premature infants can be delivered by the vacuum extractor, but it is safer not to do so.
    d. Congenital anomalies, such as hydrocephalus, make it difficult and traumatic to effect delivery by vacuum extraction.
    e. Dead fetus. Suction and traction are not efficient in this case.

Advantages

1. Some 18 lb of traction can be applied with only 1/20 the rise in intracranial pressure resulting from the use of forceps.
2. The vacuum extractor can be used before complete cervical dilatation.
3. The vacuum extractor does not encroach on the space in the pelvis, reducing the incidence of damage to maternal tissues.
4. The fetal head is not fixed by the application so it can go through the rotations that the configurations of the birth canal require. The fetal head is allowed to find the path of least resistance.
5. While it is safest to use the vacuum extractor when the head is well engaged, it can be applied to the head at a station inaccessible to forceps.

Application

The cervix should be dilated to at least 4 cm. The patient is positioned and prepared just as for a forceps delivery. The largest cup that fits is used. The lubricated cup is placed on the fetal head, over the posterior fontanelle and as close to the occiput as possible. The knob on the cup should point to the posterior fontanelle. Slowly the negative pressure is pumped up until it reaches 0.7 to 0.8 kg/cm^2. This takes 8 to 10 minutes. The apparatus is now ready for traction (Fig. 8).

Delivery

If the uterine contractions are weak, an oxytocin drip can be used. A series of tractions synchronized with the labor pains are applied, the right hand pulling the chain-tube, while the left hand presses the traction cup and the fetal head posteriorly against the sacrum. This produces a force in the direction of the birth canal. The total extraction time takes about 15 minutes, or five to 10 tractions during uterine contractions. If the cervix is not fully dilated it may take longer. The upper time limit is 30 minutes (rarely 45) to prevent damage to the baby. If delivery is not accomplished during this time, the case is considered unsuitable for vaginal delivery and cesarean section is performed. After delivery the vacuum is released and the cup removed. The large artificial caput disappears in about 10 minutes, and by the end of a week only a slight circular area of redness is seen.

Safeguards in the Use of Vacuum Extraction

1. Cephalic presentation, preferably well fixed.
2. No cephalopelvic disproportion.
3. The membranes must be ruptured.
4. Cervical dilatation must be sufficient to admit the cup. The larger cup is safer and more efficient.
5. The cup is placed as near to the occiput as possible.
6. Negative vacuum pressure must not exceed 0.7 to 0.8 kg/cm^2.
7. The cup should not remain on the fetal scalp for longer than 45 minutes. The shorter the time, the less the danger of damage to the fetal scalp.
8. Traction should be maintained at right angles to the application of the cup. The possibility of damage to the scalp is increased by diagonal or shearing forces and rocking motions.
9. Traction is exerted concomitantly with the uterine contractions and the maternal expulsive efforts.

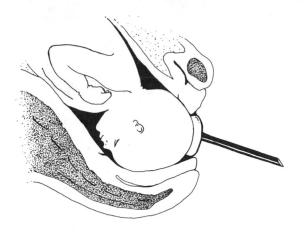

A. Traction outward and posteriorly.

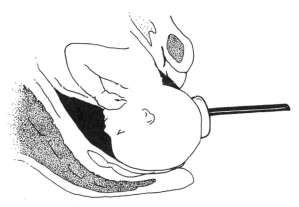

B. Traction outward and horizontally.

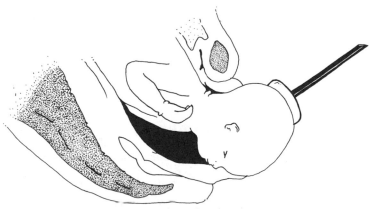

C. Traction outward and anteriorly.

FIG. 8. Vacuum extractor.

10. When insufficient time is allowed for the development of the caput within the cup there is the risk of the cup's "popping off." This accident causes tearing of the fetal scalp and should be avoided.
11. Rotation of malpositions of the head should be allowed to take place spontaneously as traction is applied. Attempts to rotate the head by turning the cup leads to avulsion injuries.
12. If advancement is not evident after three to four pulls, the procedure should be discontinued, the situation reevaluated, and a different method of delivery considered.

Complications

Maternal The incidence is low. Small lacerations of the vagina and cervix are a little more common than with spontaneous birth.

Fetal These are similar to those that occur with forceps and include:

1. A large caput, which disappears by the fourth day.
2. Abrasions, necrosis, and ulceration of the scalp at the site of application of the cup, probably as a result of the instrument's being left on too long or of improper traction. These are treated by gentle cleansing and antibiotic ointments. The skin at the site of the suction must be handled carefully to avoid rubbing off of the friable superficial layer. These areas heal without residual effects.
3. Cephalhematomas.
4. Occasional bleeding from the sagittal sinus into the subgaleal space.
5. Postnatal asphyxia.
6. Cerebral irritation related to the number of pulls, which seems to increase after five or six tractions.
7. Occasional intracranial hemorrhage.

BIBLIOGRAPHY

Dudley AG, Markham SM, McNie TM, et al: Elective versus indicated midforceps delivery. Obstet Gynecol 37:19, 1971
Niswander KR, Gordon M: Safety of the low forceps operation. Am J Obstet Gynecol 117:619, 1973
Ott WJ: Vacuum extraction. Obstet Gynecol Surv 30:643, 1975
Plauché WC: Vacuum extraction. Obstet Gynecol 52:289, 1978

25.

Anterior Positions of the Occiput: Delivery by Forceps

LOW FORCEPS DELIVERY: OCCIPUT ANTERIOR

In order to prevent the omission of essential steps, the obstetrician should train himself to perform forceps operations with a definite routine in mind. After a time these procedures become automatic. The exact details of application are described here and are not repeated in succeeding sections.

Preparations

1. The conditions and indications are rechecked to be certain that the correct procedure is being carried out.
2. The patient is placed on the delivery table with the legs in stirrups and the buttocks a little past the lower end of the table (Chap. 11, Fig. 3C).
3. Vulvar preparation is performed with green soap and water. This wash includes the upper thighs and lower abdomen.
4. If spinal or epidural anesthesia is to be used, it should have been administered by this time. If local anesthesia has been chosen, the injection is made. If general anesthesia is employed, it is administered at this point.

ANTERIOR POSITIONS OF THE OCCIPUT: DELIVERY BY FORCEPS

Orientation

VAGINAL EXAMINATION

Vaginal examination (Fig. 1A) is made to diagnose accurately the position and station of the head, whether there is flexion or extension, and the presence of synclitism or asynclitism. Since this is a low forceps procedure for occipitoanterior position, the following conditions are present:

1. The presentation is cephalic.
2. The sagittal suture is in the anteroposterior diameter of the pelvis.
3. The occiput and posterior fontanelle are next to the pubis.
4. The face and bregma are in the hollow of the sacrum.
5. The station is at least +3.

ORIENTATION AND DESIRED APPLICATION

The locked forceps are positioned outside the vagina in front of the perineum in the way there are to be when applied to the fetal head in the pelvis (Fig. 1B and C). By this simple procedure the operator fixes in his mind exactly how and where each blade should fit. In the occipitoanterior position both a perfect cephalic and an ideal pelvic application are possible (Fig. 1).

With the cephalic application:

1. The blades are over the parietal bones in an occipitomental application.
2. The front of the forceps (concave edges) point to the denominator (occiput).
3. The convex edges point to the face.

With the pelvic application:

1. The left blade is next to the left sidewall of the pelvis and the right blade near the right sidewall.
2. The concave edges point to the pubis.
3. The convex edges point to the sacrum.
4. The diameter of the forceps is in the transverse diameter of the pelvis.

LOW FORCEPS DELIVERY: OCCIPUT ANTERIOR

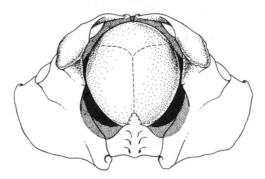

FIG. 1A. Occiput anterior (OA).

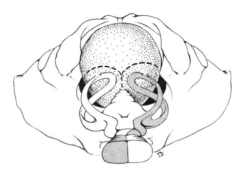

FIG. 1B and C. Low forceps, Simpson. Orientation.

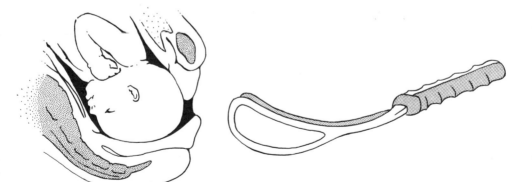

Application of Left Forceps

1. The left blade is inserted first. The handle is held by the thumb and the first two fingers of the left hand. At first the forceps is in an almost vertical position, with the handle near the mother's right groin (Fig. 2A).
2. The fingers of the right hand are placed in the vagina between the fetal head and the left vaginal wall.
3. The left blade is inserted gently into the vagina at about 5 o'clock, between the fingers and the fetal head.
4. The handle is lowered slowly to the horizontal and toward the midline; at the same time the blade is moved up by the vaginal fingers over the left side of the head, giving an occipitomental application. The blade lies between the left parietal bone and the left pelvic wall (Fig. 2B).
5. The fingers are removed and the handle is supported by an assistant, if one is available.

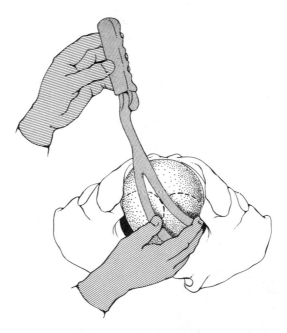

FIG. 2A. Insertion of left blade between fetal head and left side of pelvis.

Application of Right Forceps

1. The right forceps is grasped in the right hand and is held in an almost vertical position, with the handle near the mother's left groin.
2. The fingers of the left hand are inserted in the right side of the vagina between the fetal head and the vaginal wall.
3. The right blade is inserted over the left forceps between the fingers and the fetal head, at about 7 o'clock (Fig. 2C).

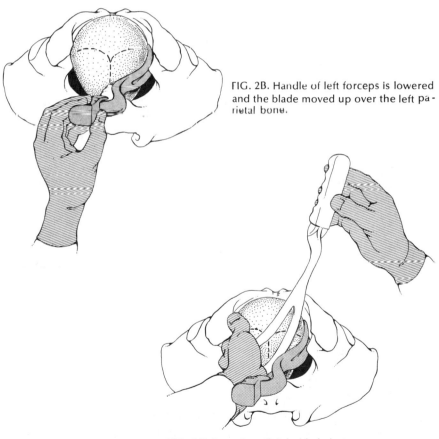

FIG. 2B. Handle of left forceps is lowered and the blade moved up over the left parietal bone.

FIG. 2C. Insertion of right blade between fetal head and right side of pelvis.

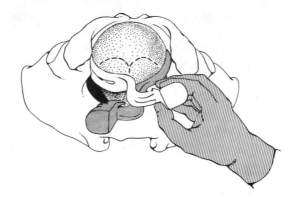

FIG. 2D. Handle of right forceps is lowered, and the blade moved up over the right parietal bone.

4. The handle is lowered to the horizontal and toward the midline. At the same time the blade is moved by the vaginal fingers up over the right side of the head to the occipitomental position. The blade fits between the right parietal bone and the right pelvic wall (Fig. 2D).
5. The fingers on the left hand are removed from the vagina, and the forceps are ready for locking.

Locking

When both blades have been applied correctly locking is easy. There should be no difficulty, and the handles must never be forced together (Fig. 3).

Extraction of the Head

PREEXTRACTION REEXAMINATION

1. Auscultation of the fetal heart is performed.
2. Vaginal examination is made to be sure that there is nothing between the forceps and the fetal head. This includes umbilical cord, cervix, and membranes.
3. Vaginal examination is performed to check the application. The blades of the forceps must be over the sides of the fetal head in a

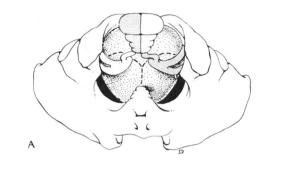

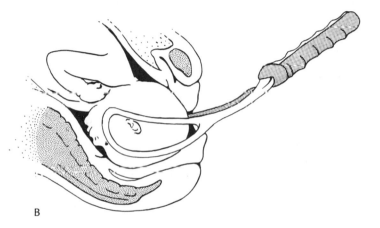

FIG. 3. OA: Locking. A and B. Forceps locked in cephalic and pelvic application.

biparietal application. The left blade should be next to the left side of the pelvis and the right blade on the right side. The concave edges of the forceps should be under the pubis and the convex edges near the sacrum. The diameter of the blades should be in the transverse diameter of the pelvis. Sometimes the blades may be a little off center, with one blade nearer the occiput and the other closer to the face. In such cases the forceps must be unlocked and the blades moved so that the application becomes symmetrical.

TRIAL TRACTION

A gentle pull on the forceps ought to bring about a small advancement of the head.

INDICATIONS FOR COMPLETE REASSESSMENT

1. When locking is difficult or impossible.
2. When trial traction fails to advance the head.
3. When vaginal examination reveals an incorrect application. The forceps should be removed and the whole situation reassessed. Reasons for the failure include:

   a. Wrong diagnosis of position
   b. Incorrect application of forceps
   c. Cephalopelvic disproportion
   d. Cervix between the blades and the head
   e. Uterine constriction ring

EXTRACTION OF THE HEAD

1. The operator sits on a stool and grasps the forceps with both hands, one hand on the handles and the other on the shanks (Chap. 24, Fig. 5A).
2. The traction must be intermittent, every 1 to 2 minutes and lasting 30 to 40 seconds.
3. Between periods of traction the forceps should be unlocked to relieve the compression of the baby's head. The fetal heart must be checked often.
4. If the patient is under general or spinal anesthesia the uterine contractions are of little help, and since the patient cannot bear down the baby is delivered by traction alone or by the assistant exerting pressure on the uterus. On the other hand, if the patient has been given a local or epidural anesthetic, traction should be made during the uterine contractions and with the patient bearing down. The combined effort makes the delivery much easier.
5. The direction of traction must follow the birth canal. First the pull should be outward and posteriorly until the occiput comes under the symphysis of the pubis and the nape of the neck pivots in the subpubic angle (Fig. 4A). In performing Pajot's maneuver, the hand on the handles makes traction in an outward direction while the hand on the shanks pulls the head posteriorly.
6. Then the direction is changed to outward and anterior to promote extension of the head. This mimics the course of events in spontaneous birth (Fig. 4B).
7. In all primigravidas and in most multiparas an episiotomy should be made before the baby is extracted and the perineum overstretched.

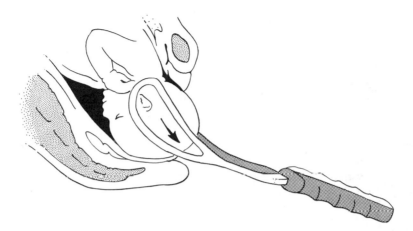

A. Traction is made outward and posteriorly until the nape of the neck is under the pubic symphysis.

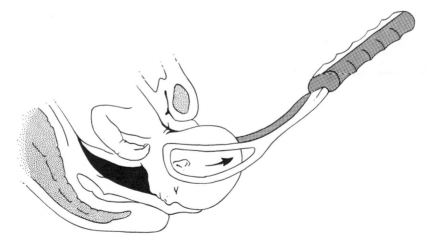

B. The direction of traction is changed to outward and anteriorly to promote extension of the head.

FIG. 4. OA: Traction with forceps.

BIRTH OF THE HEAD AND REMOVAL OF FORCEPS

Birth of the head and removal of the forceps can be accomplished in two ways:

1. Traction with the forceps is continued, and by a process of extension the forehead, face, and chin are born over the perineum. The forceps are now out of the vagina and slip off the head easily.
2. When the head is crowning, the forceps are removed by a process that is the reverse of their application. First the handle of the right blade is raised toward the mother's left groin and the blade slides around the head and out of the pelvis (Fig. 5A). Then the same is done with the left forceps by raising the handle toward the right groin (Fig. 5B). Once this has been accomplished the head is delivered by the modified Ritgen maneuver. Removing the forceps has the advantage of reducing the circumference of the part passing through the introitus by 0.50 to 0.75 cm.

Lacerations of the vagina, cervix, and uterus must be ruled out by careful examination after all forceps deliveries. If tears are found they are repaired.

LOW FORCEPS DELIVERY: OCCIPUT ANTERIOR

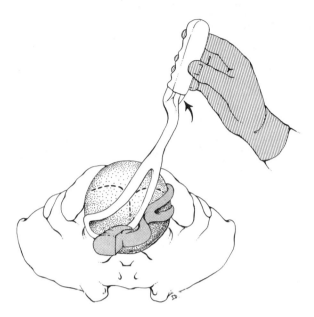

A. Removal of right forceps.

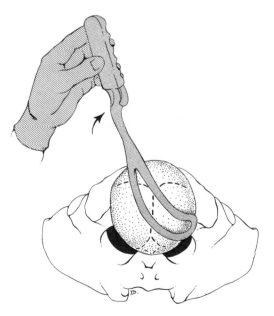

B. Removal of left forceps.

FIG. 5. OA.

FORCEPS DELIVERY: LOA

Orientation

VAGINAL EXAMINATION

1. The presentation is cephalic.
2. The sagittal suture is in the right oblique diameter of the pelvis.
3. The posterior fontanelle is in the left anterior quadrant of the pelvis (Fig. 6A).
4. The bregma is in the right posterior quadrant.
5. The station is 0 to +3 in most cases.

ORIENTATION AND DESIRED APPLICATION
The aim is for a perfect cephalic application.

1. The blades are over the parietal bones in an occipitomental application.
2. The concave edges point to the occiput.
3. The convex edges point to the face.

The pelvic application is not perfect.

1. The diameter of the forceps is in the left oblique diameter of the pelvis.
2. The left blade is in the left posterior quadrant.
3. The right blade is in the right anterior quadrant.
4. The concave edges point anteriorly and to the left.
5. The convex edges point posteriorly and to the right.
6. This can be a low to mid forceps, depending on the exact station of the head.

FORCEPS DELIVERY: LOA

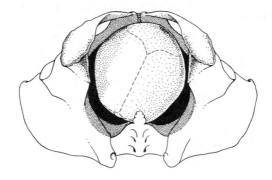

FIG. 6A. Left occiput anterior (LOA).

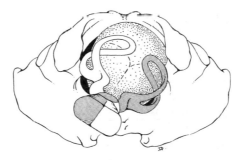

FIG. 6B. Low forceps, Simpson. Orientation.

Application of Forceps

1. The left forceps is inserted into the vagina at 5 o'clock so that it lies over the left parietal bone in an occipitomental application and in the left posterolateral quadrant of the pelvis (Fig. 7A).
2. The right blade is inserted into the vagina at 7 o'clock (Fig. 7B).
3. It is then moved anteriorly around the fetal head so that it lies over the right parietal bone in an occipitomental application, and in the right anterior quadrant of the pelvis.
4. The forceps are now locked, and vaginal examination is made to be sure that the application is correct. If not, the forceps are unlocked and the necessary adjustments made (Fig. 7C).
5. The cephalic application is ideal; the pelvic application is not, for the diameter of the blades is in the oblique diameter of the pelvis.

Rotation and Extraction

1. Traction is made in an outward and posterior direction until the occiput comes under the symphysis and the nape of the neck pivots in the subpubic angle.
2. In many cases as traction is being made the head rotates spontaneously from the LOA to the OA position. If this does not occur the operator must rotate the occiput 45° to the anterior at the same time that he is exerting traction (Fig. 7D).
3. Once the nape of the neck pivots in the subpubic angle, the direction is changed from outward and posterior to outward and anterior so that the head is born over the perineum by extension (Fig. 4B).

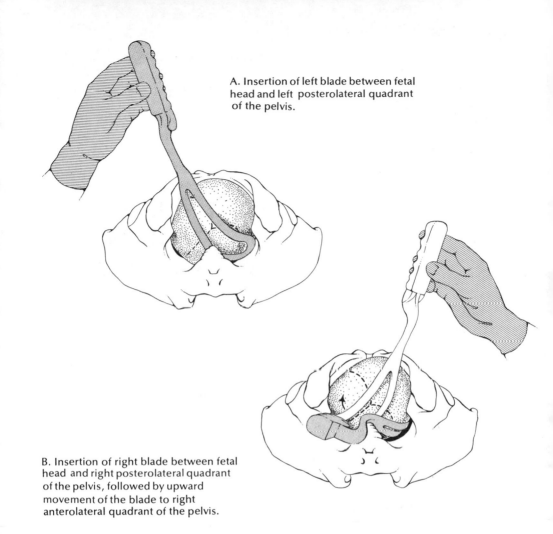

A. Insertion of left blade between fetal head and left posterolateral quadrant of the pelvis.

B. Insertion of right blade between fetal head and right posterolateral quadrant of the pelvis, followed by upward movement of the blade to right anterolateral quadrant of the pelvis.

C. Locking of forceps in cephalic application.

D. Head is rotated from LOA to OA. It is now ready for extraction.

FIG. 7.   LOA: application of forceps.

26.

Arrested Transverse Positions of the Occiput

Transverse arrest high in the pelvis is managed best by cesarean section. However, when the head is low and there is no disproportion, vaginal delivery by forceps is preferable. This can be accomplished in two ways: (1) application of forceps in the LOT position, rotation with forceps to OA, followed by extraction—always a midforceps operation; or (2) manual rotation of the head 90° to the occipitoanterior position, LOT to LOA to OA. The head is then extracted with forceps as an occiput anterior. Sometimes the rotation can be carried out only 45°, LOT to LOA. The forceps are applied to the LOA, and rotation and extraction are completed.

FORCEPS ROTATION AND EXTRACTION: LOT

Orientation

VAGINAL EXAMINATION

1. The presentation is cephalic.
2. The sagittal suture is in the transverse diameter of the pelvis.
3. The posterior fontanelle and occiput are on the left side at 3 o'clock: LOT (Fig. 1A).
4. The bregma and face are on the right side at 9 o'clock.
5. This situation is associated frequently with the military attitude, so the bregma and the posterior fontanelle may be at almost the same level in the pelvis (neither flexion nor extension).
6. The baby's right ear is next to the bladder, and the left one near the rectum.
7. Asynclitism is common, and the sagittal suture may be nearer the

FORCEPS ROTATION AND EXTRACTION: LOT

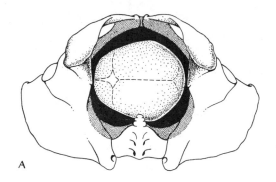

A

FIG. 1A. Left occiput transverse.

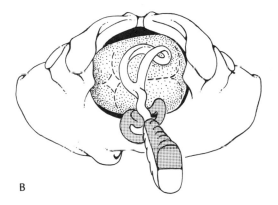

B

FIG. 1B and C. Midforceps, Simpson. Orientation.

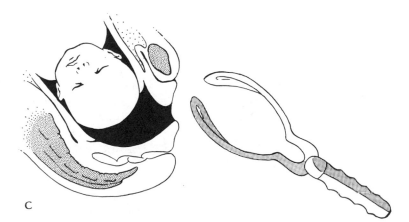

C

pubis (posterior asynclitism) or closer to the sacral promontory (anterior asynclitism).
8. The station in the majority of cases is +1 or +2.
9. Molding and caput succedaneum may obscure the landmarks.

ORIENTATION AND DESIRED APPLICATION
The aim is for an ideal cephalic application (Figs. 1B and C, 2E).

1. The front of the forceps (the concave edges) is pointing toward the denominator (the occiput).
2. The blades are over the parietal bones in an occipitomental application.

The pelvic application is not ideal.

1. The diameter of the blades is in the anteroposterior diameter of the pelvis (instead of the transverse).
2. The anterior (right) blade is between the pubis and the fetal head (instead of being next to the pelvic side wall).
3. The posterior (left) blade is between the sacrum and head.
4. The concave edges of the blades point to the left side of the pelvis.
5. The convex edges point to the right side.

Application of Forceps

We apply the anterior blade first, for two reasons: (1) Any difficulty in application is with the anterior blade. Hence there is no point in placing the posterior blade into the vagina until we are certain that the anterior one can be put in place correctly. (2) The posterior blade occupies space and, if put in first, gets in the way and makes application of the anterior forceps more difficult.

The anterior blade (for LOT it is the right) is inserted into the vagina between the posterior parietal bone (left) and the sacrum (Fig. 2A). The next step is to make the forceps wander around the fetal head into position between the anterior parietal bone (right) and the pubis (Figs. 2B and C). This is accomplished by manipulating the blade with the fingers in the vagina, and the handle with the other hand. There are two ways in which this maneuver can be accomplished:

1. The blade can be moved over the baby's face. With the left hand in the vagina manipulating the blade and the right hand on the handle, the blade is moved over the baby's face into position between the anterior parietal bone and the pubis. The advantage

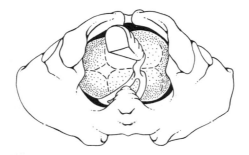

A. Insertion of anterior (right) blade between posterior parietal bone and sacrum.

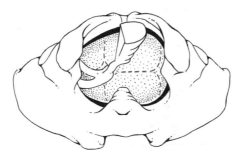

B. The blade is wandered anteriorly so that it lies between the face and the pelvic wall.

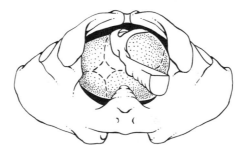

C. The blade is wandered further until it lies between the anterior parietal bone and the pubis.

FIG. 2. Forceps application and rotation: LOT to OA.

of this method is that the smaller face offers less resistance than the bulky occiput and there is less danger of damaging the maternal tissues. The disadvantage is that should the head move with the forceps the occiput rotates posteriorly.

2. The blade can be moved around the occiput. The right hand is placed in the vagina to manipulate the blade, and the left hand is on the handle. The blade is moved gently around the occiput and into position between the anterior parietal bone and the pubis. The advantage of this method is that should the head turn with the forceps, the occiput moves anteriorly, a desirable effect. The drawback is that the bulkiness and hardness of the occiput makes less room for the blade, and there is greater danger of maternal lacerations than when the blade is wandered around the face.

The posterior blade (for LOT it is the left) is inserted into the vagina between the posterior parietal bone (left) and the sacrum (Fig. 2D). The forceps are locked, and the application is checked to be certain that a good biparietal application has been achieved (Fig. 2E).

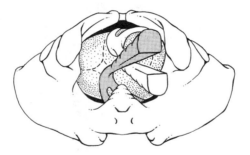

D. The posterior (left) blade is inserted between the posterior parietal bone and the sacrum.

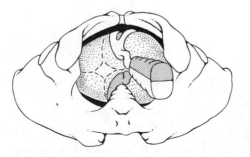

E. LOT: The forceps are locked in a cephalic application.

FIG. 2. (cont.) Forceps application and rotation: LOT to OA.

Rotation and Extraction

With the handles making a wide arc the head is rotated 90° to the anterior, LOT to LOA to OA (Fig. 3). Now the occiput is under the pubis, the face is next to the sacrum, and the sagittal suture is in the anteroposterior diameter of the pelvis. The ideal cephalic application has been maintained. The pelvic application is also good, since the diameter of the forceps is in the transverse diameter of the pelvis, the concave edges point to the pubis, the convex edges lie in the hollow of the sacrum, and the sides of the blades lie next to the side walls of the pelvis.

The head is extracted as an occipitoanterior. Traction is outward and posterior until the occiput comes under the pubis and the nape of the neck pivots in the subpubic angle. The direction is then changed to outward and anterior, so that by extension the forehead, face, and chin are born over the perineum.

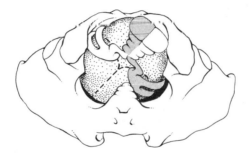

FIG. 3A. Anterior rotation: LOT to LOA (45°).

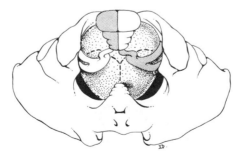

FIG. 3B. Anterior rotation: LOA to OA (45°). The head is ready for extraction.

MANUAL ROTATION AND FORCEPS EXTRACTION: LOT

1. With the patient in the lithotomy position, the operator stands facing the perineum and inserts the right hand into the vagina. The fetal head is grasped with the four fingers over the posterior parietal (left) bone and the thumb over the anterior parietal (right) bone (Fig. 4A).
2. By pronating the arm, the operator turns the fetal head 90° to the anterior, LOT to LOA to OA (Fig. 4B).
3. Forceps are then applied in the OA position, and the head is extracted as an occiput anterior.
4. ROT is managed in the same way, except that the left hand is used and the rotation is ROT to ROA to OA.

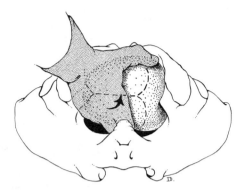

A. Grasping the head with the right hand.

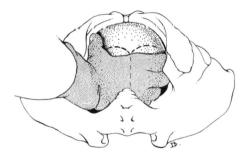

B. LOT to OA (90°).

FIG. 4. Manual rotation: LOT to OA.

27.

Arrested Posterior Positions of the Occiput

Persistent occipitoposterior arrest high in the pelvis is managed best by cesarean section. However, when the head is low and there is no disproportion, vaginal delivery with forceps should be carried out. There are several techniques for accomplishing this safely.

FORCEPS DELIVERY FACE TO PUBIS: OCCIPUT POSTERIOR

Occasionally the head seems to fit the pelvis better with the occiput posterior. This is so, for example, in some anthropoid pelves. When this is the case and especially when the vertex is at or near the perineum, it is wiser to follow nature's lead and deliver the head to pubis.

ORIENTATION

VAGINAL EXAMINATION

1. The presentation is cephalic (Fig. 1A).
2. The sagittal suture is in the anteroposterior diameter of the pelvis.
3. The posterior fontanelle and occiput are in the hollow of the sacrum.
4. The bregma and face are anterior, under the pubis.
5. The station is +1 to +3.

ORIENTATION AND DESIRED APPLICATION
    The cephalic application is not perfect but is satisfactory (Figs. 1B and C).

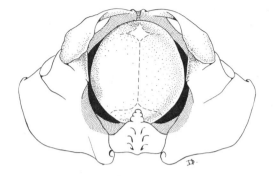

FIG. 1A. Occiput posterior.

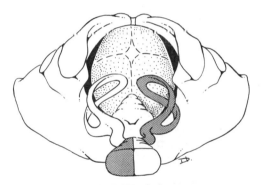

FIG. 1B and C. Simpson forceps. Orientation.

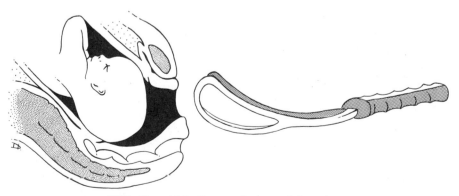

FIGS. 1B and 1C. Simpson forceps. Orientation.

1. The blades are over the parietal bones in an occipitomental application. The left blade is on the right parietal bone, and the right blade is on the left parietal bone.
2. The front of the forceps (concave edges) point to the face. In an ideal cephalic application they point to the occiput.
3. The convex edges point to the occiput. In the ideal application they point to the face.

The pelvic application is perfect.

1. The diameter of the forceps is in the transverse diameter of the pelvis.
2. The sides of the blades are next to the sidewalls of the pelvis, the left blade near the left side and right blade near the right side.
3. The concave edges point to the pubis.
4. The convex edges point to the sacrum.
5. This may be low to midforceps, depending on the exact station of the head.

APPLICATION OF FORCEPS

1. The left blade is inserted gently into the vagina at about 5 o'clock (Fig. 2A).
2. It is then moved anteriorly so that it lies between the right parietal bone and the left side of the pelvis (Fig. 2B).
3. The right blade is inserted (over the left) into the vagina at about 7 o'clock (Fig. 2B).
4. It is then moved anteriorly so that it fits between the left parietal bone of the fetal head and the right side of the pelvis.

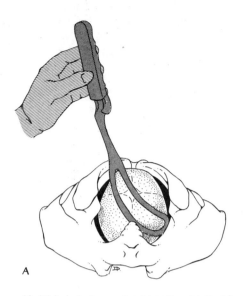

A. Insertion of left blade between fetal head and left side of pelvis.

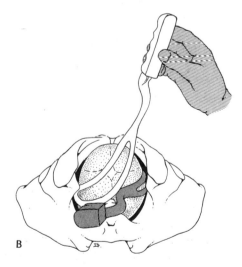

B. Handle of left blade is lowered and the blade moved up over the right parietal bone. Insertion of right blade between fetal head and right side of pelvis.

FIG. 2. OP: application of forceps.

5. The forceps are locked, and vaginal examination is made to be certain that the application is correct and that there are no obstacles to extraction. The application is biparietal. The concave edges of the blades point to the pubis and the fetal face, while the convex edges point to the sacrum and the occiput (Figs. 2C and D).

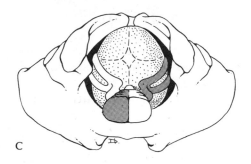

C and D. Forceps locked in biparietal application.

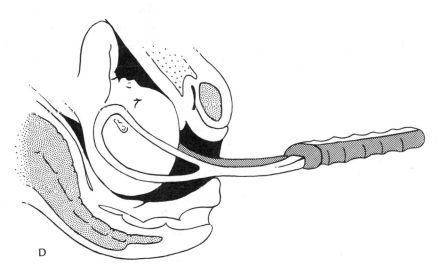

FIG. 2. (cont.) OP: application of forceps.

EXTRACTION OF THE HEAD

1. Traction is made outward and posteriorly until the area between the bregma and the nasion lies under the pubic arch (Fig. 3A).
2. Delivery is by one of two methods:
    a. The direction is changed to outward and anterior (Fig. 3B); as the handles of the forceps are raised, the occiput is born over the perineum by flexion. The forceps then slips off the head.
    b. The direction is changed to outward and anterior until the occiput is on the perineum. The forceps are removed by raising first the right handle toward the left groin so that the blade slips around the head and out of the vagina. Then the left handle is raised toward the right groin so that the left blade slides out. By a modified Ritgen maneuver flexion is increased until the occiput has cleared the perineum completely.
3. The head then falls back in extension; and the nose, face, and chin are delivered under the pubis.
4. If the head cannot be delivered as a posterior presentation without using an excessive amount of force, this method of delivery should be abandoned and an anterior rotation of the occiput carried out.
5. Since the diameter distending the perineum (biparietal, 9.5 cm) is larger than in anterior positions (bitemporal, 8.0 cm), lacerations are more extensive and an adequate episiotomy should be made.

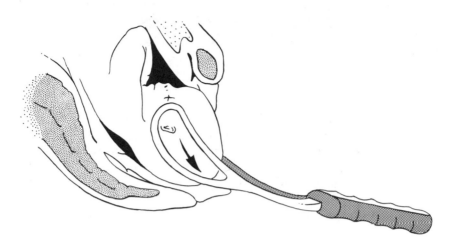

A. Traction is made outward and posteriorly until the area between the bregma and nasion lies under the pubic arch.

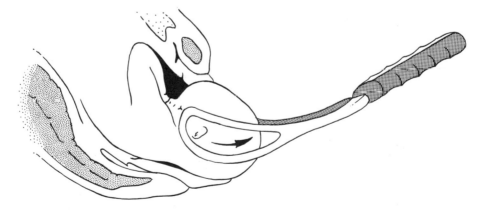

B. Traction is made outward and anteriorly to promote flexion.

FIG. 3. Extraction face to pubis, OP.

FORCEPS ROTATION: ROP TO OP AND EXTRACTION FACE TO PUBIS

Orientation

VAGINAL EXAMINATION

1. The presentation is cephalic.
2. The sagittal suture is in the right oblique diameter of the pelvis.
3. The posterior fontanelle is in the right posterior quadrant of the pelvis (Fig. 4A and 5C).
4. The bregma is in the left anterior quadrant.
5. The station is usually 0 to +2.

ORIENTATION AND DESIRED APPLICATION

The cephalic application is not perfect but is satisfactory (Fig. 4B).

1. The blades are over the parietal bones in an occipitomental application. The left blade is on the right parietal bone, and the right blade is on the left parietal bone.
2. The front of the forceps (concave edges) point to the face. In an ideal cephalic application they point to the occiput.
3. The convex edges point to the occiput. In the ideal application they point to the face.

The pelvic application is oblique.

1. The diameter of the blades is in the left oblique diameter of the pelvis.
2. The left blade is in the left posterior quadrant of the pelvis.
3. The right blade is in the right anterior quadrant.
4. The concave edges point anteriorly and to the left.
5. The convex edges are posterior and to the right.

FORCEPS ROTATION: ROP TO OP AND EXTRACTION FACE TO PUBIS

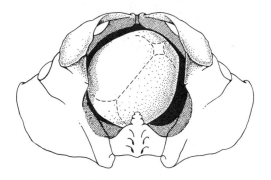

FIG. 4A. Right occiput posterior (ROP).

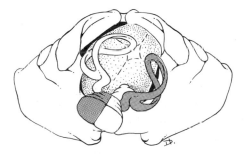

FIG. 4B. Midforceps, Simpson. Orientation.

Application of Forceps

1. The left blade is inserted gently into the vagina at about 5 o'clock, so that it lies between the right parietal bone and the left posterolateral wall of the pelvis (Fig. 5A).
2. The right blade is inserted over the left into the vagina at about 7 o'clock (Fig. 5B).
3. It is then moved anteriorly about 90° around the fetal head so that it fits between the left parietal bone and the right anterolateral wall of the pelvis.
4. The forceps are now locked, and vaginal examination is performed to make sure that the application is correct. If it is not, the forceps are unlocked and the necessary adjustments made (Fig. 5C).

Rotation and Extraction

1. The head is rotated 45° from **ROP** to **OP**, so that the occiput is in the hollow of the sacrum and the face under the pubis (Fig. 5D).
2. Traction is made outward and posteriorly until the area between the bregma and the nasion lies under the pubic arch.
3. The direction is then changed to outward and anterior, and as the handles of the forceps are raised the occiput is born over the perineum by flexion. The forceps are then removed.
4. Details of the technique for extracting the head are included in the previous section dealing with face to pubis delivery.

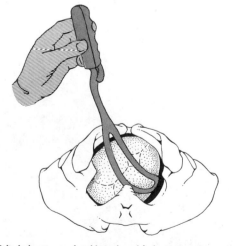

A. Insertion of left blade between fetal head and left posterolateral quadrant of pelvis.

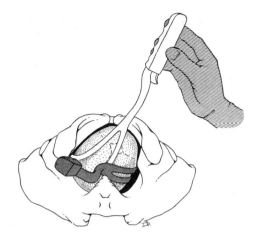

B. Handle of left blade is lowered. Insertion of right blade between fetal head and right posterolateral quadrant of pelvis, followed by upward movement of the blade to right anterolateral quadrant of pelvis.

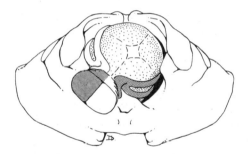

C. Locking of forceps in biparietal application.

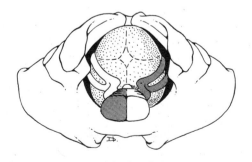

D. Posterior rotation ROP to OP (45°).

FIG. 5. ROP: forceps rotation to OP.

MANUAL ROTATION TO THE ANTERIOR

Orientation

VAGINAL EXAMINATION

1. The presentation is cephalic.
2. The sagittal suture is in the right oblique diameter of the pelvis.
3. The posterior fontanelle is in the right posterior quadrant of the pelvis (Fig. 6A).
4. The bregma is in the left anterior quadrant.
5. The station is usually 0 to +2.

Rotation is accomplished by one of two methods: (1) manual rotation of the head and shoulders (the Pomeroy maneuver); or (2) manual rotation of the head.

Pomeroy Maneuver: ROP

1. The operator places his left hand into the posterior part of the vagina between the head and the sacrum and past the fetal head into the uterus, so that the fingertips grasp the anterior shoulder and the head lies in the palm of the hand (Fig. 6B).
2. By pressure upward on the anterior shoulder (as the hand is pronated), the body and head are turned anteriorly (Fig. 6C).

The advantage of this maneuver is that since the body has been rotated, the head does not slip back to its original position. To ensure against this happening the head may be overrotated, ROP to LOA.

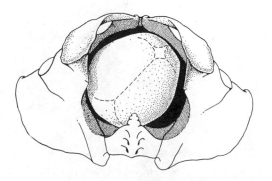

A. Right occiput posterior.

MANUAL ROTATION TO THE ANTERIOR

The disadvantage is that the head must be dislodged to the point of disengagement so that the hand can reach the shoulder. There is danger that the umbilical cord may prolapse or that the head may be extended and may not reengage properly.

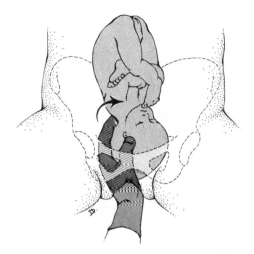

B. Fingers of the left hand are placed behind the anterior shoulder.

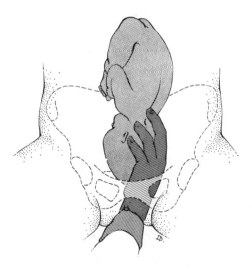

C. Anterior rotation of the shoulders and head, ROP to LOA.

FIG. 6. ROP: Pomeroy maneuver.

Manual Rotation of Occiput to Anterior: ROP

1. After the patient is anesthetized the operator inserts the left hand in the vagina and grasps the fetal head, placing the thumb on the anterior parietal (left) bone and the fingers on the posterior parietal (right) bone. The left hand is better for ROP and the right for LOP (Figs. 7A and B).
2. First the head is flexed.
3. Then the head is rotated anteriorly to the occiput anterior position by pronating the hand in the vagina: ROP to ROT to ROA to OA (Figs. 7C through E).
4. At the same time the operator turns the body in the identical direction by applying pressure with his other hand on the shoulders or breech through the maternal abdomen.

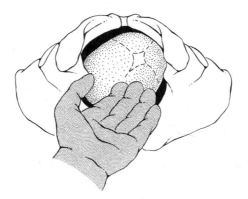

A. Orientation, left hand.

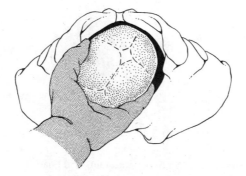

B. Left hand grasps the head; the thumb is on the anterior parietal (left) bone, and the fingers are on the posterior parietal (right) bone.

MANUAL ROTATION TO THE ANTERIOR

This method is safe for the baby and for the mother. However, when the fit between baby and pelvis is snug or when the head is impacted, it is difficult to obtain a good grasp of the head and manual rotation may be impossible. Furthermore, the shoulders do not always rotate with the head, and sometimes when the head is released by the operator's hand it returns to the original posterior position. Despite these disadvantages manual rotation is so safe and so free from vaginal tears that it should be tried before resorting to more complicated methods.

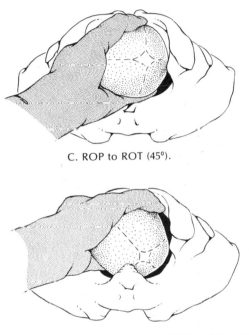

C. ROP to ROT (45°).

D. Manual rotation using left hand: ROT to ROA (45°).

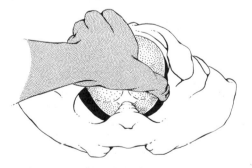

E. Manual rotation using left hand: ROA to OA (45°). Head ready for extraction.

FIG. 7. ROP: manual rotation to OA.

Sometimes complete rotation to the OA position is not possible. In such cases forceps are applied to the head in the new position (ROT or ROA), rotation to OA is achieved with the forceps, and the head is extracted.

DELIVERY

Once manual rotation of the head to the occipitoanterior has been accomplished, two methods of delivery are available: Originally the patient was permitted to awaken from the anesthetic and the onset of labor was awaited, the hope being that spontaneous delivery would take place. Today we believe that, once the indications for interference are present, the baby should be born without delay. Hence manual rotation is followed by extraction with forceps in the new position.

DOUBLE APPLICATION OF FORCEPS: ROP (MODIFIED SCANZONI MANEUVER)

A double application of forceps for the treatment of occipitoposterior positions was performed by William Smellie during the 18th century. In 1830 Scanzoni revived, improved, and popularized the maneuver, which has since been associated with his name. Bill further modified operation, and his technique is the one that we use today.

Orientation

VAGINAL EXAMINATION

1. The presentation is cephalic.
2. The sagittal suture is in the right oblique diameter of the pelvis.
3. The posterior fontanelle is in the right posterior quadrant of the pelvis (Fig. 8A).
4. The bregma is in the left anterior quadrant.
5. The station is usually 0 to +2.

ORIENTATION AND DESIRED APPLICATION
The cephalic application is not perfect but is satisfactory.

1. The blades are over the parietal bones in the occipitomental application. The left blade is on the right parietal bone, and the right blade is on the left parietal bone (Fig. 8B and 9C).

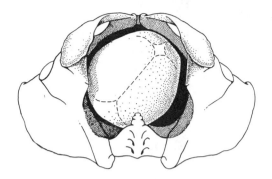

A. ROP orientation.

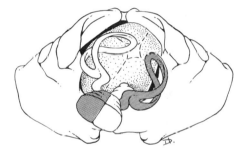

B. Midforceps, Simpson. Orientation.

FIG. 8. Scanzoni maneuver.

2. The front of the forceps (concave edges) point to the face. In an
   ideal cephalic application they point to the occiput.
3. The concave edges point to the occiput. In the ideal application
   they point to the face.

The pelvic application is oblique.

1. The diameter of the blades is in the left oblique diameter of the
   pelvis.
2. The left blade is in the left posterior quadrant of the pelvis.
3. The right blade is in the right anterior quadrant.
4. The concave edges point anteriorly and to the left.
5. The convex edges are posterior and to the right.

Application of Forceps

1. The left blade is inserted gently into the vagina at about 5 o'clock, so that it lies between the right parietal bone and the left postero-lateral wall of the pelvis (Fig. 9A).
2. The right blade is inserted into the vagina at about 7 o'clock (Fig. 9B).
3. It is then moved anteriorly about 90° around the fetal head so that it fits between the left parietal bone and the right antero-lateral wall of the pelvis.
4. The forceps are now locked, and vaginal examination is performed to make sure that the application is correct. If it is not, the forceps are unlocked and the necessary adjustments made (Fig. 9C).

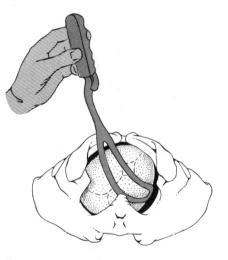

A. Insertion of left blade between fetal head and left posterolateral quadrant of pelvis.

DOUBLE APPLICATION OF FORCEPS: ROP (MODIFIED SCANZONI MANEUVER)

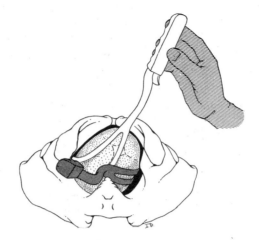

B. Handle of left blade is lowered. Insertion of right blade between fetal head and right posterolateral quadrant of pelvis, followed by upward movement of blade to right anterolateral quadrant of pelvis.

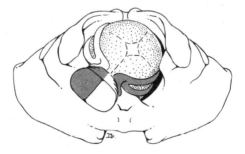

C. Locking of forceps in biparietal application.

FIG. 9. Scanzoni maneuver: application of forceps: ROP.

Rotation: ROP to OA

1. After the forceps are locked the handles are raised toward the opposite groin, in ROP toward the left groin. This maneuver favors flexion of the head (Fig. 10A).
2. Without traction the handles are carried around in a large circle so that they point first to the left groin (ROP), next toward the left thigh (ROT; Fig. 10B), then toward the left ischial tuberosity (ROA; Fig. 10C), and finally toward the anus and floor (OA; Fig. 10D). With the wide sweep of the handles the blades turn in a small arc and do not deviate from the same axis during the process of rotation. The fetal head turns with the use of very little force on the part of the operator.
3. The rotation is continued until the occiput lies under the symphysis pubis and the sagittal suture is in the anteroposterior diameter of the pelvis. The extent of the rotation is 135°, and the sequence is ROP to ROT to ROA to OA. The relationship of the forceps to the fetal head has not changed, but now the concave edges of the blades are posterior and the convex edges are anterior. The forceps are upside down, and the pelvic curve of the blades is the reverse of the curve of the maternal pelvis. This situation is not suitable for extracting the head, and adjustments are necessary.

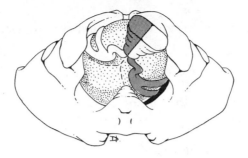

A. ROP: head is flexed by raising the handles of the forceps.

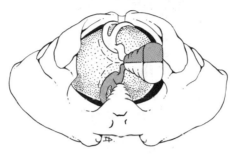

B. Anterior rotation by forceps: ROP to ROT (45°).

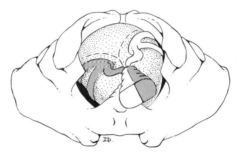

C. ROT to ROA (45°).

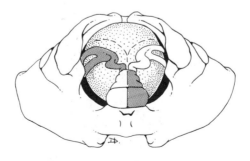

D. ROA to OA (45°).

FIG. 10. Scanzoni maneuver: Rotation.

Removal of Forceps

1. Before removing the forceps a small amount of traction is made, not with the idea of delivering the head but simply to fix it in its new position.
2. The forceps are unlocked.
3. The right forceps is removed first by depressing the handle further so that the blade slides around the head and out of the vagina (Fig. 11A).
4. Then the left forceps is removed in the same way (Fig. 11B).

A vaginal examination is performed in the new OA position (Fig. 11C).

1. The sagittal suture is in the anteroposterior diameter of the pelvis.
2. The occiput is under the pubis.
3. The face is near the sacrum.

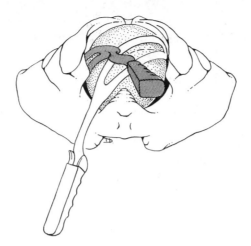

A. Removal of right blade.

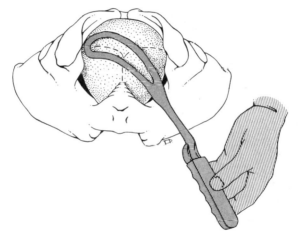

B. Removal of left blade.

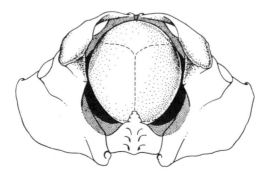

C. New position: **OA**

FIG. 11. Scanzoni maneuver: Forceps removal.

Reapplication of Forceps

1. The left blade is inserted between the fetal head and the left posterolateral quadrant of the pelvis (Fig. 12A).
2. The handle is lowered to the horizontal and the blade moved over the left parietal bone.
3. The right blade is inserted between the fetal head and the right posterolateral quadrant of the pelvis (Fig. 12B).
4. The handle is lowered to the horizontal and the blade moved over the right parietal bone.
5. The forceps are locked in a biparietal cephalic and pelvic application (Fig. 12C).
6. Then the head is extracted in the usual way.

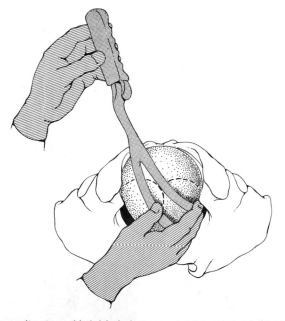

FIG. 12A. Reapplication of left blade between fetal head and left side of pelvis.

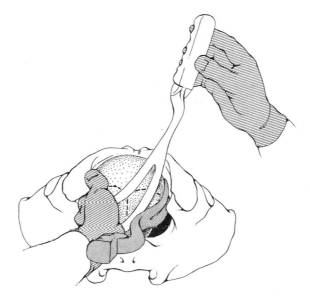

FIG. 12B. Reapplication of right blade between fetal head and right side of pelvis.

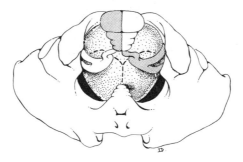

FIG. 12C. Locking of forceps in biparietal cephalic and pelvic application.

Alternate Method of Removing and Reapplying Forceps Using Two Sets

Occasionally the shoulders do not rotate with the head and there is a tendency for the head to turn back to the ROP position once the forceps are removed (Fig. 13A). This can be prevented by employing two sets of forceps in the following way:

1. The right blade (upside down) is removed from the left side of the pelvis (Fig. 13B). An assistant holds the original left blade in place preventing the head from turning back.
2. The left blade from the new set is then inserted right side up into the left side of the maternal pelvis in the usual manner (Fig. 13C).
3. The left upside down blade is removed from the right side of the pelvis (Fig. 13D). The head is prevented from turning back by the new left blade, which is held by an assistant.
4. The right blade of the new set is now inserted into the vagina (Fig. 13E).
5. The forceps are now in a correct application and are locked (Fig. 13F).
6. Extraction is carried out in the usual way.

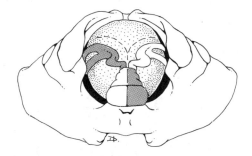

A. New position: OA. Forceps upside down.

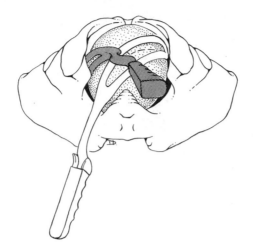

B. Removal of right Simpson forceps from left side of pelvis

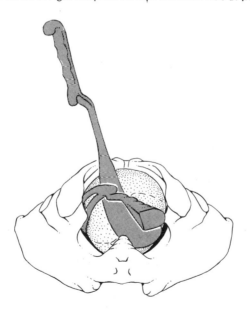

C. Insertion of left Tucker-McLane forceps between fetal head and left side of pelvis. The left Simpson is still in place.

FIG. 13. Two-forceps maneuver.

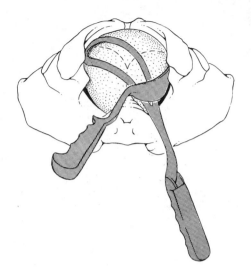

D. Removal of left Simpson forceps from right side of pelvis.

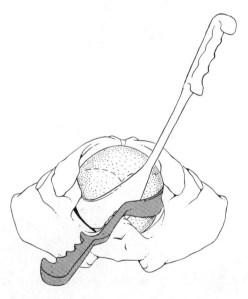

E. Insertion of right Tucker-McLane forceps between fetal head and right side of pelvis.

FIG. 13 (cont.).

DOUBLE APPLICATION OF FORCEPS: ROP (MODIFIED SCANZONI MANEUVER)

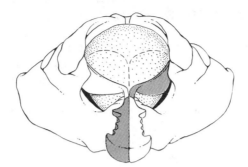

F. Locking of Tucker-McLane forceps in biparietal cephalic and pelvic application.

The risk of extensive vaginal lacerations, claimed by some authors to be inherent in the Scanzoni maneuver because of the long forceps rotation, has been exaggerated greatly. As long as the operation is performed gently and slowly a minimal amount of damage occurs. Many of the extensive vaginal tears and vesical and rectal fistulas occurred in cases of definite disproportion, where vaginal delivery should never have been carried out.

As the following translation of Scanzoni's article reveals, Scanzoni described the rotation of the head only as far as the ROT or ROA position.

> The head stands with the forehead turned toward the front and left so that the sagittal suture passes in the right oblique diameter; the left blade is applied in front of the left sacroiliac synchrondrosis, the right behind the right obturator foramen: with this the transverse diameter of the forceps is placed in the left oblique diameter of the pelvis, their concave edges and tips are turned to the anterior circumference of the left lateral hemisphere of the pelvis, and so also with the forehead. An eighth of a circle is now described with the instrument, directed from left to right, whereby the right blade comes to rest under the symphysis and the left in the hollow of the sacrum; and in this way the head is rotated, the earlier standing forehead is moved to the middle of the left lateral wall of the pelvis, and the sagittal suture is placed parallel with the transverse diameter of the pelvis.
>
> Now both blades of the forceps are removed and again applied, so that the left blade comes to lie behind the left obturator foramen, the right in the front of the right sacroiliac ligament, whereupon by the next rotation the occiput is brought completely under the pubic arch.

MAUGHAN MANEUVER: ROP

1. The left forceps blade is placed upside down in the right postero-lateral part of the vagina so that it lies over the occiput. The concave side of the blade points posteriorly and the convex side anteriorly (Fig. 14A).
2. The blade is wandered anteriorly so that it sweeps by the occiput, catches the anterior fetal ear, and rotates the ear to a position directly behind the symphysis pubis. The sequence is ROP to ROT (45°). The sagittal suture is now in the transverse diameter of the pelvis (Fig. 14B).
3. The second blade is inserted between the fetal head and the sacrum so that it lies over the posterior ear (Fig. 14C).
4. The forceps are then locked, each blade resting over an ear.
5. The head is rotated slowly 90° so that the occiput is placed behind the symphysis. The sequence is ROT to ROA to OA.
6. The head is then extracted as an occipitoanterior.

This maneuver for rotation of the fetal head is primarily one of a single-forceps blade application, applied upside down to the opposite side of the maternal pelvis (i.e., in right occipitoposterior, the left blade to the right side of the pelvis) in such fashion that, on anterior sliding movement, it sweeps over the occiput and, catching on the anterior fetal ear, rotates it to a position directly behind the symphysis pubis. The movement of this blade into place is therefore completely in the direction that rotation of the fetal head is intended, without upward displacement of the head.

KEY IN LOCK MANEUVER OF DeLEE

This is a multiple application method. The forceps are applied in the transverse diameter of the pelvis so that each blade lies next to the corresponding side of the maternal pelvis. Since application to the fetal skull is often not ideal, this operation must be performed delicately, with the least possible compression being applied to the baby. The head is pushed up a short distance in the axis of the birth canal and rotated gently, so that the small fontanelle is brought anteriorly about 5°. This is accomplished by sweeping the handles of the forceps through an arc of 10° outside the pelvis. The head is then pulled down in the pelvis, a little less than it was pushed up, to fix it in its new position. The forceps are loosened and returned to the transverse diameter of the pelvis, but the head is

KEY IN LOCK MANEUVER OF DeLEE

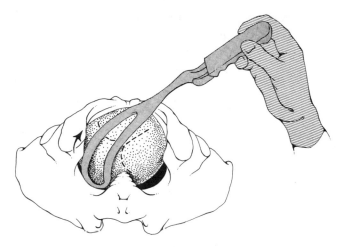

A. ROP. Left forceps blade inserted upside down over the occiput.

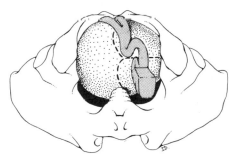

B. Forceps blade moved anteriorly under the pubis; head rotates ROP to ROT.

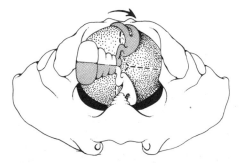

C. Posterior blade inserted between parietal bone and sacrum. Forceps locked in biparietal cephalic application. Arrow shows direction of further rotation ROT to OA.

FIG. 14. Maughan maneuver.

maintained in its new position. The head is then pushed up and rotated another 5°. These small rotations are continued until eventually the head is in the anterior position and the front (concave side) of the forceps points properly to the symphysis pubis and also to the fetal occiput. The head is then extracted in the usual way.

28.

Arrested Face
Presentations

FORCEPS EXTRACTION: MENTUM ANTERIOR

Orientation

VAGINAL EXAMINATION

1. The presentation is cephalic (Fig. 1A).
2. The long axis of the face is in the anteroposterior diameter of the pelvis.
3. The chin is under the pubic symphysis.
4. The forehead is toward the sacrum.

ORIENTATION AND DESIRED APPLICATION

The aim is for a biparietal cephalic application (Fig. 1B and 2A).

1. The front of the forceps (concave edges) point toward the denominator (the chin).
2. The blades are over the parietal bones in a mentooccipital (reverse occipitomental) application.

The pelvic application is correct.

1. The diameter of the blades is in the transverse diameter of the pelvis.
2. The sides of the blades are next to the corresponding side walls of the pelvis.
3. The concave edges point to the pubis.
4. The convex edges are in the hollow of the sacrum.

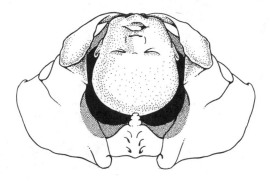

FIG. 1A. Face presentation: Mentum anterior.

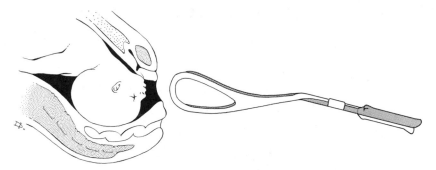

FIG. 1B. Face presentation: Kjelland forceps.

Application of Forceps

1. The left blade is inserted into the vagina at about 5 o'clock and is moved around the face slightly until it lies between the right cheek and the left wall of the pelvis.
2. The right blade is inserted into the vagina at about 7 o'clock and is moved around the face until it lies between the left cheek and the right wall of the pelvis.
3. The forceps are locked, and vaginal examination is made to be sure that the application is correct and that no adjustment is necessary (Fig. 2A).

Extraction of the Head

1. The handles of the forceps are depressed toward the floor to deflex the head completely.

FORCEPS EXTRACTION: MENTUM ANTERIOR

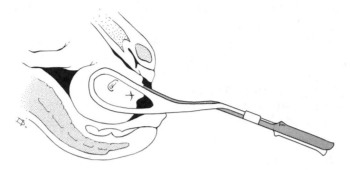

A. Locking of forceps. Beginning traction in the axis of the birth canal.

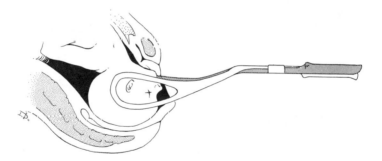

B. Horizontal traction.

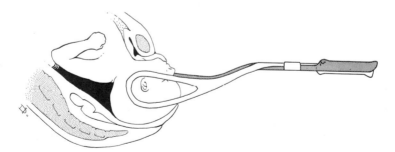

C. Delivery by flexion of the head.

FIG. 2. Mentum anterior.

2. Traction is made in an outward, horizontal, and slightly posterior direction until the chin appears under the symphysis pubis and the submental region of the neck impinges in the subpubic angle (Fig. 2B).
3. With further descent the face and forehead appear, and the direction of traction is changed to outward and anterior. This brings about both descent and flexion, and the vertex and occiput are born over the perineum (Fig. 2C).
4. Since a large diameter is being born over the perineum, an episiotomy is advisable.

FORCEPS ROTATION AND EXTRACTION: MENTUM POSTERIOR

Because the bulk of the head is in the anterior quadrant of the pelvis, the usual application is not practical and the forceps are applied upside down. Because of their small pelvic curve the Kjelland forceps are valuable for this operation, but any instrument can be used.

Orientation

VAGINAL EXAMINATION

1. The long axis of the face is in the anteroposterior diameter of the pelvis (Fig. 3).
2. The chin is in the hollow of the sacrum.
3. The forehead is under the pubic symphysis.

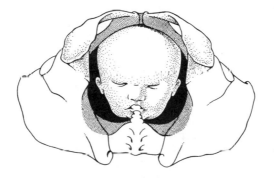

FIG. 3. Mentum posterior (MP) orientation. Face presentation.

ORIENTATION AND DESIRED APPLICATION
The cephalic application is biparietal.

1. The front of the forceps (concave edges) points to the denominator, the chin (Fig. 4A and B).
2. The blades are over the parietal bones.

The pelvic application is upside down.

1. The diameter of the blades is in the transverse diameter of the pelvis.
2. The sides of the blades are next to the opposite side walls of the pelvis: left blade next to the right wall, and right blade near the left wall.
3. The concave edges point to the sacrum.
4. The convex edges point to the pubis.

Application of Forceps Upside Down

1. The right blade is inserted first. Its handle is grasped by the left hand and is held a little below the vagina and near the mother's right thigh. The convex edge of the blade is anterior.
2. The right blade is inserted into the vagina between the left side of the face and the left wall of the vagina.
3. The left blade is inserted next. Its handle is grasped by the right hand and is held a little below the vagina and near the mother's left thigh. The convex edge is anterior (upside down).
4. The left blade is introduced into the right side of the vagina between the right side of the face and the right pelvic wall.
5. The forceps are locked, and vaginal examination is made to be sure that the application is correct (Fig. 4B).

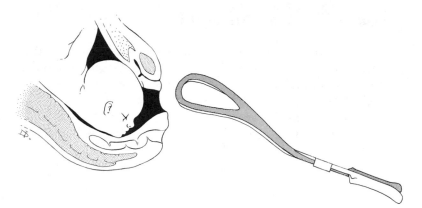

A. Kjelland forceps upside down.

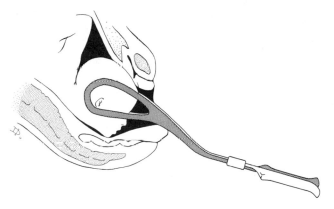

B. Forceps locked, upside down.

FIG. 4. MP orientation.

Rotation to Anterior: MP to MA

1. The face is then rotated 180° with the forceps: MP to RMP to RMT to RMA to MA. The chin is now under the pubis, and the forehead is in the hollow of the sacrum (Fig. 5).
2. The cephalic application has been maintained.
3. The pelvic application is now right side up, with the concave edges of the forceps next to the pubis and the convex edges near the sacrum.

Extraction of the Head

1. Vaginal examination is made to check the application.
2. Traction is made in an outward and posterior direction until the chin appears under the symphysis and the submental region of the neck impinges in the subpubic angle.
3. With further descent, the face and forehead appear and the direction of traction is changed to outward and anterior. This brings about both descent and flexion, and the vertex and occiput are born over the perineum.
4. Because of the large diameter being delivered, an episiotomy is essential.

FORCEPS ROTATION AND EXTRACTION: MENTUM POSTERIOR

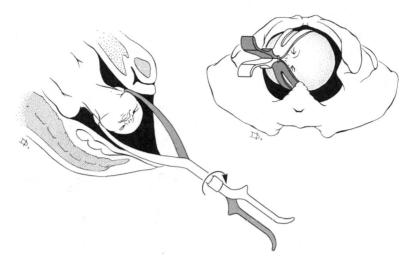

A. Anterior rotation with forceps: MP to RMT.

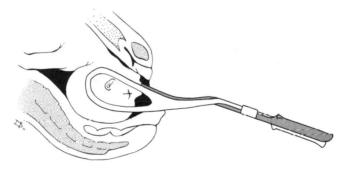

B. Anterior rotation with forceps: RMT to MA.

FIG. 5.

29.

Breech: Delivery of the Aftercoming Head by Forceps

While any type of forceps can be used for this procedure, the Piper forceps, which was designed especially for this operation, is best. The handles are depressed below the arch of the shanks, the pelvic curve is reduced, and the shanks are long and curved. These features make this instrument easier to apply to the aftercoming head.

FORCEPS DELIVERY

Orientation

VAGINAL EXAMINATION

1. The long axis of the head is in the anteroposterior diameter of the pelvis.
2. The occiput is anterior.
3. The face is posterior.

ORIENTATION AND DESIRED APPLICATION

1. The cephalic application is biparietal and mentooccipital, with the front of the forceps (concave edges) toward the occiput and the convex edges toward the face.
2. The pelvic application is good, with the diameter of the forceps in the transverse diameter of the pelvis, the concave edges pointing toward the pubis and the convex edges toward the sacrum. The sides of the blades are next to the side walls of the pelvis.

Application of Forceps

1. An assistant lifts the baby's body slightly (Fig. 1A), but not too much, for the structures in the neck are damaged by excessive stretching. The lower and upper limbs and the umbilical cord are kept out of the way.
2. The handle of the left blade is grasped in the left hand.
3. The right hand is introduced between the head and the left posterolateral wall of the vagina.
4. The left blade is then inserted between the head and the fingers into a mentooccipital application.
5. The fingers are removed from the vagina, and the handle is steadied by an assistant.
6. The handle of the right blade is grasped with the right hand.
7. The left hand is introduced between the head and the right posterolateral wall of the vagina.
8. The right blade is introduced between the head and the fingers into a mentooccipital application.
9. The fingers are removed from the vagina.
10. The forceps are locked (Fig. 1B), and vaginal examination is made to be certain that the application is correct.

Extraction of the Head

1. Traction is outward and posterior until the nape of the neck is in the subpubic angle.
2. The direction is then changed to outward and anterior, and the face and forehead are born over the perineum in flexion.
3. An episiotomy should be used.

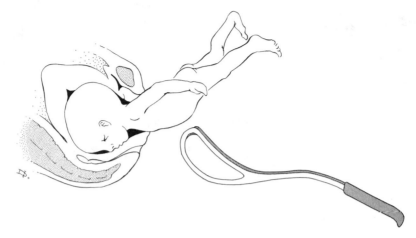

A. Orientation: Piper forceps.

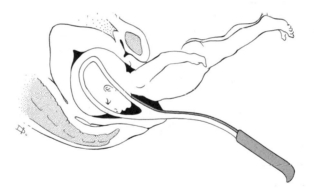

B. Piper forceps locked in cephalic application. Beginning traction.

FIG. 1. Breech presentation.

30.

Version and Extraction

DEFINITIONS

Version is an operation by which the fetus is turned in utero for the purpose of changing the presentation.

CEPHALIC VERSION   This results in a cephalic presentation.

PODALIC VERSION   This results in a breech.

EXTERNAL VERSION   All manipulations are done through the abdominal wall.

INTERNAL VERSION   The operation is performed with the hand or fingers inside the uterus. In most cases the intrauterine manipulations are furthered by the other hand acting through the abdominal wall.

EXTRACTION   This is the operative and immediate forceful delivery of the child.

EXTERNAL VERSION

Indications

Cephalic version is used to (1) turn a breech to a cephalic presentation, or (2) change a transverse lie to a cephalic presentation. Podalic version is used to turn a transverse lie to a breech presentation. This is done only when cephalic version has failed.

Prerequisites

Certain conditions must be present before external version is attempted:

1. There must be a single pregnancy.

388

2. Accurate diagnosis of the fetal position is of prime importance.
3. Fetopelvic disproportion should be ruled out.
4. The presenting part must not be deeply engaged.
5. The fetus must be freely movable.
6. There must be intact membranes with a good quantity of amniotic fluid.
7. Uterine relaxation is essential.
8. The maternal abdominal wall must be lax and thin enough to permit manipulations.
9. If possible the placenta should be located.
10. The best time for external version is between 32 and 36 weeks.

Contraindications

1. Deep engagement of the breech in the pelvis
2. Gross congenital abnormalities of the fetus
3. Intrauterine fetal death
4. Multiple pregnancy
5. Premature rupture of the membranes
6. Antepartum bleeding
7. Uterine scars, e.g., previous cesarean section
8. Cases in which vaginal delivery is not intended
9. Preeclampsia and hypertension

Dangers

1. Unexplained fetal death may follow version.
2. Fetal bradycardia is noted in many cases immediately following the version, although almost all heart rates return to normal within 3 minutes.
3. The position achieved by the version may be worse than the original one. For example, little has been gained by changing a breech to a brow presentation.
4. There is danger of injury to the umbilical cord and interference with the uteroplacental circulation.
5. There may be prolapse of the umbilical cord.
6. Induction of premature labor may take place.
7. There may be premature separation of the placenta from the uterine wall.
8. Premature rupture of the membranes may occur after version.

Technique

PREPARATION

1. The patient lies on her back on a firm table with the abdomen uncovered. To help relax the abdominal wall muscles, a pillow is put under the head, and the hips and knees are flexed.
2. Placing the woman in slight Trendelenburg position (hips higher than the shoulders) for 15 to 20 minutes may help dislodge the presenting part and so make the version easier.
3. The bladder should be empty.
4. If the mother's abdomen or the operator's hands are moist, powder should be sprinkled on the abdomen.
5. The diagnosis must be precise. The presentation should be confirmed by x-ray or ultrasound, and the location of the placenta demonstrated by ultrasound.

ANESTHESIA

There is considerable controversy about the use of an anesthetic agent in the performance of version. There is no doubt that it is easier to perform the operation when the patient is asleep and completely relaxed. On the other hand, it increases the danger of injury. When the patient is awake, her complaints of pain serve as an indication that the manipulations are too vigorous and that it is wise to be more gentle or to stop.

Bonnar, in a study of 500 cases, came to the conclusion that version under anesthesia does not reduce perinatal morality. The lower death rate after successful version is achieved at the expense of those babies who died as a result of the procedure. Version under anesthesia is indicated only when the possibility of perinatal mortality from breech birth is greater than 2.0 percent.

PROCEDURE

1. The operator stands at the patient's side.
2. The fetal heart is checked frequently before, during, and after the procedure. If at any time there is irregularity or a marked change in the rate, the operation is discontinued.
3. One hand is placed on the head and the other on the breech.
4. The presenting part is dislodged from the pelvis (Fig. 1A).
5. The head is moved toward the pelvis and the breech toward the fundus to achieve a transverse lie (Fig. 1B). This position is maintained while the fetal heart is ausculted.
6. If the fetal heart rate is slow or irregular, the baby is turned back to the original position.

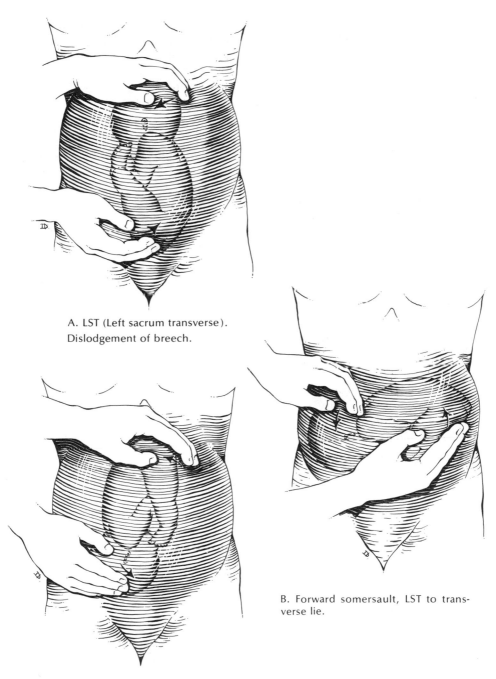

A. LST (Left sacrum transverse).
Dislodgement of breech.

B. Forward somersault, LST to transverse lie.

C. Forward somersault completed,
transverse lie to ROT.

FIG. 1. External version.

7. If the heart is normal the version is continued until the head is over the pelvis and the breech is in the fundus (Fig. 1C).
8. If at this point the baby's heart is abnormal, the fetus must be returned to its primary position.
9. After the version is complete and the fetal heart is noted to be normal, the head should be pushed into the pelvis to try and prevent recurrence of the malpresentation. Unfortunately and despite all efforts, this often happens.
10. Version must never be forced. If the procedure cannot be performed easily and gently, it should be abandoned or postponed.

DIRECTION OF VERSION

The fetus is turned in the direction in which it is easier to move it, with either the occiput or the face leading the way. It is important that flexion of the head be maintained during the procedure. It is simpler to preserve flexion of the head by the backward somersault (occiput first), but there is more danger of the legs tangling with the umbilical cord. With the forward somersault (face first) there is less chance of the legs causing trouble, but it is more difficult to keep the head flexed.

CAUSES OF FAILED OR DISCONTINUED VERSION

1. Large fetus and/or small amount of amniotic fluid
2. Fetal bradycardia
3. Maternal obesity
4. Uterine malformation
5. Maternal bleeding
6. Unknown

INTERNAL PODALIC VERSION

Internal version is always podalic. With a hand inside the uterus it is feasible to grasp the feet and turn the baby to a footling breech. When the feet have been brought through the introitus the version is complete.

Indications

1. When the situation of the mother or fetus is such that immediate rapid delivery is essential
2. Prolapse of the umbilical cord

3. In compound presentations where the arm is prolapsed below the head and cannot be pushed out of the way
4. Delivery of the second twin if it has not engaged within 30 minutes of the birth of the first
5. Transverse or oblique lie

Prerequisites

1. Accurate diagnosis of position of the child is essential.
2. The child must be alive. There is no point is submitting the mother to a dangerous procedure if the baby is dead.
3. The presenting part should not be deeply engaged.
4. The pelvis must be large enough to permit the passage of the fetal head, i.e., no disproportion.
5. The cervix must be open enough to admit the hand.
6. If extraction is to follow the version, the cervix must be dilated fully.
7. The uterus must not be in tetanus nor be too tightly coapted around the child. The baby must be freely movable.
8. Membranes should be intact or recently ruptured. There must be sufficient amniotic fluid to permit turning.

Contraindications

1. Contracted pelvis with fetopelvic disproportion. It is pointless to perform podalic version if there is not enough room for the head to come through.
2. An incompletely dilated or a rigid cervix.
3. A spastic uterus, which does not relax even under anesthesia. A spastic uterus not only makes version difficult or impossible but increases greatly the danger of uterine rupture.
4. Danger of uterine rupture. When the patient has been in labor for a long time with the lower uterine segment thinned out and with a high retraction ring, any intrauterine manipulations carry a grave danger of uterine rupture.
5. Rupture of the membranes. Once the membranes have been ruptured for a long time (over 1 hour) and the amniotic fluid has drained away, version is difficult, and the attempt carries with it the risk of uterine rupture and fetal death.
6. Uterine scar from previous cesarean section or extensive myomectomy.

Dangers

MATERNAL DANGERS

1. Inherent dangers of deep anesthesia
2. Rupture of the uterus
3. Lacerations of the cervix
4. Abruptio placentae
5. Infection following the intrauterine manipulations

FETAL DANGERS

1. Asphyxia from cord prolapse or compression
2. Anesthetic depression, causing asphyxia
3. Asphyxia from placental separation
4. Intracranial damage and hemorrhage
5. General trauma from the difficult procedure

Technique

PREPARATION

1. The patient is placed in the lithotomy position with the buttocks a little past the end of the table.
2. The bladder is catheterized. The rectum should be empty.
3. An intravenous infusion with a large bore needle is set up.
4. Crossmatched blood should be available.
5. The patient is anesthetized deeply.

PROCEDURE

1. The introitus and vagina are lubricated with green soap or dettol.
2. One hand is placed on the uterine fundus to steady the uterus and the baby.
3. The other hand is placed through the cervix into the uterine cavity.
4. When the operator is ready for immediate action, the membranes are ruptured.
5. The fetal head is displaced upward out of the pelvis if the presentation is cephalic.

6. With the intrauterine hand, both feet are grasped if possible
(Fig. 2A). If both feet are not attainable, then one foot is grasped.
The operator must make sure that he has a foot and not a hand.
7. The feet are pulled slowly toward the pelvic inlet (Fig. 2B).

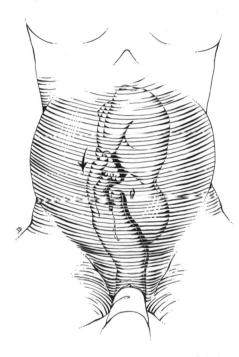

A. Cephalic presentation. Grasping both feet.

B. Downward traction on feet. Upward
pressure on head. Cephalic presentation converted to footling breech.

FIG. 2. Internal podalic version.

8. With the outer hand the head is pushed gently toward the fundus.
9. When possible the baby should be turned so that the back remains anterior and the head in flexion.
10. When the knees have reached the introitus, version is complete.
11. If there is no need for immediate delivery, the patient is permitted to recover from the anesthesia and to resume labor.

EXTRACTION FOLLOWING VERSION

If there is an indication for immediate delivery, and this is so in most cases where internal version is performed, the baby is extracted as a footling breech. This procedure is described in Chapter 18.

CESAREAN SECTION OR VERSION AND EXTRACTION

In the days when cesarean section was fraught with great danger to the mother, version and extraction was employed frequently in the management of various obstetric difficulties. The improvement in surgical technics, discovery of antibiotics, advances in anesthesia, and availability of blood for transfusion have decreased the fetal and maternal mortality and morbidity associated with abdominal delivery to a point where cesarean section is preferable by far to version and extraction. The use of the latter procedure is limited today to situations of an emergent nature, where immediate delivery of the baby is essential.

BIBLIOGRAPHY

Bradley-Watson PJ: The decreasing value of external cephalic version in modern obstetric practice. Am J Obstet Gynecol 123:237, 1975
Ranney B: The gentle art of external cephalic version. Am J Obstet Gynecol 116:239, 1973

31.

Obstetric Analgesia and Anesthesia

Pain is one of Nature's defense mechanisms, a warning of danger. In pregnancy it tells the woman that she is having uterine contractions. A painless labor is as treacherous as a silent coronary thrombosis. However, once labor has been diagnosed and proper care instituted, pain has served its purpose; it then becomes appropriate to offer the woman relief. In 1847 Sir James Young Simpson introduced anesthesia into obstetric practice. Intermittently inhaled ether and then chloroform were used to relieve the pains of the final stages of labor and delivery. Many new techniques have been evolved, but the perfect method of abolishing the pain of childbirth has not been achieved.

CAUSES OF PAIN DURING LABOR

1. Myometrial anoxia: Contraction of a muscle during a period of relative anoxia causes pain. When uterine relaxation between contractions is insufficient to allow adequate oxygenation, the severity of pain is increased.
2. Stretching of the cervix: Cervical stretching causes pain that is felt mainly in the back.
3. Pressure on the nerve ganglia adjacent to the cervix and vagina.
4. Traction on the tubes, ovaries, and peritoneum.
5. Traction on and stretching of the supporting ligaments.
6. Pressure on the urethra, bladder, and rectum.
7. Distention of the muscles of the pelvic floor and perineum.

INNERVATION OF PELVIC STRUCTURES

Uterus and Cervix

The sensation of pain (caused by myometrial contractions and cervical dilatation) passes by sensory sympathetic pathways to the area of the uterosacral ligaments, and thence via the uterine, pelvic, hypogastric, and aortic plexuses into the dorsal roots of the 11th and 12th thoracic segments and into the spinal cord. The motor nerves are also sympathetic. They start in the 10th, 11th, and 12th ventral rami and pass through the aortic, hypogastric, pelvic, and uterine plexuses to terminate in the uterus.

Vagina, Vulva, and Perineum

The pudendal nerve is the main supply of the perineum. It arises from the anterior branches of the second, third, and fourth sacral nerves. These join into a single trunk 0.5 to 1.0 cm proximal to the ischial spine. The nerve passes through the greater sciatic foramen, somewhat diagonally across the posterior surface of the sacrospinous ligament, medial to the pudendal vessels, to enter the lesser sciatic foramen. As the nerve passes medial and posterior to the inferior tip of the spine, it enters the pudendal canal and proceeds to the lower edge of the urogenital diaphragm. The nerve is blocked most easily where it lies close to the tip of the ischial spine.

The pudendal nerve divides into three main branches: (1) the inferior hemorrhoidal nerve, (2) the dorsal nerve of the clitoris, and (3) the perineal nerve. The inferior hemorrhoidal nerve supplies the lower rectum, the external sphincter ani, and the skin anterior and lateral to the anus. In 50 percent of cases this nerve arises as a separate branch from the fourth sacral nerve and is not part of the pudendal trunk. In these cases it lies close to the pudendal nerve medial to the ischial spine. The dorsal nerve of the clitoris supplies that organ and the area around it. The perineal nerve is the largest branch. It supplies the superficial structures of the vulva and the skin, fascia, and deep muscles of the perineum.

While the main sensations of pain are carried by the pudendal nerve, a few impulses pass via the posterior femoral cutaneous nerve into the second, third, and fourth sacral nerves, and the ilioinguinal nerve into the first lumbar segment.

PAIN DURING THE STAGES OF LABOR

First Stage Pain is caused mainly by uterine contractions, thinning of the lower segment of the uterus, and dilatation of the cervix.

Second Stage Pain results from two sources. The first is the stretching of the vagina, vulva, and perineum; and the second is the contracting myometrium.

Third Stage   Pain is caused by passage of the placenta through the cervix, plus that produced by the uterine contractions.

OBJECTIVES AND METHODS

Objectives for the mother include:

1. Relief of pain
2. Freedom from fear
3. Some degree of amnesia
4. Safe and relatively painless delivery

Objectives for the infant are:

1. To improve the progress of labor
2. To make the delivery less traumatic

Objectives for the obstetrician must include:

1. More deliberate management of labor
2. Reduction of pressure from patient and relatives to do something prematurely
3. Optimum conditions at delivery

Methods of achieving objectives are:

1. Prenatal training for childbirth, which dissipates fear and tension
2. Sedation by the use of drugs such as barbiturates and tranquilizers
3. Analgesia by narcotics such as morphine and Demerol
4. Amnesia, provided specifically by scopolamine (hyoscine) but also to a lesser degree by sedatives and analgesics
5. Anesthesia (absence of all sensation) by a wide variety of agents: inhalant, local, intravenous, and conduction techniques.

Criteria for Ideal Method

The method must ensure that:

1. The health of the mother is not endangered.
2. No harm comes to the fetus. Drugs given to the mother cross the placenta and reach the infant; varying degrees of respiratory de-

pression result and the baby may be apneic at birth. Some babies are lethargic after birth and require stimulation in the nursery. The long-term effects of narcosis on the infant's brain must be considered as well.

3. The agent has the ability to abolish or diminish pain and the memory of suffering.
4. The efficiency of the uterine contractions is not decreased. This could cause prolonged labor during the first and second stages and atonic postpartum hemorrhage in the third.
5. The ability of the patient to cooperate intelligently with the medical and nursing staff is maintained.
6. There is no need for operative interference solely because of the anesthesia.
7. The method is reasonably simple to use.

There is no system of analgesia and anesthesia available which fulfills all these criteria. Compromises are made, but safety must never take second place to efficiency. As a general rule most anesthetists prefer regional to general anesthesia for patients undergoing vaginal delivery because there is less danger of aspiration of gastric contents and because judiciously used regional anesthesia has little effect on the baby. Fifty percent of obstetrical anesthetic deaths are related to general anesthesia and are most often directly attributable to the aspiration of gastric contents.

GENERAL DATA ON USES OF ANALGESIA AND ANESTHESIA

1. There is wide variation in the degree of analgesia and anesthesia, ranging from the minimal dosage designed to take the edge off the pain to the complete abolition of sensation.
2. The smallest effective amount is best.
3. Unless there is a contraindication, the request of the patient for relief should not be refused.
4. Given too soon or in excessive dosage, analgesic preparations interfere with uterine contractions and delay labor. Prescribed at the proper time, pain is relieved and labor may be speeded up by the relaxation of tension.
5. The widespread use of episiotomy has increased the need for anesthesia.
6. Certain anesthetics—such as spinals, epidurals, or general anesthesia—given too soon increase the incidence of forceps extractions.

7. Premature infants are exceedingly susceptible to narcotics of any kind, and best results are attained when the mother is given no narcotics and no general anesthesia.
8. The quality and quantity of nursing supervision determine to an extent the drugs that can or cannot be used safely. Since some agents cause excitement, patients receiving them must be under constant observation.
9. The availability of the obstetrician is important in deciding what drugs can be given. Remote control is never as successful as personal management.
10. The availability of a trained anesthetist is essential if complicated techniques are to be employed.

TRAINING FOR CHILDBIRTH

The purpose of training for childbirth is to prepare a woman for labor and delivery so that she approaches the end of her pregnancy with knowledge, understanding, and confidence rather than apprehension and fear. She should be assured that relief will be provided should pain be excessive and that the modern obstetric armamentarium is available to ensure the safety of herself and her unborn child.

One of the first modern advocates of natural childbirth was Grantly Dick-Read. He described the "fear-tension-pain" cycle and hypothesized that fears regarding labor produced tension in the circular muscle fibers of the lower part of the uterus. As a result the longitudinal muscles of the upper part of the uterus have to act against resistance, causing tension and pain. Dick-Read's solution to this problem was to counteract the socially induced expectations regarding labor by providing mothers-to-be with information and assurance to the effect that labor does not have to be painful.

Velvovsky and his followers in the Soviet Union denied that labor was inherently painful. Based on the work of the physiologist Pavlov, they worked out a training procedure designed to inhibit the experience of pain at the cortical level. This is known as the psychoprophylactic method. Lamaze, originator of the Lamaze method, is the best known proponent in the Western world.

Aims of Prenatal Training

1. The apprehension of young women caused by the exaggerated tales of horror told by multiparas is counteracted.

2. The patient is given an opportunity to gain confidence: The facts of childbirth are explained, and the methods available to relieve pain are described.
3. Exercises are taught which strengthen certain muscles and relax others.
4. The patient is trained in breath control.
5. The patient is never told that labor and delivery are painless. On the contrary, it is emphasized that analgesia and anesthesia are available should they be needed or desired.
6. It is important that the patient not be placed in competition with other women or with an ideal analgesia-free labor and delivery. Too many women who do need assistance are left with a feeling of failure and remain emotionally disturbed.
7. While patients should be encouraged to take part in the training classes, reluctant women must never be forced to participate.
8. Constant emphasis is placed on the fact most labors are normal.
9. The program has two parts. The education and exercises are beneficial to all. Whether an individual is desirous of or able to carry on without drugs can be decided only during labor.

Whenever possible the patient should be in a private labor room, with an attendant at all times. This may be her husband, some other relative, a friend, a nurse, or her doctor. Peace and quiet in the labor suite are essential. Nothing that might worry the patient should be said in her hearing. Women in labor read erroneous and worrisome significance into innocent remarks. Unruly and noisy patients should be kept out of earshot, since nothing frightens a woman in labor as much as hearing another's screams.

Achievements of Trained Childbirth

Claims regarding the beneficial effects of trained childbirth include the following:

Psychologic Effects Decreased perception of pain, increased cooperation of the patient during labor, reduced incidence of postpartum depression, and a more positive attitude toward future pregnancy.

Obstetric Benefits There is a reduction in the need for analgesia and anesthesia, forceps, episiotomy, and cesarean section. The length of labor is reduced and the blood loss is less than in untrained patients.

Benefits to the Child   There is an increase in the oxygenation of fetal blood, quicker initiation of spontaneous respiration, less need for resuscitation, and decrease in the incidence of neonatal morbidity and mortality.

It is unfortunate that opinion regarding training for childbirth has undergone a steady polarization almost since its introduction. On the one hand it has been acclaimed as one of the most significant advances of modern medicine. On the other hand it has been denigrated as primitive and medically unacceptable. Taken as a whole, the reported studies suggest that training for childbirth brings a number of important physical and psychologic benefits to mother and child. The achievements seem impressive. However, critical analysis of these studies reveals that most of them do not meet the most fundamental requirements of the scientific method, including appropriate control groups, double-blind techniques, and statistical tests to rule out chance.

Nevertheless, because training programs can do no harm, because the probability is strong that they are helpful, and because patients and their spouses enjoy the experience, it is our feeling that prenatal classes should be encouraged.

RELIEF OF PAIN DURING THE FIRST STAGE OF LABOR

It is not possible to guarantee complete analgesia and amnesia for the entire labor, and this promise should never be made to the patient. Excessively deep analgesia not only carries risks to mother and child but can complicate the progress and management of labor. However, pain can be relieved safely to a degree that the patient's strength is conserved, she can maintain control, and the apprehension of her family is allayed.

Each patient is handled individually. The types and amount of therapy depend on the patient's personality as well as on the efficiency of the labor. In many cases labor is so short that a single administration of an analgesic is enough to carry the patient to the point of delivery. In difficult labors where multiple doses are required, the program of analgesia and amnesia must be planned carefully. Multiparas generally need less support than primigravidas. The complete personal supervision of the obstetrician is necessary in proportion to the degree of perfection required of the results.

During the first stage of labor the main objectives are the production of analgesia (relief of pain) and amnesia (loss of memory). Since it is not safe to give doses of narcotics large enough to produce both analgesia and amnesia, scopolamine has been added to enhance the amnesia. Unfortunately, drugs that encourage amnesia sometimes lead to excitement and even delirium.

Narcotics

MORPHINE
Morphine has been used in obstetrics for many years. The dose is 10 mg (1/6 grain). Because of the danger of fetal narcosis it is prescribed less frequently today during labor. It is useful to relieve postpartum pain.

Effects on the Mother   The threshold for pain is elevated. Fear and anxiety are replaced by feelings of indifference; and lethargy and sleep are induced.

Effects on the Fetus   Effect on the fetus depends on the time relationship of administration to delivery. The action on the fetus of 10 mg given intramuscularly to the mother reaches a peak in 1.5 hours. Administration within 3 hours of birth is dangerous. The risk of fetal narcosis is increased by general anesthesia and traumatic delivery. Morphine is especially bad for premature infants.

Effect on Labor   The effect on labor varies greatly. Sometimes it weakens or stops uterine contractions. In other cases it improves labor, especially in the colicky uterus where after a rest the pattern of the contractions becomes more efficient and coordinated.

DEMEROL (PETHIDINE, MEPERIDINE)
Demerol is a synthetic preparation with a mild atropine-like action. It is an excellent analgesic for labor. The patient is able to rest between her contractions and can cooperate. The dose is 100 mg given every 3 to 4 hours. Few patients receive more than 200 mg. The analgesic effect is almost equivalent to 10 mg of morphine, but the duration is a little shorter.

Effects on the Mother   The analgesic effect is good. Transient euphoria and restlessness may occur, although lethargy, mental impairment, and sleep are less than with morphine. The efficiency is increased when combined with scopolamine.

Effects on the Fetus   The effect on the fetus is related to the dosage. Respiratory depression is less than with morphine, but it can be serious. The greatest effect on the fetus is reached at 1.5 hours after intramuscular injection. Testing of the newborn's orientation reflexes demonstrated that infants whose mothers had received meperidine during labor performed less efficiently than those whose mothers had been given no medication. The former remained drowsy and less responsive. The best antidote to meperidine appears to be levallorphan. It has no depressive effect when an excessive amount of meperidine is not present.

Effect on Labor   Effect on labor is not marked. The action on the uterine contractions is less than with morphine. Often the good relaxation achieved with Demerol seems to speed up cervical dilatation.

Amnesia

SCOPOLAMINE (HYOSCINE)
Scopolamine hydrobromide is an amnesic, the effect of which is achieved without loss of consciousness. It is administered with an analgesic. The dose varies from 1/250 to 1/100 grain (0.25 to 0.60 mg).

Effects on the Mother   Scopolamine does not affect the pain threshold. Pain is felt, but the memory of it is fragmentary or absent. With large doses amnesia is complete. The patient becomes drowsy and may lose touch with her surroundings. A varying degree of restlessness and even delirium can occur. Because of this fact, constant supervision and sometimes actual physical restraint are necessary. Scopolamine has an action similar to atropine and causes dryness of the mouth and throat. There are no aftereffects, but there is great individual variation in response to the drug.

Effects on the Fetus   Although scopolamine crosses the placenta, no ill effects on the fetus have been noted.

Effect on Labor   There is no prolongation of labor or increase in operative deliveries.

Barbiturates

The barbituric acid derivatives have been used in obstetrics since 1924. They are employed mainly for their hypnotic property and to a lesser degree to produce amnesia. While they can be used for purposes of analgesia, the large doses required to do so produce respiratory depression in both mother and child. Pentobarbital and secobarbital are popular today.

Effects on the Mother Barbiturates are hypnotics; therefore in small doses (200 mg) they induce lethargy and sleep. The drug can be given orally as soon as good labor is established, and it takes effect in 20 to 30 minutes. Fear and apprehension are replaced by an attitude of indifference and freedom from anxiety. Sometimes a mood of elation develops and there is release of inhibitions; some patients become overactive to the point of extreme excitement. There is little effect on the pain threshold as long as the patient remains conscious.

Effects on the Fetus The drug crosses the placenta and can cause prolonged respiratory depression in the baby. The action on the fetus outlasts that on the mother; some babies exhibit lethargy and sleepiness long after birth. There is an especially great danger in premature babies.

Effect on Labor Excessive amounts of barbiturates can prolong labor. Impairment of uterine activity is related closely to the dosage. The cooperation of the patient may be lost.

Tranquilizers

The ataractics or tranquilizers are depressants of the central nervous system, but they differ from the hypnotics in acting primarily at the subcortical level, affecting the structures concerned with emotion. The most effective drugs are the phenothiazine derivatives, including promazine (Sparine), chlorpromazine (Thorazine), and promethazine (Phenergan). In the usual doses these drugs have tranquilizing and analgesic effects, but in large doses they are hypnotic.

When used with barbiturates or hypnotics the ataractic drugs have an additive or even a potentiating effect. The amount of a sedative or narcotic needed to produce a desired effect is reduced when a phenothiazine derivative is given with it.

The chief objections to the use of these drugs are the side effects, especially hypotension, which does not respond well to vasopressors. In some cases delay in the onset of respiration and crying has been reported in the newborn. These drugs should not be employed when the baby is premature.

DIAZEPAM (VALIUM)

Diazepam is an excellent tranquilizer and muscular relaxant. It has been used widely to induce sedation and repose during labor, and it is efficient in the management of preeclampsia and eclampsia.

However, it has been noted that the infants of mothers who were treated with large doses of diazepam during the 24 to 48 hours before delivery manifested symptoms of (1) hypotonia, (2) hypothermia, (3) low Apgar scores, (4) impaired metabolic response to cold stress, (5) neurologic or respiratory depression, (6) apneic spells, and (7) reluctance to feed. A total dose of 30 mg or less in the 15 hours preceding delivery has little effect on the infant's state. Larger amounts, however, do cause the above symptoms.

Diazepam and its metabolite (N-methyl diazepam) cross the placenta and tend to accumulate in the fetus, especially in the heart, lungs, and brain. Within 12 minutes the concentration in the fetal circulation equals that in the maternal plasma. With time the plasma levels in the fetus are higher than in the mother. The newborn metabolizes and excretes diazepam and N-methyl diazepam at a lower rate than do children and adults. Once accumulated in the fetus, these substances are released slowly over a period of 8 to 10 days.

Paracervical Block

Paracervical block is an effective, easily performed method of achieving relief of pain during the first stage of labor. Here the sensation of pain (caused by uterine contractions and cervical dilatation) passes by sensory and sympathetic pathways to the area of the uterosacral ligaments, through the pelvic and hypogastric plexuses, to the lower rami of the 11th and 12th thoracic vertebrae. For this type of pain paracervical block works well.

During the second stage of labor, pain (produced by distention of the vagina and vulva) is transmitted via the sensory fibers of the pudendal nerves to the second, third, and fourth sacral vertebrae. Paracervical block is ineffective in this area, and other types of anesthesia are needed.

TECHNIQUE

The injection is made transvaginally into the posterolateral fornices, thus blocking the sensory pathways at the junction of the uterosacral ligaments with the cervix. The procedure can be carried out in the patient's bed, but it is done more accurately on the delivery table. The block is instituted during the active phase of labor, with the cervix at least 3 to 4 cm dilated.

The equipment consists of a 20 gauge needle, 13 to 18 cm long, with a sheath or needle guide of such length that about 1.5 cm of the tip of the needle protrudes when it is inserted up to its hub. The needle sheath is guided by the fingers into the vagina and placed in the fornix just lateral to the cervix, at a tangent to the presenting part (Fig. 1). The needle (with attached syringe) is introduced through the guides until the point rests against the mucosa. With quick, slight pressure the needle is pushed through the mucosa to a depth of 6 to 12 mm. Aspiration is performed to guard against direct intravascular injection. If no blood comes back, the desired amount of anesthetic solution is injected. It is advisable to wait a few minutes after the injection of one side. The fetal heart is auscultated. If it is normal the other side is injected. If fetal bradycardia occurs the procedure should be discontinued. Mepivacaine (Carbocaine), lidocaine (Xylocaine), and procaine (Novocaine) in 1 percent concentrations are effective. Mepivacaine seems to have a longer lasting effect.

The sites of injection vary. Some workers inject the solution at 3 and 9 o'clock. Others give several injections at 3, 4, 8, and 9 o'clock. In any case, 10 ml is given on each side in single or multiple doses.

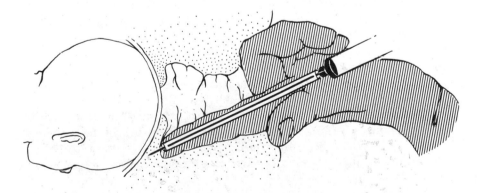

FIG. 1. Paracervical block.

EFFECTIVENESS

Most patients experience complete or partial relief from pain almost immediately. They remain alert and cooperative. The block gives relief for about 1 hour. In many cases a single block remains effective until the cervix is fully dilated. In others a second block is necessary.

Other forms of anesthesia are required for the actual delivery. Pudendal block or direct infiltration of the perineum are effective and safe.

EFFECT ON LABOR

Opinions vary concerning the effect of paracervical block on labor. Some state that labor is shortened, some say it is inhibited, while others feel that the effect varies from one patient to the next and is not predictable. The anesthetized patient may be unaware of strong uterine contractions, and oxytocin augmentation must be used with care, lest the uterus rupture.

MATERNAL COMPLICATIONS

1. Transient numbness and paresthesias of one or both lower extremities is common. This is the result of the local anesthetic spreading to the sciatic nerve or part of the lumbosacral plexus.
2. Rapid absorption or intravascular injection causes dizziness, euphoria, anxiety, shaking movements, and rarely convulsions.
3. Occasionally there is transient hypotension.
4. A hematoma may form at the site of injection.
5. A rare case of parametritis has been reported.

FETAL COMPLICATIONS

Changes in the fetal heart rate occur in about 30 percent. These include: (1) tachycardia over 160 per minute, (2) bradycardia between 100 and 120, and (3) bradycardia under 100. This last group, making up about 5 percent, is considered to be significant.

A hypothetical explanation is that the initial bradycardia is caused by a direct effect of the anesthetic on the fetal myocardium, the central nervous system, or both. If the bradycardia is not severe, nothing else happens. If the bradycardia is marked and prolonged, it causes hypoperfusion of the fetal tissues and hypoxia. Recovery of the fetus from the transient myocardial depression is represented by a phase of tachycardia. High levels of the drug in the blood can be correlated with the fetal bradycardia, fetal acidosis, and neonatal depression.

There are several ways by which the anesthetic may reach the fetal circulation:

1. The needle, if placed too deeply or in the wrong direction, may penetrate the cervix or lower uterine segment with the possibility of direct injection into the fetus.
2. There is danger of injecting the anesthetic into the myometrium, leading to massive absorption into the placental area.
3. Significant amounts of anesthetic solution are placed near the uterine arteries; since diffusion can occur across the arterial wall, large amounts of anesthetic have direct access to the intervillous pool.
4. Any material absorbed via the maternal venous system is slow to reach the fetus; this then is an unlikely route.
5. The injected fluid may compress the uterine vessels, reducing the blood flow and leading to hypoperfusion of the maternal side of the placenta.

Changes in the fetal heart rate are seen more often in (1) primigravidas, (2) infants weighing less than 2,500 g, and (3) when fetal distress was already present. There is no association with maternal premedication, fetal position or presentation, or the state of the membranes.

In most reports the incidence of asphyxia in the newborn following paracervical block-induced bradycardia is not higher than the general incidence, which suggests that the bradycardia is not a sign of asphyxia. However, cases have been documented, especially when the fetal heart rate was below 100, in which the rate of neonatal depression and low Apgar scores is increased. Further study indicated that this is seen mainly in babies born within 30 minutes of the block's administration. Infants delivered after 30 minutes, when the fetal heart had returned to normal, showed no ill effects in most instances. The fetus thus appears to tolerate the anesthetic better than the neonate. The bradycardia following paracervical block must be differentiated from that secondary to anoxia. Usually drug induced bradycardia occurs within 20 minutes, lasts only for 1 to 15 minutes, and is not affected by the uterine contractions. A fall in the fetal scalp pH in association with fetal heart rate (FHR) patterns of late deceleration suggests that the fetus is becoming asphyxiated.

Effects are related to dosage. Fetal bradycardia is unusual as long as the fetal blood levels are lower than those of the mother. A 1 percent solution is safest. The dose of local anesthetic should not exceed 300 mg, and several minutes should elapse between the injections on the two sides while the FHR is observed. The point of the needle should be placed just under the mucosa.

PRECAUTIONARY MEASURES

1. Paracervical block is unlikely to cause the intrauterine death of a healthy fetus, but it may do so when the fetus is already compromised. Hence this technic should not be used in cases of placental insufficiency and other high-risk situations.
2. The block should not be given if delivery is anticipated within 30 minutes.
3. If bradycardia does occur, the infant must not be delivered as an emergency. It is better to wait 30 minutes until the fetal heart rate is normal.
4. Pitocin is used with caution. The uterus may become hypertonic; since the patient feels no pain, the excessive contraction is missed by the attendants.
5. Vaginal bleeding is a contraindication to paracervical block.
6. The block should not be used when there is a history of sensitivity to local anesthetics.
7. The procedure is not safe in the presence of vaginal infection.

Lumbar Epidural Block

This technique is described later in this chapter.

RELIEF OF PAIN DURING THE SECOND STAGE OF LABOR

The essential requirements for a method of easing pain during this stage are:

1. Short induction
2. Rapid elimination and return to consciousness
3. Safety for mother and child
4. No diminution of uterine activity
5. Simple administration when possible.

Methods in common use include the inhalant gases, perineal infiltration, pudendal block, saddle block, and epidural anesthesia. Methods used for analgesia during the first stage, such as continuous epidural anesthesia, may be enough to carry the patient through the second stage, but in most cases supplementary anesthesia is needed.

During the late first and second stages of labor the patient can be given the inhalant gases to promote analgesia. The gas is given only during the contraction and in small concentration; the patient remains conscious. As the head is being born the plane of anesthesia must be deepened to eliminate the severe pain as the presenting part passes through the introitus.

Inhalant Anesthesia

NITROUS OXIDE AND OXYGEN

Pleasant to take and nonflammable, nitrous oxide gas is efficient in supplying analgesia during the last part of the first stage, as well as light analgesia and anesthesia during the second and third stages. Deep anesthesia requires the addition of one of the anesthetic vapors, nitrous oxide being used for the induction.

Effects on the Mother   There are a number of effects:

1. Nitrous oxide is soluble in the tissues and diffuses rapidly so that both induction and recovery are rapid.
2. It is nontoxic, and the patient feels well after the administration is discontinued. The gas can be given for long periods.
3. It is used as an analgesic by giving it to the patient with each pain, so relief is achieved quickly. The patient is told to take three breaths and to hold the third as she bears down.
4. The depth of the anesthesia can be altered quickly.
5. As the head is being born one of the rapidly acting vapors (Trilene, cyclopropane, Fluothane) must be added to deepen the anesthesia.
6. With safe mixtures of nitrous oxide and oxygen the degree of relaxation is not enough to perform difficult maneuvers such as forceps extractions or versions.
7. Unless anoxia is produced there is no untoward effect on the circulatory, respiratory, or nervous systems.
8. The disadvantage is that a 4:1 mixture of nitrous oxide/oxygen is needed to produce first plane anesthesia. Deepening the anesthesia by reducing the percentage of oxygen carries the risk of anoxia and is dangerous.

ETHER

Given by the simple open drop method ethyl ether has a wide margin of safety for the mother. It does not produce analgesia without anesthesia and cannot be given intermittently with the contractions as can nitrous oxide.

Effects on the Mother These are both good and bad:

1. It does not damage the liver.
2. At levels used for obstetrics, the respiratory or circulatory systems are not depressed.
3. Once induction has been accomplished by nitrous oxide, a small concentration of ether is enough to maintain the anesthesia.
4. Ether is irritating to the respiratory passages and causes much secretion, making prolonged induction unpleasant to the patient.
5. The delayed recovery period is associated with nausea and vomiting.

Effects on the Baby Ether crosses the placental barrier. Its elimination from mother and child are slow, and if deep and prolonged anesthesia is required the baby becomes depressed.

Effect on Labor Enough relaxation of the myometrium is attainable to permit intrauterine manipulations. This relaxation can persist into the third stage with resultant hemorrhage from an atonic uterus. When enough ether is given for complete anesthesia, the strength of the uterine contractions is reduced.

CYCLOPROPANE
Cyclopropane is a useful and potent anesthetic.

Advantages There are several:

1. It is given with a high concentration of oxygen, thus lessening the danger of respiratory depression. Mixtures of 10 percent cyclopropane and 90 percent oxygen are enough to induce first plane anesthesia, while 13 to 25 percent cyclopropane provides moderate muscle relaxation.
2. It takes 12 to 15 minutes for the fetal concentration to reach the same level as in the mother. If the baby is born within 8 minutes of the onset of anesthesia, it is not profoundly depressed.
3. It acts rapidly—two or three breaths achieve analgesia, while four to five permit episiotomy.
4. All levels of anesthesia can be attained.
5. It is eliminated rapidly, so recovery is complete soon after the anesthetic is discontinued.
6. It is pleasant to take.

Disadvantages   Included are:

1. It is extremely flammable and even explosive.
2. It should be used only by expert anesthetists.
3. Cardiac arrhythmias, fibrillation, and, rarely, cardiac arrest occur more often than with other anesthetic agents. The danger is increased if pituitary extracts and adrenaline have been used.
4. There is increased bleeding from incised wounds, but excessive uterine hemorrhage is related to the depth of the anesthesia.

HALOTHANE: FLUOTHANE

Fluothane is a liquid the anesthetic potency of which is twice that of chloroform and four times that of ether. It acts so rapidly that an excessive depth of anesthesia can be produced before the inexperienced person realizes it. Since the margin of safety is small, observation must be constant; only trained anesthetists should use this drug.

This is a pleasant anesthetic for the patient. Induction and recovery are so short that coughing or vomiting is seen rarely. It is not inflammable and not explosive.

Fluothane has an effect on the myometrium comparable to that of chloroform. Complete uterine relaxation is attainable quickly. Fluothane may have a place when intrauterine manipulations are to be performed, or in emergencies such as prolapse of the cord, where rapid anesthesia and relaxation of muscle is essential. However, because of its effect on the myometrium, an increased incidence of atonic postpartum hemorrhage has been reported.

Aspiration of Vomitus During Anesthesia

Aspiration of vomitus and the resultant pulmonary infection is a great danger. Because of delayed emptying during labor there is often undigested food, fluid, and gas in the stomach at delivery. Regurgitation and vomiting may take place. While the patient is recovering from the anesthetic, the cough reflex is poor and aspiration is especially dangerous at this time. Women in labor should be given no solid food and a limited amount of clear fluids. If hydration is a problem glucose solution should be infused by vein.

When vomiting does occur the patient must be placed in Trendelenburg position to promote postural drainage, and the airway must be cleaned with an efficient suction machine. If the patient has eaten a large meal within 6 hours of delivery, inhalation anesthesia is unwise.

Aspiration during or following anesthesia can be divided into two groups.

ASPIRATION OF PARTICULATE MATTER

Regurgitation and aspiration of particulate material produces the classic picture of bronchial obstruction and atelectasis. This is an acute, serious, and dramatic situation which, if not treated rapidly and effectively, can lead to the patient's choking and then death. The condition develops quickly and diagnosis is easy. Treatment includes postural drainage, removal of the debris with suction, and when necessary bronchoscopy to reestablish patency of the airway. Antibiotics are given to control pulmonary infection.

MENDELSON'S SYNDROME

This is produced by the aspiration, often silent, of highly acidic gastric fluid, resulting in a chemical or allergic tracheitis and pneumonitis. The bronchiolar spasm and the peribronchial congestive and exudative reaction interferes with the pulmonary circulation to a degree that cardiac failure may supervene. The patient develops pulmonary edema with the production of large amounts of pink, frothy sputum, progressively worsening cyanosis, tachycardia, tachypnea, and hypotension. The massive outpouring of fluid may lead to hypovolemic shock. The patient becomes restless and agitated. Diffuse bronchi are heard on ausculation and x-ray of the chest reveals mottled densities.

Prevention of Mendelson's Syndrome

1. Since anxiety increases gastric acidity, patients due to undergo surgery need adequate sedation.
2. Since lack of food increases gastric acidity, excessive periods of fasting before surgery should be avoided.
3. The role of gastric acidity has been established clearly in the condition of aspiration pneumonitis. It has been suggested that the patient at risk be defined as that patient who has at least 25 ml of gastric juice of pH below 2.5 in the stomach at delivery. Therefore, anything that either raises the gastric pH to above 2.5 or reduces the volume of gastric fluid to below 25 ml can reduce the number of patients at risk. Each patient in labor is given an oral dose of 15 to 30 ml of liquid magnesium trisilicate every 2 to 3 hours during labor and 45 to 60 minutes before elective cesarean section.
4. There must be alertness to the problem during and following anesthesia. Careful monitoring is essential in the recovery room.
5. Proper intubation during anesthesia is important.
6. The avoidance of general anesthesia for vaginal and abdominal deliveries may be the most efficient measure for the prevention

of aspiration. Certainly, inhalation anesthesia should not be used if the patient has eaten recently.

Treatment of Mendelson's Syndrome

1. Irrigation of the tracheobronchial tree is performed using 250 to 400 ml of normal saline to dilute and wash out the acidic aspirant.
2. Bronchoscopy is unnecessary unless obstruction is suspected, but prompt suctioning decreases the amount of gastric juice and removes bits of food and particulate epithelial matter from the pharynx.
3. The administration of 100 percent oxygen by positive pressure is the mainstay of supportive therapy.
4. Hydrocortisone, 1 g every 6 hours, is given intravenously for 1 to 2 days. This is followed by 1 g daily for another 1 to 3 days.
5. The patient is monitored by serial hematocrits and central venous pressure determinations when necessary.
6. Plasma or high molecular substitutes may be needed to replace the lost blood volume.
7. Excessive fluids may aggravate the pulmonary edema, and diuretics are useful on such cases.
8. Digitalization may be needed.
9. Antibiotics are used to prevent infection.

Prognosis In most cases recovery will be rapid, with noticeable improvement within 12 hours and functional clearing in 24 hours. Radiologic changes will remain for several days following clinical recovery.

Local Anesthesia

The two methods of local anesthesia are (1) direct infiltration of the perineal tissues and (2) pudendal nerve block. Local anesthesia is one of the best choices for obstetrics, but nervous, high-strung women and impatient doctors are not associated with a high rate of success.

ADVANTAGES

1. The technique is simple. The obstetrician should administer the drug himself.
2. There are no ill effects on the vital organs; respiratory function is not depressed; and fatalities (with the exception of the rare drug allergy) are almost unknown. It is useful for women with heart disease, tuberculosis, and similar diseases.
3. The baby's vital functions are not affected; it is not narcotized; and the respiratory center is not depressed. It is a good method for premature infants.
4. There is no nausea or vomiting.
5. The cough reflex is not depressed, and there is no danger of aspirating vomitus.
6. The mother is awake during the delivery.
7. There is no interference with uterine contractions, and therefore postpartum bleeding is minimal.
8. Since the baby is not affected there is no need to hurry, and the delivery can be performed gently and carefully.
9. Postpartum nursing care is easy.
10. There is little or no effect on other parts of the body, and the vital centers are not depressed. Under proper control the complications are minimal.

DISADVANTAGES

1. Not every patient is suitable.
2. The technique does not work in every case. Practice is needed to acquire proficiency.
3. In rare instances the needle breaks.
4. Care must be taken not to inject into a blood vessel, since intravenous injection may cause convulsions, cardiac arrest, or even death.
5. The rare person is allergic to the anesthetic agent, and every patient should be asked about a history of drug sensitivity.
6. Carelessness in technique may lead to sepsis.
7. A blood vessel may be torn during the procedure, leading to formation of a hematoma.
8. Only perineal pain is relieved. The discomfort from the uterine contractions continues.
9. If extensive operative work is necessary, additional anesthesia (usually inhalatory) must be administered.

Direct Infiltration Anesthesia

The main purpose of perineal infiltration is to permit incision and repair of episiotomy, as well as suturing of lacerations (Fig. 2).

TECHNIQUE

1. Because of its rapid and profound action we prefer 1 percent Xylocaine (lidocaine hydrochloride). Procaine or Metycaine can also be used. For the average case 30 to 50 ml of solution is sufficient.
2. Either of two approaches may be used:
   a. The needle is inserted at the posterior fourchette and the injections made laterad.
   b. The needle is inserted at a point halfway between the anus and the ischial tuberosity and the injections made toward the midline.
3. With a small 25 gauge needle a wheal is made by injecting a small amount of the solution into the skin at the point where the needle is to be inserted.
4. The needle is then changed to a No. 20, which is inserted through the wheal. Multiple injections are made into the subcutaneous tissue, muscles, and fascia.
5. The area to be anesthetized is triangular in shape, the angles being the clitoris, the perianal region, and the point halfway between the anus and the tuberosity.

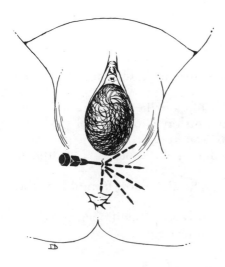

FIG. 2. Local anesthesia: direct infiltration.

6. During the procedure the plunger of the syringe must be pulled back repeatedly to be sure that the needle is not in a blood vessel.
7. Adequate anesthesia is achieved in about 5 minutes.

ADVANTAGES
1. The technique is simple; no special anatomic knowledge is necessary.
2. The rate of success is almost 100 percent.
3. The injection can be made at any time, even when the head is on the perineum.

DISADVANTAGES
Complete perineal anesthesia is not achieved. Only the infiltrated areas are affected.

Pudendal Nerve Block

The time of administration of pudendal anesthesia is important to its success. Once the head or breech is distending the perineum, it is too late. In primigravidas the injection is made when the cervix is fully dilated and the presenting part is at station +2. In multiparas the anesthetic is given when the cervix is dilated 7 to 8 cm. Pudendal anesthesia is sufficient for spontaneous delivery or low forceps extraction, for breech deliveries, and for episiotomy and repair of lacerations. Many obstetricians combine pudendal block with local infiltration, described above.

PERCUTANEOUS TRANSPERINEAL APPROACH

The anesthetic agent (1 or 2 percent Xylocaine, procaine, or Mety-caine) is injected around the pudendal nerve through a 5-inch 20-gauge needle. After a wheal has been raised the needle is inserted through the skin midway between the anus and the ischial tuberosity. With a finger in the vagina as a guide (some prefer to put the finger in the rectum), the needle is directed through the ischial fossa toward the posterior surface of the ischial spine. As the needle nears the spine the vaginal finger directs it posteriorly toward the inferior tip of the spine and into the pudendal canal (Fig. 3). When the needle is in the canal, free from muscle and ligament, it can be moved back and forth without resistance. If it is not in the correct place it must be withdrawn 3 to 4 cm and reinserted. One method of ensuring correct location of the needle tip is to aspirate the pudendal vessels. Once this is accomplished the needle is withdrawn from the blood vessel and reinserted medially, where the pudendal nerve lies.

The anesthetic solution (10 ml) is deposited; 3 ml is injected beneath the inferior tip of the spine. The needle is then introduced a little deeper, and another 3 ml is placed into the canal just under the superior tip of the spine. The needle is then inserted a little beyond the spine into the greater sciatic notch, where 4 ml is injected. This last injection catches the inferior hemorrhoidal nerve in the patient where it arises as a separate branch from the fourth sacral nerve. Effective anesthesia is achieved in about 15 minutes.

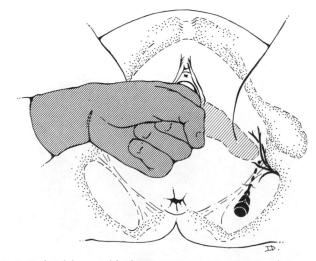

FIG. 3. Pudendal nerve block: percutaneous transperineal approach.

TRANSVAGINAL TECHNIQUE

The vaginal route is simple, effective, and safe. The ischial spine is palpable easily through the vagina, and the point where the sacrospinous ligament is attached to it serves as the landmark to locate the pudendal nerve.

A 10- or 20-ml syringe with a 5-inch 20-gauge needle is used. The left pudendal nerve is anesthetized first. The ischial spine is located with the vaginal fingers (left hand). The syringe is held in the right hand. The needle is placed in the groove formed by the apposition of the first and second fingers of the left hand, or the tip of the needle may be pressed against the ball of the index finger. Protected by the fingers the needle is placed into the vagina to the tip of the ischial spine (Fig. 4). The syringe is held above the left hand so that the needle can be directed laterally and downward to enter the vaginal mucosa over the sacrospinous ligament and posterior and medial to the tip of the ischial spine. The needle is inserted into the sacrospinous ligament and 3 ml is injected. The needle is pushed deeper; as it enters the loose tissue behind the ligament, resistance ceases and the fluid flows in easily. Aspiration is attempted to guard against the needle's being in a blood vessel, and then 7 to 8 ml is injected behind the ligament. The needle is withdrawn and the procedure repeated on the right side.

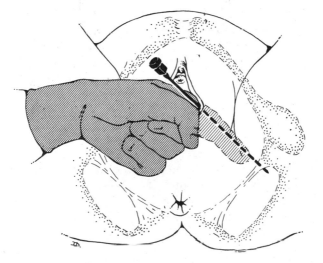

FIG. 4. Pudendal nerve block: transvaginal route.

Continuous Lumbar Epidural Analgesia and Anesthesia

Most of the pain of the first stage of labor is conducted from the uterus via the sympathetic pathways to the 11th and 12th thoracic segments. During this stage it is not only unnecessary but undesirable to block the sacral roots. To do so would prematurely relax the muscles of the pelvic floor and interfere with flexion and rotation of the baby's head as it passes through the birth canal. Later the pain caused by the distention of the perineum by the presenting part can be relieved by anesthetizing the sacral segments.

Subarachnoid blocks (spinal anesthesia) cause marked motor paralysis, the ability of the patient to bear down is poor or absent, and operative delivery is necessary. With epidural injection, solutions are used which are strong enough to block the small pain fibers but not the large motor nerves. Hence the patient feels no pain but is able to cooperate well during the delivery, bearing down when asked to do so. Sometimes the patient loses the urge to bear down and must be told when she is having a contraction and instructed to force down. This occurs after the perineal dose has taken effect.

TECHNIQUE

While a single shot epidural block is effective for the delivery, the continuous method is better as it provides analgesia for the greater part of the labor as well. The needle is inserted in the epidural (or extradural) space; it does not enter the spinal canal.

The patient lies on her side. A No. 17 Tuohy needle (some anesthetists prefer an 18-gauge, thin-walled, short-leveled needle) is inserted into the second or third lumbar interspace with the orifice of the needle pointing toward the head. Epidural puncture is made using the loss of resistance technic. A dose of 5 to 10 ml of the anesthetic solution is injected into the epidural (extradural) space. A vinyl plastic catheter is inserted through the needle, which is removed over the catheter. The patient is turned on her back and another 3 to 5 ml of solution is injected. This is to avoid the pooling of the agent on one side and consequent unilateral analgesia. Usually, subjective relief of pain starts to develop within 3 to 5 minutes, and maximal effect is present in 8 to 15 minutes. If there is no evidence of analgesia by 10 minutes, it is likely that the drug was injected outside of the epidural space. When the analgesic effect wears off, more solution is injected through the catheter. The optimal time to institute this analgesic method is when labor is well established in the active phase, and the cervix is dilated to 4 to 6 cm in primigravidas and 3 to 4 cm in multiparas.

Satisfactory drugs include buvipacaine (Marcaine) (0.25 to 0.5 percent), lidocaine (0.5 to 1.0 percent), and mepivacaine (0.5 to 1.0 percent). The lower strengths are preferable, and only when these are ineffective are the stronger concentrations employed. Marcaine produces analgesia for 2.5 to 3 hours. To avoid interference with the uterine contractions and to obviate paralysis of the perineal muscles (which would interfere with the mechanism of internal rotation of the fetal head), two approaches are available. One is to use segmental epidural block so that the sacral nerves are spared. The other is to employ a low concentration of local anesthetic. This is sufficient to provide relief of pain from uterine contractions without producing significant block of the motor nerves.

As the cervix becomes fully dilated and the head descends, the patient feels pain in the lower pelvis and rectum. The last injection (perineal dose) is given after internal rotation is complete and just prior to delivery. Higher concentrations are used to assure perineal relaxation. In some cases it is advantageous to sit the patient up for 5 minutes, or to position her at a 45° angle, to allow the anesthetic solution to descend to the sacral roots. If the block interrupts the afferent sacral nerves the patient may lose the urge to bear down. However, she will respond to encouragement to bear down when the contraction sets in.

ADVANTAGES

1. Almost the entire labor can be made pain-free. In a difficult case epidural analgesia brings about a marked change for the better in the patient's general condition and morale. In addition, the relatives are placated.
2. The effect can be maintained as long as necessary.
3. The level of anesthesia is controllable by posture.
4. The mother is alert and cooperative. She retains the ability to bear down. Delivery may be spontaneous, but even if forceps are used the patient can help by pushing down while the operator is exerting traction.
5. The anesthesia is complete and brings about good relaxation. It permits operative deliveries to be performed carefully and without haste.
6. Epidural techniques are of value in trials of labor. Should cesarean section be necessary the same anesthetic is used.
7. There are no postspinal headaches.
8. There is no effect on the fetus, unless marked hypotension occurs.

DISADVANTAGES

1. There is danger of masking the strength of the uterine contrac-

tions to the point where uterine rupture occurs. This risk is increased by the use of oxytocin.

2. Significant hypotension, a drop of 20 mm Hg systolic or diastolic, occurs in close to one-third of patients. The epidural anesthetic causes sympathetic blockade, leading to vasodilation, visceral pooling of blood, decreased peripheral resistance, reduced venous return, and a decrease of cardiac output. The consequent decrease in uterine and placental perfusion may affect the fetus. The supine position may aggravate the problem. The patient should be placed on her left side.

3. FHR patterns may be affected. In most cases epidural anesthesia has no adverse effects on the fetus. Occasionally late decelerations are noted. These may result from a toxic effect of the local anesthetic on the fetus, but it is more likely to represent an effect of hypoxia resulting from decreased maternofetal exchange.

4. Accidental intravascular injection or too rapid absorption may cause twitching, convulsions, or loss of consciousness.

5. The dura may be punctured. Because of the large size of the Tuohy needle severe headache may result.

6. Rarely, there is infection at the site of injection.

7. A few patients have reported backache.

8. In a few cases the catheter has broken and a small piece is left in situ. It causes no ill effects.

9. Occasionally the uterine contractions become weaker and less frequent. An oxytocin infusion then improves the labor and brings about good progress.

10. With large doses the patient loses the desire and the ability to bear down. The increased use of midforceps constitutes the most significant complication of the second stage.

CONTRAINDICATIONS

1. Rapid, easy labor
2. Diseases of the central nervous system
3. Spinal lesions
4. Patients receiving anticoagulant therapy
5. Patients who have an hemorrhagic diathesis
6. Hypotension
7. The low back pain syndrome
8. Skin infection
9. Opposition from the patient

SAFEGUARDS AND PRECAUTIONS

1. The dosage is half that required for surgery.
2. The injection is not made during a uterine contraction because the solution is forced too high.
3. Oxygen should be available with means of applying positive pressure for artificial respiration.
4. Intravenous fluids and vasopressors must be at hand in case there is hypotension.
5. An intravenous barbiturate must be prepared for treating the patient should convulsions result from accidental intravascular injection.
6. During the delivery the mother is given oxygen by mask to increase the blood levels, thereby providing the baby with as much oxygen as possible.

Spinal Anesthesia: Saddle Block

Saddle block is a low spinal anesthetic confined to the perineal area. In practice the region of anesthesia is a little more widespread than the saddle area, but this does not interfere with the aims of the technique. With the addition of glucose to the anesthetic agent the solution is made hyperbaric. The subarachnoid injection is made with the patient in a sitting position, so that the heavy solution gravitates downward. The length of time that the patient sits up determines the level of anesthesia. Five minutes is sufficient. In this way complete anesthesia of the perineal region is attained, the perineal muscles are relaxed, and there is partial loss of sensation in the abdomen and thighs. The sympathetic fibers that carry the feeling of pain from the uterus are blocked, and the pains of labor are relieved or abolished. The injection must not be made during a contraction because the agent would be forced to too high a level.

While uterine contractions do not cease and there is no increase in uterine atony and postpartum hemorrhage, effective progress of labor halts, so this anesthetic is used terminally. The patient is not able to deliver the baby herself, and extraction with forceps is necessary. Hence the anesthetic can be given only when labor has reached the point where easy low forceps can be performed. The cervix must be fully dilated.

ADVANTAGES AND DISADVANTAGES

Terminal spinal is an excellent anesthetic, especially for difficult deliveries, since it provides good anesthesia and excellent relaxation and is easier to administer than epidural anesthesia.

However, spinal anesthesia has certain disadvantages that limit its field of usefulness:

1. Postspinal headaches, which occur in almost 10 percent, can cause prolonged discomfort.
2. Bladder dysfunction is frequent.
3. Occasionally paresthesias of the lower limbs and abdomen develop, and sometimes there is a temporary loss or diminution of sensation in these areas.
4. Unilateral footdrop has occurred.
5. A rare complication is nerve damage, such as chronic progressive adhesive arachnoiditis or transverse myelitis. These lead to paralysis of the lower part of the body.
6. Several deaths have been reported, although their exact mechanism is not known.
7. In a few instances the anesthetic solution has risen in the subarachnoid space high enough to produce difficulty with respiration.
8. The incidence of forceps deliveries is increased.
9. Patients with bleeding problems or shock should not be given this type of anesthesia.

ANESTHESIA FOR CESAREAN SECTION

There is no single "best" anesthesia for cesarean section. Every method has its good and bad features. The choice of the technique to be employed is based on the indication for the operation, the presence of general maternal problems (e.g., heart disease, pulmonary complications), the condition of the fetus, and the availability of trained personnel. The three main types of anesthesia used today are local, spinal or epidural, and general.

Local Anesthesia

Several agents are available, among them procaine (Novocain) as a 0.5 percent solution, lidocaine (Xylocaine), and mepivacaine (Carbocaine). Addition of adrenaline to make a dilution of 1:200,000 delays absorption and prolongs the effect of the anesthetic. About 300 ml of the solution is used.

TECHNIQUE

Atropine 0.4 mg is given as premedication 30 minutes before surgery. In nervous patients this may be combined with 50 mg of Demerol.

A skin wheal is made just below the umbilicus with a 25-gauge needle. A 20-gauge needle, 4 inches long, is used to inject the solution intradermally and subcutaneously down to the pubic symphysis for a distance of about 3 cm on each side of the midline. After a few minutes have passed the skin and subcutaneous tissue are incised. The tissue must be handled gently and a minimum amount of traction exerted.

The anterior sheath of the rectus muscle is infiltrated in the same way, in the midline and out to the sides to block the nerves at the lateral margins of the recti. A large amount of solution is placed in the suprapubic region, since this is the area of highest sensitivity. The fascia is then incised.

The peritoneum is anesthetized and opened to expose the uterus. About 50 to 60 ml of anesthetic is injected under the bladder flap and spread with the fingers under the bladder and to the sides. The bladder peritoneum is cut and pushed caudad.

The uterus is then opened, the baby extracted, the placenta removed, and the incision closed. The nervous patient may be put to sleep with Pentothal just prior to incision of the uterus.

ADVANTAGES

Except for the rare instance of sensitivity to the anesthetic agent or intravascular injection, this method is completely safe for the mother. There is also no ill effect on the fetus (no respiratory depression).

DISADVANTAGES

1. The patient must be prepared to accept this type of anesthetic. It is not suitable for the nervous or hyperexcitable woman.
2. The method is time-consuming and is not good for cases in which rapid operating is necessary.
3. The surgeon must be gentle, patient, and willing to accept slow operating.

General Anesthesia

TECHNIQUE

1. Atropine 0.4 mg is given intramuscularly 30 to 60 minutes prior to surgery.

2. An intravenous infusion of 5 percent glucose in water is set up.
3. Anesthesia is insitituted with 250 mg of Pentothal (2.5 percent solution).
4. Succinylcholine 100 mg is given intravenously to promote muscle relaxation.
5. An endotracheal tube is inserted.
6. The anesthesia is maintained by intermittent positive pressure with nitrous oxide and oxygen.
7. Muscle relaxation is achieved by a succinylcholine drip.
8. Two to three minutes prior to delivery of the baby the amount of nitrous oxide is reduced, and oxygen and succinylcholine are continued.
9. No more Pentothal is given until the umbilical cord is clamped, at which time the agent can be injected to deepen the level of anesthesia if this is desired.
10. Timing is important, and to avoid respiratory depression in the infant at least 10 minutes should elapse between injection of the Pentothal and the uterine incision.

ADVANTAGES

1. It is highly acceptable to the patient.
2. There is no hypotension.
3. It is effective in cases of hemorrhage or fetal distress, when speed is important.
4. Fetal depression or asphyxia are rare.

DISADVANTAGES

1. The timing must be accurate or fetal depression may occur.
2. An experienced anesthesiologist is essential to success.

Lumbar Epidural and Spinal Anesthesia

TECHNIQUE
This has been described in a previous section.

ADVANTAGES
The use of drugs that depress the infant can be avoided. In those cases in which a trial of labor is being carried on under epidural analgesia, the same anesthetic can be continued for the cesarean section.

DISADVANTAGE

Maternal hypotension is frequent and may be accompanied by fetal bradycardia.

PREMATURE INFANTS

Premature babies have a low resistance to sedatives, analgesics, and general anesthetics. Small amounts of these agents (whose effects on term babies may be minor) depress the respiratory center of the small fetus to the extent of causing severe apnea and asphyxia. Delay in the onset of breathing can result in anoxic brain damage.

We avoid prescribing sedatives and analgesics during labor and where possible do not employ general anesthesia for the delivery. If the patient is able to carry on, we deliver the baby under local infiltration or perineal block. In cases where the pains of labor are severe and the patient needs help, a continuous lumbar epidural block is instituted. This relieves or abolishes the pain of labor and is an excellent anesthetic for the actual delivery. As the baby is being born the mother is given oxygen by mask. In this way the respiratory center of the fetus is protected during both labor and delivery.

MEDICAL COMPLICATIONS OF PREGNANCY

1. *Preeclampsia and eclampsia:* For vaginal delivery regional anesthesia is best. Epidural is good. For cesarean section either regional block or balanced general anesthesia is satisfactory.
2. *Diabetes:* In general regional anesthesia is best both for vaginal delivery and cesarean section.
3. *Cardiac disease:* Epidural is best for vaginal delivery. General anesthesia is preferred for cesarean section.

BIBLIOGRAPHY

Baggish MS, Hooper S: Aspiration as a cause of maternal death. Obstet Gynecol 43:327, 1974

Beck NC, Hall D: Natural childbirth. Obstet Gynecol 52:371, 1978

Bloom SL, Horswill CW, Curet LB: Effects of paracervical blocks in the fetus during labor: a prospective study with the use of the direct fetal monitoring. Obstet Gynecol 114:218, 1972

Brackbill Y, Kane J, Maniello RL, Abramson D: Obstetric meperidine usage and assessment of neonatal state. Anesthesiology 40:116, 1974

OBSTETRIC ANALGESIA AND ANESTHESIA

Crcc JE, Meyer J, Hailey DM: Diazepam in labor: its metabolism and effect on the clinical condition and thermogenesis of the newborn. Br Med J 3 Nov 76:251

Johnson WL, Winter WW, Eng M, et al: Effect of pudendal, spinal, and peridural block anesthesia on the second stage of labor. Am J Obstet Gynecol 113:116, 1972

LeHew WL: Paracervical block in obstetrics. Am J Obstet Gynecol 113:1079, 1972

Mandelli M, Morselli PL, Nordio S, et al: Placental transfer of diazepam and its disposition in the newborn. Clin Pharmacol Ther 17:564, 1975

Morrison JC, Wiser WL, Rosser SI, et al: Metabolites of meperidine related to fetal depression. Am J Obstet Gynecol 115:1132, 1973

Ranney B, Stanage WF. Advantages of local anesthesia for cesarean section. Obstet Gynecol 45:163, 1975

Roberts RB, Shirley MA: The obstetrician's role in reducing the risk of aspiration pneumonitis. Am J Obstet Gynecol 124:611, 1976

Wingate, MB, Wingate L, Iffy L, et al: The effect of epidural analgesia upon fetal and neonatal status. Am J Obstet Gynecol 119:1101, 1974

32.

Postpartum Hemorrhage

The term postpartum hemorrhage, in its wider meaning, includes all bleeding following the birth of the baby: before, during, and after the delivery of the placenta. By definition, loss of over 500 ml of blood during the first 24 hours constitutes postpartum hemorrhage. After 24 hours it is called late postpartum hemorrhage. The incidence of postpartum hemorrhage is about 10 percent.

At normal delivery an average of 200 ml of blood is lost. Episiotomy raises this figure by 100 ml and sometimes more. Pregnant women have an increased amount of blood and fluid, enabling the healthy patient to lose 500 ml without serious effect. To the anemic patient, however, an even smaller amount of bleeding can be dangerous.

CLINICAL FEATURES

Clinical Picture

The clinical picture is one of continuing bleeding and gradual deterioration. The pulse becomes rapid and weak; the blood pressure falls; the patient turns pale and cold; and there is shortness of breath, air hunger, sweating, and finally coma and death. A treacherous feature of the situation is that because of compensatory vascular mechanisms the pulse and blood pressure may show only moderate change for some time. Then suddenly the compensatory function can no longer be maintained, the pulse rises quickly, the blood pressure drops suddenly, and the patient is in shock. The uterus can fill up with considerable blood, which is lost to the patient even though there may be little external hemorrhage.

Danger of Postpartum Hemorrhage

The danger of postpartum hemorrhage is twofold. First, the resultant anemia weakens the patient, lowers her resistance, and predisposes to puerperal infection. Second, if the loss of blood is not arrested, death will be the final result.

Studies of Maternal Deaths

Studies of maternal deaths show that women have died from continuous bleeding of amounts which at the times were not alarming. It is not the sudden gush that kills, but the steady trickle. In a large series of cases Beacham found that the average interval between delivery and death was 5 hours 20 minutes. No woman died within 1 hour 30 minutes of giving birth. This suggests that there is adequate time for effective therapy if the patient has been observed carefully, the diagnosis made early, and proper treatment instituted.

ETIOLOGY

The causes of postpartum hemorrhage fall into four main groups.

Uterine Atony

The control of postpartum bleeding is by contraction and retraction of the myometrial fibers. This causes kinking of the blood vessels and so cuts off flow to the placental site. Failure of this mechanism resulting from disordered myometrial function is called uterine atony and is the main cause of postpartum hemorrhage. While the occasional case of postpartum uterine atony is completely unexpected, in many instances the presence of predisposing factors alerts the observant physician to the possibility of trouble.

1. Uterine dysfunction: Primary uterine atony is an intrinsic dysfunction of the uterus.
2. Mismanagement of the placental stage: The most common error is to try to hurry the third stage. Kneading and squeezing the uterus interferes with the physiologic mechanism of placental detachment and may cause partial placental separation with resultant bleeding.

3. Anesthesia: Deep and prolonged inhalation anesthesia is a common cause. There is excessive relaxation of the myometrium, failure of contraction and retraction, uterine atony, and postpartum hemorrhage.
4. Ineffective uterine action: Ineffective uterine action during the first two stages of labor is likely to be followed by poor contraction and retraction during the third stage.
5. Overdistention of the uterus: The uterus that has been overdistended by conditions such as large baby, multiple pregnancy, and polyhydramnios has a tendency to contract poorly.
6. Exhaustion from prolonged labor: Not only is the tired uterus likely to contract weakly after delivery of the baby, but the worn-out mother is less able to stand loss of blood.
7. Multiparity: The uterus that has borne many children is prone to inefficient action during all stages of labor.
8. Myomas of the uterus: By interfering with proper contraction and retraction, uterine myomas predispose to hemorrhage.
9. Operative deliveries: This includes operative procedures such as mid forceps and version and extraction.

Trauma and Lacerations

Considerable bleeding can take place from tears sustained during normal and operative deliveries. The birth canal should be inspected after each delivery so that the sources of bleeding can be controlled.

Sites of hemorrhage include:

1. Episiotomy. Blood loss may reach 200 ml. When arterioles or large varicose veins are cut or torn the amount of blood lost can be considerably more. Hence bleeding vessels should be clamped immediately to conserve blood.
2. Vulva, vagina, and cervix.
3. Ruptured uterus.
4. Uterine inversion.
5. Puerperal hematomas.

In addition, other factors operate to cause an excessive loss of blood where there is trauma to the birth canal. These include:

1. Prolonged interval between performance of the episiotomy and delivery of the child.
2. Undue delay from birth of the baby to repair of the episiotomy.

3. Failure to secure bleeding vessel at the apex of the episiotomy.
4. Neglecting to inspect upper vagina and cervix.
5. Nonappreciation of the possibility of multiple sites of injury.
6. Undue reliance on oxytocic agents accompanied by too long a delay in exploring the uterus.

Retained Placenta

Retention in the uterus of part or all of the placenta interferes with contraction and retraction, keeps the blood sinuses open, and leads to postpartum hemorrhage. Once part of the placenta has separated from the uterine wall, there is bleeding from that area. The part of the placenta that is still attached prevents proper retraction, and bleeding goes on until the rest of the organ has separated and is expelled.

The retention of the whole placenta, part of it, a succenturiate lobe, a single cotyledon, or a fragment of placenta can cause postpartum bleeding. In some cases there is placenta accreta. There is no correlation between the amount of placenta retained and the severity of the hemorrhage. The important consideration is the degree of adherence.

Bleeding Disorders

Any of the hemorrhagic diseases (blood dyscrasias) can affect pregnant women and occasionally are responsible for postpartum hemorrhage.

Afibrinogenemia or hypofibrinogenemia may follow abruptio placenta, prolonged retention in utero of a dead fetus, and amniotic fluid embolism. One etiologic theory postulates that thromboplastic material arising from the degeneration and autolysis of the decidua and placenta may enter the maternal circulation and give rise to intravascular coagulation and loss of circulating fibrinogen. The condition, a failure of the clotting mechanism, causes bleeding that cannot be arrested by the measures usually employed to control hemorrhage.

INVESTIGATION

1. To obtain a reasonable idea of the amount of blood lost, an estimate is made and the figure doubled.
2. The uterine fundus is palpated frequently to make certain it is not filling up with blood.

3. The uterine cavity is explored both for placental remnants and for uterine rupture.
4. The vulva, vagina, and cervix are examined carefully for lacerations.
5. The pulse and blood pressure are measured and recorded.
6. A sample of blood is observed for clotting.

TREATMENT

Prophylaxis

1. Every pregnant woman should know her blood group.
2. Antepartum anemia is treated.
3. Certain patients are susceptible to and certain conditions predispose to postpartum hemorrhage. These include:
   a. Multiparity of more than five babies
   b. History of postpartum hemorrhage or manual removal of the placenta
   c. Abruptio placentae
   d. Placenta previa
   e. Multiple pregnancy
   f. Polyhydramnios
   g. Intrauterine death with prolonged retention of the dead fetus
   h. Prolonged labor
   i. Difficult forceps delivery
   j. Version and extraction
   k. Breech extraction
   l. Cesarean section
4. In cases where uterine atony is anticipated, an intravenous infusion is set up before the delivery and oxytocin added to ensure good uterine contractions. This is continued for at least 1 hour post partum.
5. Excessive and prolonged inhalatory anesthesia should be avoided.
6. As long as the child is in good condition and there is no need for rapid extraction, the body is delivered slowly. This facilitates placental separation and permits the uterus to retract sufficiently to control bleeding from the placental site.
7. Once the placenta has separated it should be expelled.
8. Squeezing or kneading the uterus before the placenta has separated is traumatic and harmful.
9. One of the ergot preparations or oxytocin is given after delivery

of the placenta to ensure good uterine contraction and retraction.
10. Careful postpartum observation of the patient is made, and the uterine fundus is palpated to prevent its filling with blood. The patient remains in the delivery room for at least 1 hour post partum.
11. Fibrinogen studies are done in cases of placental abruption and retained dead fetus.
12. When hemorrhage is anticipated adequate amounts of blood should be cross-matched and available.

Supportive Measures

1. The key to successful treatment is the transfusion of blood. The amount must be adequate to replace at least the amount lost. Usually a minimum of 1 liter is needed, and it is given quickly. When response to blood replacement is not satisfactory the following conditions must be considered:
   a. Continued unappreciated ooze
   b. Bleeding into an atonic uterus
   c. Silent filling of the vagina
   d. Bleeding behind and into a uterine pack
   e. Hematoma formation
   f. Intraperitoneal bleeding as with ruptured uterus
   g. Afibrinogenemia or hypofibrinogenemia
   h. Bacteremic shock
2. Until blood is available plasma expanders are used.
3. If the blood pressure is falling, the foot of the table is elevated.
4. General anesthesia should be discontinued and oxygen given by face mask.
5. Warmth is provided by blankets.
6. Morphine is given by hypodermic injection.
7. If afibrinogenemia is present, fibrinogen is administered intravenously; 2 to 6 g is injected. Because of the danger of serum hepatitis following the use of fibrinogen, the patient is given gamma globulin.

Placental Bleeding

In the presence of excessive bleeding associated with the third stage, no time should be wasted. Manual removal of the placenta is carried out immediately and oxytocics given. The uterus should not be manhandled in efforts to squeeze out the placenta.

Uterine Atony

UTERINE MASSAGE   The uterine fundus is massaged through the abdomen.

ERGOMETRINE   Ergometrine 0.125 or 0.25 mg is given intravenously and/or 0.5 mg intramuscularly.

OXYTOCIN   Oxytocin can be given intramuscularly, but the best method is by an intravenous drip with 5 or 10 units of oxytocin in a liter of 5 percent glucose in water. This is run at a speed sufficient to keep the uterus contracted.

UTERINE EXPLORATION   Manual exploration of the uterus is carried out, and blood clots and fragments of placenta and membrane are removed.

LACERATIONS   The cervix, vagina, and vulva are examined for lacerations.

UTERINE COMPRESSION   Bimanual compession of the uterus (Fig. 1) is a valuable method of controlling uterine atonic bleeding. One hand is placed in the vagina against the anterior wall of the uterus. Pressure is exerted against the posterior aspect of the uterus by the other hand through the abdomen. With a rotatory motion the uterus is compressed and massaged between the two hands. This provides twice the amount of uterine stimulation that can be achieved by abdominal massage alone. In addition, compression of the venous sinuses can be effected and the flow of blood reduced. As part of this procedure, the atonic uterus is elevated, anteverted, and anteflexed.

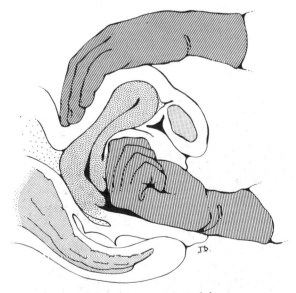

FIG. 1. Bimanual compression of the uterus.

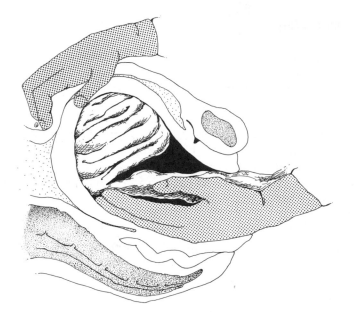

FIG. 2. Packing of the uterus.

UTERINE PACKING Packing the uterine cavity is a controversial subject (Fig. 2). Most authorities condemn its use in that the procedure is unphysiologic. Up to this point attempts had been made to empty the uterus; now it is to be filled. It is unlikely that a uterus that does not respond to powerful oxytocic drugs will be stimulated to contract by the gauze pack. It is impossible to pack an atonic uterus so tightly that the blood sinuses are closed off. The uterus simply balloons and fills up with more blood. Thus the packing not only does no good but is dangerous in that it leads to a false sense of security by obscuring the flow of blood. Ten yards of 3-inch packing gauze absorbs 1,000 ml of blood. Furthermore, packing favors infection.

Despite these antipacking arguments, many obstetricians believe that it is worth trying to control bleeding by this method before more radical measures are employed. The patient must be observed carefully. Deterioration of the vital signs, ballooning of the uterus, or continuation of the bleeding are signs that the pack is ineffective and must be removed. Packing must be done properly. One or two 5- or 10-yard rolls of gauze are needed. With one hand on the abdomen the operator steadies the uterine fundus, while the pack is pushed through the cervix and into the cavity of the uterus with the fingers of the other hand. The gauze is placed first into one corner of the uterus and then the other, so coming down the cavity from side to side. The uterus must be packed tightly. Then the vagina is packed. A large, firm pad is placed on the abdomen above the uterus, and a tight abdominal and perineal binder is applied. The gauze packing is removed in 12 hours.

COMPRESSION OF AORTA In thin women compression of the aorta against the spine may slow down the bleeding.

HYSTERECTOMY If the bleeding continues, the abdomen must be opened and hysterectomy performed. Deaths following and during hysterectomy have been reported; these resulted from delaying the operation until the patient was nearly moribund. Performed in time, hysterectomy is effective and lifesaving.

LIGATION OF UTERINE ARTERIES Since most of the uterine blood is supplied by the uterine arteries, their ligation can control postpartum hemorrhage. The collateral supply is sufficient to maintain the viability of the organ. The abdomen is opened, the uterus is elevated by the surgeon's hand, and the area of the uterine vessels are exposed. Using a large needle and No. 1 chromic catgut, the suture is placed through the myometrium of the lower segment of the uterus, 2 to 3 cm medial to the vessels. It is brought out through the avascular area of the broad ligament. A substantial amount of myometrium is included in the suture to occlude some of the inferior coronary branches of the uterine artery. In most cases the uterine vein is also ligated, but the hypertrophied ovarian veins drain the uterus adequately. The vessels are ligated, but not divided. Recanalization will take place in most cases. The uterus becomes blanched with a pink hue, and bleeding subsides. Subsequent menstruation and pregnancy are unaffected. Transvaginal ligation of the uterine arteries is a blind and hazardous procedure which is not recommended.

LIGATION OF INTERNAL ILIAC ARTERIES Internal iliac artery ligation may be performed in any situation in which pelvic bleeding is uncontrollable. Collateral circulation is so extensive that the pelvic arterial system is never deprived of blood, and there is no necrosis of any of the pelvic tissue. Entry into the abdomen is made by a midline or transverse incision. First the common iliac artery and its bifurcation into the external and internal iliac arteries is palpated and visualized through the posterior peritoneum. The ureter crosses anterior to the bifurcation of the common iliac artery, and it must be identified to prevent its being damaged. The posterior peritoneum is tented and incised in a longitudinal direction, beginning at the level of the origin of the internal iliac artery and extending caudad for 4 to 6 cm. This incision is lateral to the ureter and medial to the internal iliac artery. The ureter usually remains attached to the medial flap of peritoneum. Both the external and internal iliac arteries must be identified to be certain that the correct vessel is tied. Care is taken to avoid injury to the veins. Two No. 2-0 silk sutures are placed around the internal iliac artery 1 cm apart and then tied. The procedure is repeated on the other side.

Umbrella Pack Following Total Hysterectomy

Described by Logothetopulos in 1925, the umbrella pack (Fig. 3) is of value in desperate situations where, after hysterectomy, pelvic bleeding is uncontrollable even by such drastic measures as ligation of the internal iliac arteries.

TECHNIQUE

1. The outside of the pack is a 24-inch square piece of nonadhesive nylon (or cotton).
2. Into the center of this cloth is placed 15 to 20 yards of firm, non-compressible 2-inch gauze packing.
3. The four corners of the cloth are brought together to form a funnel-shaped sling, similar to a parachute, with the gauze packing inside.
4. The end of the gauze packing put in last is left protruding through the funnel.
5. The pack is placed in the true pelvis (the uterus having been removed previously) with the tail coming out through the vagina.
6. Traction on the tail pulls the bolus snugly into the pelvis, compressing the bleeding points. An intravenous bottle containing 1,000 ml of fluid is attached to the tail to provide traction. Sometimes two bottles are needed.
7. Traction is maintained for 24 hours. The pack is left in for 36 hours.
8. The pack is removed by pulling on the end of the gauze which is outside the vagina. Once the gauze is removed the nylon cloth container collapses and comes out easily.

Insertion of the pack is accomplished in one of two ways. Using the abdominal technique (Fig. 3) the pack is formed outside the patient and is inserted via the abdominal incision. A dressing forceps is passed up through the vagina, the tail of the pack is grasped, and it is pulled down and out. For the vaginal application the nylon square (Fig. 4) is held in front of the vulva, and its center is pushed up gradually through the vagina and into the pelvis by packing the gauze into the cloth, using a ring forceps (Fig. 5).

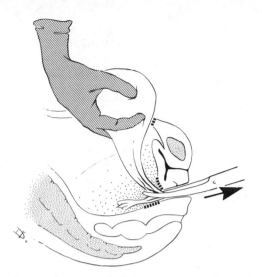

FIG. 3. Umbrella pack. Insertion through abdominal incision during laparotomy. The tail of the pack is pulled down through the vagina.

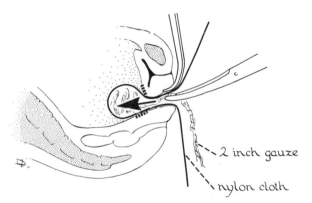

FIG. 4. Umbrella pack. Insertion thorugh vagina. The gauze is packed inside the nylon cloth.

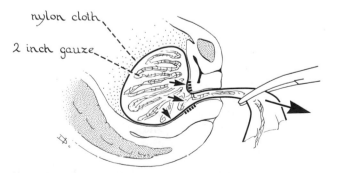

FIG. 5. Umbrella pack in place. Traction on the tail of the pack compresses the bleeding points.

COMPLICATIONS

1. Tangling of the gauze within the cloth makes its removal difficult.
2. The cloth may stick to the raw surfaces of the pelvis. Hence non-adherent nylon is best.
3. In rare cases the flow of urine is obstructed.
4. Serious infection has not been encountered; but where life-threatening hemorrhage is present, infection is a secondary consideration.

Lacerations

1. Rupture of the uterus necessitates laparotomy with either repair of the tear or hysterectomy.
2. Lacerations of the cervix, vagina, and vulva are repaired and the bleeding controlled with figure-8 sutures.
3. In some cases the bleeding from the vaginal tears cannot be controlled with sutures. Where there are large varicosities each passage of the needle through the tissue seems to provoke fresh bleeding. In such cases the vagina should be packed firmly with gauze that is left in for 24 hours.
4. Rarely, bleeding from a small superficial laceration in the lower uterine segment can be controlled by packing.

PITUITARY INSUFFICIENCY

Insufficiency of the anterior lobe of the pituitary gland was described by Simmonds in 1914. In 1937 Sheehan described the syndrome in women of childbearing age. Symptoms include:

1. Mammary involution and failure to lactate.
2. Weakness and lethargy
3. Hypersensitivity to cold
4. Diminished sweating.
5. Excessive involution of the uterus.
6. Atrophy of the external genitalia.
7. Amenorrhea or oligomenorrhea.
8. Loss of body hair, including the pubic area.
9. Absence of menopausal symptoms.

The condition is initiated by severe shock, the result of massive hemorrhage. The pituitary gland undergoes ischemia followed by necrosis. From 5 to 99 percent of the anterior lobe may be affected. As long as 10 percent of the gland is left in a functioning state, the patient will be in a reasonably normal condition. In severe cases death may occur. In less acute situations the patient can live for years in a subnormal state, a prey to infection.

The exact nature of the vascular disturbance is not known. Possible conditions include:

1. Arterial spasm
2. Arrest of the portal circulation of the pituitary
3. Coagulation in the capillaries
4. Venous thrombosis
5. Disseminated intravascular coagulation.

LATE POSTPARTUM HEMORRHAGE

Late postpartum hemorrhage is the loss of 500 ml of blood after the first 24 hours and within 6 weeks. While most of these episodes occur by the 21st day, the majority take place between the fourth and ninth postpartum days. The incidence is around 1 percent.

Nonuterine Bleeding

In a few cases the origin is the cervix, vagina, or vulva. Local infection leads to sloughing of sutures and dissolution of thrombi, with hemorrhage at the site of the episiotomy or lacerations. The amount of blood lost depends on the size of the vessels. Treatment includes cleaning out infected debris, suturing bleeding points, and if necessary, pressure packing the vagina. Blood transfusion is given as needed.

Uterine Bleeding

ETIOLOGY

1. Retained fragments of placenta
2. Intrauterine infection
3. Subinvolution of the uterus and the placental site
4. Uterine myoma, especially when submucous
5. Tendency to recurrence
6. Sometimes the use of estrogens to inhibit lactation

MECHANISM OF BLEEDING

The exact sequence of events is not known, but some type of sub-involution is present. Three probable factors are: (1) late detachment of thrombi at the placental site, with reopening of the vascular sinuses; (2) abnormalities in the separation of the decidua vera; and (3) intrauterine infection, leading to dissolution of the thromboses in the vessels. The basic mechanism is similar, regardless of whether placental tissue has been retained.

CLINICAL PICTURE

The amount of bleeding varies. Most of these patients require hospitalization and many need blood transfusion. A few go into shock.

TREATMENT

1. Oxytocics are given.
2. If bleeding continues, curettage is performed carefully, so as not to perforate the soft uterus. In many cases no placental tissue is found, the histologic examination showing organized blood clot, decidual tissue, or fragments of muscle. The results of curettage are satisfactory regardless of whether placenta was present. Removal of the inflamed tissue with its superficial bleeding vessels permits the uterus to contract around the deeper, healthier vessels, thus producing more effective hemostasis.
3. Blood is replaced by transfusion.
4. Antibiotics are given to control infection.
5. Repeat curettage may be necessary.
6. If all else fails, hysterectomy is performed.

BIBLIOGRAPHY

Hester JD: Postpartum hemorrhage and re-evaluation of uterine packing. Obstet Gynecol 45:501, 1975
Moszkowski EF: Postpartum pituitary insufficiency. South Med J 66:878, 1973
O'Leary JL, O'Leary JA: Uterine artery ligation for control of post cesarean section hemorrhage. Obstet Gynecol 43:849, 1974
Rome RM: Secondary postpartum hemorrhage. Br J Obstet Gynecol 82:289, 1975

33.

Antepartum Hemorrhage

Hemorrhage in the latter part of pregnancy poses a serious threat to the health and life of both mother and child. Placenta previa and abruptio placentae make up the vast majority of these cases.

CLASSIFICATION

1. Placenta previa
2. Abruptio placentae (premature separation)
3. Vasa previa
4. Rupture of marginal sinus
5. Local lesions
6. Idiopathic: no discoverable cause.

PLACENTA PREVIA

In this condition the placenta is implanted in the lower uterine segment and lies over or near the internal os of the cervix. It is in front of the presenting part of the fetus. The incidence is 1:200 pregnancies.

Etiology

The etiology is unknown, but placenta previa is more common in multiparas and when the placenta is large and thin. It is thought that when the endometrium and decidua of the upper segment of the uterus are deficient, the placenta spreads over more of the wall of the uterus in an effort to obtain an adequate supply of blood.

445

Classification

PLACENTA PREVIA

1. *Total or central:* The entire internal os of the cervix is covered by placenta (Fig. 1A).
2. *Partial:* Part of the internal os of the cervix is covered by placenta (Fig. 1B).
3. *Marginal:* The placenta extends to the edge of the cervix, but does not lie over the os (Fig. 1C). When the cervix effaces and dilates in late pregnancy, a marginal placenta previa may be converted into the partial variety.

LOW-LYING PLACENTA

The placenta is in the lower uterine segment, but does not encroach on the internal os of the cervix (Fig. 1D).

Clinical Manifestations

The main or only symptom is painless vaginal bleeding. In most cases the bleeding is unprovoked, but it may be preceded by trauma or coitus. The first hemorrhage is almost never catastrophic. It may stop and start again later. Sometimes there is a continuing trickle of blood so that the patient becomes anemic. A feature of placenta previa is that the degree of anemia or shock is equivalent to the amount of blood lost.

Source of the Bleeding

As the lower segment of the uterus develops and the cervix effaces and dilates, there is a degree of separation of the placenta from the wall of the uterus. This is associated with rupture of the underlying blood vessels. If these are large the bleeding will be profuse.

Associated Conditions

1. Failure of engagement.
2. Abnormal presentations, such as breech and transverse lie, are more common, probably because the placenta occupies the lower part of the uterus.

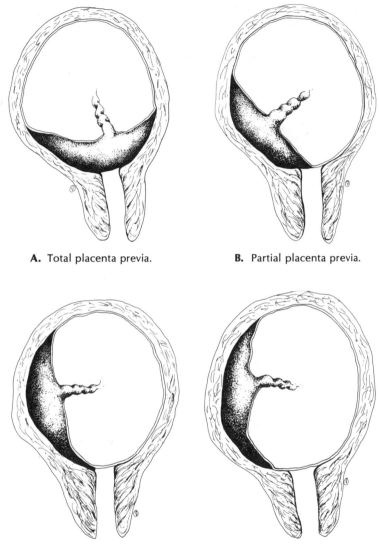

A. Total placenta previa.   **B.** Partial placenta previa.

C. Marginal placenta previa.   **D.** Low lying placenta.

FIG. 1. Placenta previa.

3. Congenital fetal anomalies.
4. Placenta accreta. The incidence is higher than when the placenta is implanted in the upper segment of the uterus.
5. Postpartum hemorrhage is seen more often.

Physical Findings

1. The patient feels no pain, unless labor has begun.
2. The uterus is soft and not tender.
3. The presenting part is high.
4. The fetal heart is usually present.
5. Shock is rare.

Placental Localization

1. Ultrasonic examination is safest and accurate.
2. Radioactive isotope. This method is accurate and safe for the fetus.
3. Soft tissue x-ray may locate the placenta but is not as reliable as the above techniques.

ABRUPTIO PLACENTAE

This condition, known also as premature separation of the placenta, involves the detachment of the placenta from the wall of the uterus. Abruptio placentae is initiated by hemorrhage into the decidua basalis which divides, leading to separation of the part of the placenta adjacent to the split. A hematoma forms between the placenta and the uterus.

In most cases the bleeding progresses to the edge of the placenta. At this point it may break through the membranes and enter the amniotic cavity or, more often, the blood tracks down between the chorion and the decidua vera until it reaches the cervix, and then comes out of the vagina. Occasionally there is extensive extravasation of blood into the myometrium, a condition described as uteroplacental apoplexy, or Couvelaire uterus. The incidence of abruptio placentae is around 1:200 pregnancies.

Etiology

The cause of placental abruption is not known. The condition is associated with the following:

1. Hypertensive disorders of pregnancy.
2. Overdistension of the uterus, including multiple pregnancy and polyhydramnios.
3. Trauma.
4. Short umbilical cord.

Classification

DEGREE OF SEPARATION OF THE PLACENTA

1. *Total:* Fetal death is inevitable.
2. *Partial:* The fetus has a chance. Separation of more than 50 percent of the placenta is incompatible with fetal survival.

LOCATION OF THE BLEEDING

1. *External or apparent* (Fig. 2A). The blood may be bright red or dark and clotted. The pain is mild unless the patient is in labor. The degree of anemia and shock is equivalent to the apparent blood loss.
2. *Internal or concealed:* There is little vaginal bleeding. The blood is trapped in the uterus. The pain is severe and the uterus is hard and tender. The fetal heart is absent. The degree of shock is greater than expected for the amount of visible bleeding.
3. *Mixed or combined:* All varieties of the above groups are seen.

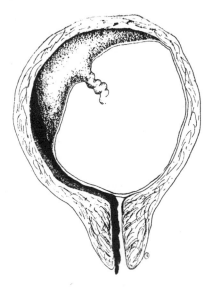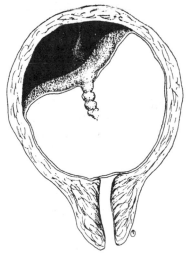

A. External or apparent.   **B.** Internal or concealed.

FIG. 2. Abruptio placentae.

Clinical Picture

This depends on the location of the blood and the amount lost. The latter may be small or large enough to lead to maternal death. The clinical triad includes abdominal pain, uterine tenderness with high tonicity, and vaginal bleeding. The uterus may have a board-like rigidity and may enlarge as blood accumulates in the cavity. Often the patient is in labor. The fetal heart tones may be absent. When the blood loss is great hypovolemic shock supervenes.

Complications

1. Hemorrhagic shock is due to blood loss, apparent or concealed.
2. Disseminated intravascular coagulation. Thromboplastin from the decidua and amniotic fluid enters the circulation and leads to hypofibrinogenemia.
3. Postpartum hemorrhage is caused both by the failure of the uterus to contract properly and by the coagulopathy.
4. Renal lesions. Ischemic necrosis of the kidneys, acute tubular necrosis, and/or bilateral cortical necrosis leads to renal shutdown.
5. Sheehan's syndrome results from ischemic necrosis of the anterior lobe of the pituitary gland as a consequence of shock.

Painless Abruption

Several cases have been reported of separation of a posteriorly implanted placenta, severe enough to cause fetal death, but differing from the usual clinical presentation in that the only symptoms are vaginal bleeding and backache. The uterus is not tender, relaxes between contractions if the patient is in labor, and allows for easy palpation and auscultation of the fetus. The diagnosis depends on the demonstration, by ultrasound, of a posterior, upper segment, placental implantation.

VASA PREVIA

Vasa previa refers to the presentation of fetal blood vessels across the internal os of the cervix. The condition is associated with a low-lying placenta and a velamentous insertion of the umbilical cord. In the latter the umbilical cord inserts into the membranes, and the branching vessels run between the amnion and the chorion before joining the placenta. Unprotected by Wharton's jelly, the blood vessels are vulnerable. If they are compressed the fetus becomes asphyxiated. If they are ruptured the fetus exsanginates. In either case fetal death occurs frequently. Vasa previa is rare, occurring in less than 1:5,000 deliveries. However, in association with velamentous insertion of the cord the incidence is 1:50.

Clinical Picture

The two symptoms are (1) fetal bradycardia when the vessels are compressed and (2) vaginal hemorrhage when the vessels are torn.

Antepartum diagnosis is uncommon and here lies the main problem. When labor has started and the cervix opens, leaving the membranes unsupported, rupture of the vasa previa is almost inevitable. Once hemorrhage has occurred there is little hope for the fetus unless the origin of the blood is suspected and rapid treatment instituted.

Diagnosis

1. *Fetal heart rate:* Vasa previa may be suspected when each episode of vaginal bleeding is followed by irregularities of the fetal heart.
2. *Vaginal examination:* The vessels may be felt by the fingers. The condition may be confused with presentation of the umbilical cord.
3. *Amnioscopy:* The blood vessels may be seen.
4. *Kleihauer test:* This procedure demonstrates the presence of fetal red blood cells and establishes that the bleeding is of fetal origin.
5. *Cesarean section:* Severe fetal bradycardia may lead to emergency cesarean section without the diagnosis being made until after the operation.

RUPTURE OF MARGINAL SINUS

The marginal sinus rims the circumference of the placenta and is one of the channels by which blood from the intervillous spaces is returned to the maternal circulation. Normally it is torn during the third stage of labor as the placenta separates from the wall of the uterus.

Occasionally the marginal sinus ruptures in the third trimester of pregnancy. The etiology is unknown. The clinical picture is that of mild, painless bleeding, unaccompanied by uterine rigidity or changes in the fetal heart.

LOCAL LESIONS

1. Neoplasms
   a. Cervical polyp
   b. Cervical cancer
2. Infection
   a. Vaginitis
   b. Cervicitis

IDIOPATHIC

In this case no cause or reason for the bleeding is ever found. Probably it results from a slight separation of the membranes from the uterine wall. The bleeding is usually small in quantity and there is no effect on the mother, fetus, or pregnancy. Sometimes an excessive amount of bloody show is a sign of impending labor.

Treatment involves the ruling out of serious conditions, followed by expectant management. Most patients go to term.

GENERAL MANAGEMENT OF THIRD TRIMESTER BLEEDING

Preliminary Evaluation

1. The patient is admitted to hospital.
2. Blood loss is estimated.
3. Vital signs are determined.
4. The degree of shock is evaluated.
5. The hemoglobin and hematocrit are measured.
6. Clotting factors, including fibrinogen, are assayed.

Obstetric Evaluation

1. The period of gestation is calculated.
2. The abdomen is palpated for consistency and tenderness of the uterus.
3. Fetal position is determined.
4. The fetal heart is auscultated.
5. The placenta is localized by ultrasound or radioactive isotopes.

Preliminary Management

1. An intravenous infusion with a transfusion unit and a large-bore needle or intracath is set up.
2. Blood is cross-matched, at least two units.
3. The patient is kept in bed.
4. No vaginal or rectal examinations are performed at this time.

Treatment

1. If the bleeding stops and there is no recurrence for several days, and if placenta previa is not present, a speculum examination is performed to rule out local lesions. If all findings are negative, discharge of the patient from hospital is considered.
2. If the bleeding goes on, treatment of the specific condition is carried out.

DIFFERENTIAL DIAGNOSIS

	Placenta Previa	Abruptio Placentae
Onset	Quiet and sneaky	Sudden and stormy
Bleeding	External	External and concealed
Color of blood	Bright red	Dark venous
Anemia	= Blood loss	>Apparent blood loss
Shock	= Blood loss	>Apparent blood loss
Toxemia	Absent	May be present
Pain	Only labor	Severe and steady
Uterine tenderness	Absent	Present
Uterine tone	Soft and relaxed	Firm to stony hard
Uterine contour	Normal	May enlarge and change shape
Fetal heart tones	Usually present	Present or absent
Engagement	Absent	May be present
Presentation	May be abnormal	No relationship

MANAGEMENT OF PLACENTA PREVIA

Expectant Treatment

Because the first episode of bleeding is rarely catastrophic and because the fetus may be too premature to survive outside of the uterus, an attempt is made to prolong the pregnancy in the interests of the infant. A reasonable goal is 37 to 38 weeks.

1. Hospitalization. The time and amount of the next episode of bleeding are unpredictable. Therefore the patient must remain in hospital.
2. Transfusion. At least two units of blood should be available.
3. Anemia. Blood transfusion and supplements of iron are given if anemia is present.
4. Pulmonary maturity. The lecithin/sphingomyelin (L/S) ratio of the amniotic fluid helps determine the optimum time for delivery.

Termination of the Pregnancy

INDICATIONS

1. Excessive bleeding. Fetal maturity is ignored.
2. The pregnancy has reached 37 to 38 weeks and pulmonary maturity is assured.

CESAREAN SECTION
This is performed for the following indications:

1. Profuse bleeding
2. Total or partial placenta previa; certain diagnosis by ultrasound
3. Fetal distress
4. Abnormal presentation (e.g., breech, transverse lie)

DOUBLE SET-UP EXAMINATION
This procedure is carried out when the diagnosis is uncertain. The patient is taken to the operating room, where all preparations have been made for immediate cesarean section. Under anesthesia, abdominal and vaginal examinations are performed to ascertain the fetal presentation, the condition of the cervix, and the location of the placenta. Treatment is based on these findings.

Cesarean Section This is performed when the diagnosis is made of complete or partial placenta previa, when profuse bleeding is provoked by the examination, when there is fetal distress, or when the presentation is abnormal. Many obstetricians prefer the lower segment vertical uterine incision in this situation because it provides easier access to bleeding sinuses if suture is necessary and because, if the placenta is anterior, it is easier to find a path around it to extract the baby than when the incision is transverse. Some physicians perform the transverse lower segment procedure, while a few believe that the classical incision is best for placenta previa.

Induction of Labor The membranes are ruptured and an oxytocin infusion is instituted. The descent of the head, by causing pressure on the placenta, will control the bleeding from the uterine sinuses. This procedure is carried out when:

1. The bleeding is minimal.
2. The placenta covers no more than 10 percent of the internal os.
3. The cervix is effaced and at least 3 cm dilated.
4. The fetal head is in the pelvis.

Await Onset of Labor Patient is returned to the ward when:

1. No placenta previa is found
2. No indication for induction is present.

Prognosis

Mother Good as long as shock and severe anemia are prevented.

Fetus The mortality rate is around 15 percent. Factors that worsen the chances for fetal survival include:

1. Uncontrollable maternal hemorrhage and shock
2. Placental separation
3. Excessive anesthesia
4. Delivery of premature infant

Placenta Previa
First Bleed

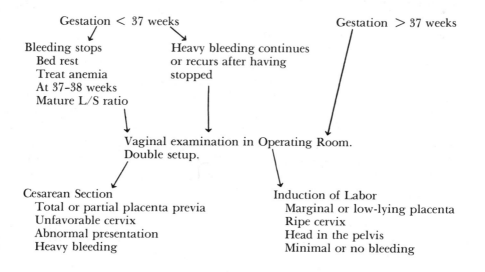

Gestation < 37 weeks   Gestation > 37 weeks

Bleeding stops   Heavy bleeding continues
  Bed rest   or recurs after having
  Treat anemia   stopped
  At 37–38 weeks
  Mature L/S ratio

Vaginal examination in Operating Room.
Double setup.

Cesarean Section   Induction of Labor
  Total or partial placenta previa   Marginal or low-lying placenta
  Unfavorable cervix   Ripe cervix
  Abnormal presentation   Head in the pelvis
  Heavy bleeding   Minimal or no bleeding

MANAGEMENT OF ABRUPTIO PLACENTAE

Initial Evaluation and Stabilization

1. History and physical examination
2. Blood for hemoglobin, hematocrit, platelets, prothrombin time, and fibrinogen
3. Intravenous line with 18-gauge needle
4. Cross-match four units of blood
5. Transfuse as necessary

Time of Delivery

Except for mild cases, when bleeding is minimal, the aim is to effect delivery as soon as possible and for the following reasons:

1. A number of intrauterine fetal deaths occur after the mother has been admitted to hospital and is awaiting delivery.
2. The neonatal mortality rises as the interval between abruption and birth is lengthened.
3. Early delivery and consequent reduction of the period of fetal hypoxia reduces both fetal and neonatal mortality.
4. In these cases the fetuses do not tolerate the process of labor too readily.

Cesarean Section

1. If the fetus is viable and the fetal heart tones are present, immediate cesarean section is justified in the interests of baby and mother. An exception to this principle would be the situation in which the cervix is at least half dilated, the head is deep in the pelvis, the position is normal, and the patient is multiparous, suggesting that birth will take place within a short time.
2. In the case of a dead fetus, cesarean section is performed only in the interests of the mother when bleeding is uncontrollable. If bleeding is minimal, labor is induced.

Induction of Labor

The membranes are ruptured artificially and an oxytocin infusion is set up. Fetal monitoring is mandatory. Induction of labor is considered under the following conditions:

1. Bleeding is minimal, suggesting a mild degree of placental separation.
2. The mother is in good condition.
3. Rapid vaginal delivery is anticipated because the patient is multiparous, the cervix is 4 to 5 cm dilated, the fetal position is normal, and the head is well into the pelvis.

Treatment of Bleeding

1. Adequate transfusion.
2. Disseminated intravascular coagulation. Delivery within 8 hours prevents this complication in most cases. If it occurs, cryoprecipitate, fibrinogen, or fresh plasma may be given once the delivery is under way.
3. Hysterectomy may be necessary if bleeding from a noncontracting uterus cannot be controlled.

Prognosis

MATERNAL

The maternal prognosis depends on (1) the extent of placental separation; (2) the blood loss; (3) whether the hemorrhage is apparent or concealed (the latter is more grave); (4) the extent of uteroplacental apoplexy; (5) the degree of interference with the clotting mechanism; and (6) the interval between the placental abruption and the institution of treatment. With proper management the mortality is less than 1 percent.

FETAL

Perinatal mortality ranges between 30 and 50 percent. The outlook for the fetus is influenced by (1) the extent of placental separation; (2) the interval between the accident and delivery; and (3) prematurity.

MANAGEMENT OF VASA PREVIA

1. In the presence of fetal bleeding immediate delivery is essential, vaginally or by cesarean section.
2. If there is no bleeding, cesarean section may be necessary, but if vaginal delivery is imminent the membranes can be ruptured away from the vessels and the baby extracted.
3. In the presence of a dead fetus, vaginal delivery is awaited.
4. Post partum the baby's blood picture must be studied, and if necessary, immediate transfusion carried out.

BIBLIOGRAPHY

Knab DR: Abruptio placentae, an assessment of the time and method of delivery. Obstet Gynecol 52:625, 1978

Pallewela CS: Antepartum diagnosis of vasa previa—report of a case causing sudden fetal death. Postgrad Med J 50:723, 1974

Quek SP, Tan KL: Vasa previa. Aust NZ J Obstet Gynaecol 12:206, 1972

34.

Episiotomy, Lacerations, Uterine Rupture, and Inversion

EPISIOTOMY

An episiotomy (perineotomy) is an incision into the perineum to enlarge the space at the outlet, thereby facilitating the birth of the child. Fielding Ould, in 1872, was probably the first obstetrician to perform an episiotomy.

Advantages to the mother include the following:

1. A straight incision is simpler to repair and heals better than a jagged, uncontrolled laceration.
2. By making the episiotomy before the muscles and fascia are stretched excessively, the strength of the pelvic floor can be preserved and the incidence of uterine prolapse, cystocele, and rectocele reduced.
3. The structures in front are protected as well as those in the rear. By increasing the room available posteriorly, there is less stretching of and less damage to the anterior vaginal wall, bladder, urethra, and periclitoral tissues.
4. Tears into the rectum can be avoided.

It is also advantageous to the child. A well timed episiotomy not only makes the birth easier but lessens the pounding of the head on the perineum and so helps avert brain damage. This is true for any baby but is especially important for those who have a low resistance to trauma, such as premature infants, babies born to diabetic mothers, and those with erythroblastosis.

Indications for episiotomy are:

1. Prophylactic: To preserve the integrity of the pelvic floor
2. Arrest of progress by a resistant perineum
   a. Thick and heavily muscled tissue
   b. Operative scars
   c. Previous well repaired episiotomy
3. To obviate uncontrolled tears, including extension into the rectum
   a. When the perineum is short, there being little room between the back of the vagina and the front of the rectum
   b. Where large lacerations seem inevitable
4. Fetal reasons
   a. Premature and infirm babies
   b. Large infants
   c. Abnormal positions such as occipitoposteriors, face presentations, and breeches
   d. Fetal distress, where there is need for rapid delivery of the baby and dilatation of the perineum cannot be awaited

There is a proper time to make the episiotomy. Made too late, the procedure fails to prevent lacerations and to protect the pelvic floor. Made too soon, the incision leads to needless loss of blood. The episiotomy is made when the perineum is bulging, when a 3 to 4 cm diameter of fetal scalp is visible during a contraction, and when the presenting part will be delivered with the next three or four contractions. In this way lacerations are avoided, overstretching of the pelvic floor is prevented, and excessive bleeding is obviated.

There are three types of episiotomy: (1) midline; (2) mediolateral, left or right; and (3) lateral episiotomy, which is no longer used (Fig. 1A).

Midline Episiotomy

TECHNIQUE

In making the incision two fingers are placed in the vagina between the fetal head and the perineum. Outward pressure is made on the perineum, away from the fetus, to avoid injury to the baby. The scissors (some prefer a scalpel) are placed so that one blade lies against the vaginal mucosa and the other on the skin. The incision is made in the midline from the fourchette almost to but not through the external fibers of the anal sphincter (Fig. 1B). The cut is in the central tendinous portion of the perineal body to which are attached the bulbocavernosus muscle in front, the superficial transverse perineal and part of the levator ani muscles at the sides, and the anal sphincter behind (Fig. 1B). This is an excellent anatomic incision.

ADVANTAGES

1. The muscle belly is not cut.
2. It is easy to make and easy to repair.
3. The structural results are excellent.
4. Bleeding is less than with other incisions.
5. Postoperative pain is minimal.
6. Healing is superior and dehiscence is rare.

DISADVANTAGES

The one drawback is that should there be extension of the incision as the head is being born, the anal sphincter is torn and the rectum entered. Although most bowel injuries heal well if repaired properly, this accident should be avoided. Median episiotomies are not ideal in the following situations:

1. Short perineum
2. Large baby
3. Abnormal positions and presentations
4. Difficult operative deliveries

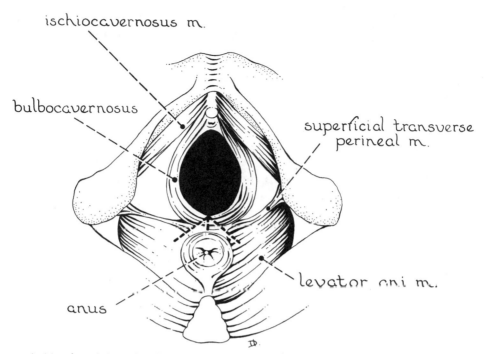

ischiocavernosus m.

bulbocavernosus

superficial transverse
perineal m.

levator ani m.

anus

A. Muscles of the pelvic floor and perineum. The sites of median and mediolateral episiotomy are shown.

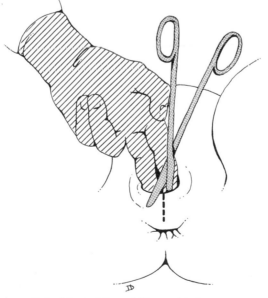

B. Incision of the midline episiotomy.

FIG. 1. Midline episiotomy.

REPAIR

Since in most cases the third stage is completed soon after the birth
of the child, the repair of the episiotomy is performed after the placenta
is delivered, the uterus contracted, and the cervix and vagina found to
be uninjured. Not only are intrauterine procedures, such as manual removal of the placenta, and intravaginal procedures more difficult to perform after the episiotomy has been closed, but the repair may be broken
down.

Except for the subcuticular layer, a medium, round needle is employed. In the deep tissues a cutting edge needle may lacerate a blood vessel and cause a hematoma. Our preference is for 000 chromic catgut.

First the vaginal mucosa is sewn together (Fig. 2A). The procedure
is begun at the top of the incision, the first bite being taken a little above
the apex to include any retracted blood vessel. The suture is tied leaving
one end long. The edges of the wound are then approximated but not
strangulated, using a simple continuous or a lock stitch to assure hemostasis. Each bite includes the mucous membrane of the vagina and the
tissue between the vagina and rectum. This reduces bleeding, eliminates
dead space, and makes for better healing. The repair is carried past the
hymenal ring to the skin edges. The last two bites include the subcutaneous tissue at the base of the episiotomy but do not come through the
skin. This end of the continuous suture may be tied, or it may be left untied and held with a hemostat.

The second stitch near the base of the wound is the crown suture
(Fig. 2B). The needle passes under the skin deeply enough to catch and
bring together the separated and retracted ends of the bulbocavernosus
muscle and fascia. The crown suture is important: If these tissues are
approximated too tightly coitus is painful, and if too loose, the introitus
gapes.

Next the transverse perineal and levator ani muscles and fascia are
approximated in the midline anterior to the rectum with three or four
interrupted sutures (Fig. 2C). One layer is enough in most cases.

Finally the incision is closed by one of several methods:

1. The skin edges are united by interrupted, or mattress, sutures
   which pass through the skin and subcutaneous tissue. These are
   tied loosely to prevent strangulation as postpartum swelling
   takes place (Fig. 2D).
2. The skin edges are approximated using a continuous subcuticular stitch on a small cutting needle, starting at the lower end
   of the incision. The first bite is taken in the subcuticular tissue
   just under but not through the skin, going from side to side until
   the base (upper end) of the wound is reached. Here it is tied sep-
   arately, or if the suture used to repair the vaginal mucosa has

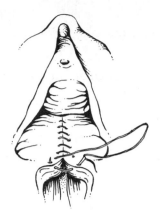

A. Closure of the vaginal mucosa by a continuous suture.

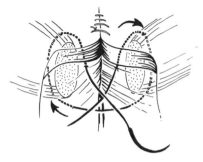

B. The crown suture, reuniting the divided bulbocavernous muscle.

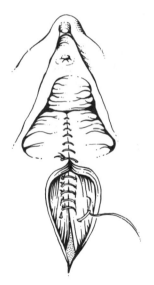

C. Drawing together the perineal muscles and fascia with interrupted sutures.

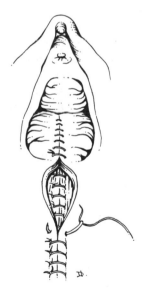

D. Approximation of the skin edges with interrupted sutures.

FIG. 2. Repair of the midline episiotomy.

465

been left untied, this suture and the subcuticular one are tied together. This completes the repair (Fig. 3D).

AFTERCARE

Aftercare of the episiotomy is essentially a matter of cleanliness. The perineum is cleaned with a mildly antiseptic solution after each urination and bowel evacuation. Heat, as from an electric bulb, may be used to dry the area and to reduce the swelling. Daily showers and washing with mild soap and water are excellent ways of keeping the perineum clean and free from irritating discharges. Several investigators have used oral proteolytic enzymes with success in reducing pain and edema.

Mediolateral Episiotomy

When a large episiotomy is needed, or when there is danger of rectal involvement, the mediolateral variety is advised. Included here are patients with short perineums, contracted outlets, large babies, face to pubis deliveries, attitudes of extension, breech births, and midforceps operations.

TECHNIQUE

The incision is made from the midline of the posterior fourchette toward the ischial tuberosity, far enough laterally to avoid the anal sphincter. The average episiotomy is about 4 cm long and may reach the fatty tissues of the ischiorectal fossa. Whether it is placed on the left or right side is unimportant.

The following structures are cut:

1. Skin and subcutaneous tissue.
2. Bulbocavernosus muscle and fascia.
3. Transverse perineal muscle.
4. Levator ani muscle and fascia. The extent to which this structure is involved is determined by the length and depth of the incision.

REPAIR

The technique is essentially the same as for the median perineotomy. The vaginal mucosa is repaired starting at the apex, and bringing together the mucous membrane and the underlying supporting tissue (Fig. 3A). The crown suture is placed carefully (Fig. 3B).

The muscles and fascia which were cut are approximated with interrupted sutures (Fig. 3C). The tissues on the medial side tend to retract, and care must be taken not to enter the rectum. Some operators prefer to

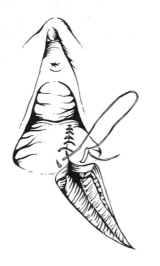

A. Closure of the vaginal mucosa by a continuous suture.

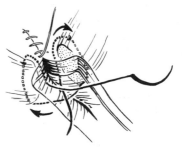

B. The crown suture.

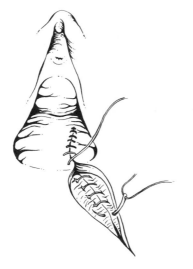

C. Drawing together the perineal muscles and fascia with interrupted sutures.

D. Approximation of the skin edges with a continuous subcuticular suture.

FIG. 3. Repair of left mediolateral episiotomy.

place these sutures, leaving them untied, before the vaginal mucosa is repaired. In many patients a single layer of four or five stitches is sufficient. When the wound is deep or when there is much bleeding two layers may be necessary, one in the muscles, and one to bring together the overlying fascia. The skin edges are joined by a subcuticular stitch beginning at the apex (Fig. 3D), or by interrupted sutures through skin and subcutaneous tissue.

Disruption of Episiotomy

ETIOLOGY
Like incisions in other parts of the body, an episiotomy may dehisce. Predisposing factors include:

1. Poor healing powers
   a. Nutritional deficiencies
   b. Anemia
   c. Exhaustion after a long and difficult labor
   d. Avascular scarred tissue
2. Failure of technique
   a. Careless approximation of the wound
   b. Incomplete hemostasis leading to hematoma formation
   c. Failure to obliterate dead space
3. Devitalization of tissue
   a. Use of crushing instruments
   b. Strangulation of tissue by tying sutures too tightly
   c. Employment of too heavy catgut
4. Infection
   a. Infected lochia in puerperal sepsis
   b. Poor technique and neglect of aseptic standards
   c. Proximity of the rectum
   d. Extension of the incision into or passage of the needle through the bowel
   e. Sepsis in a hematoma
   f. Improper postpartum cleanliness

CLINICAL COURSE
The episiotomy becomes extremely painful, tender, swollen, red, and indurated. The patient may or may not have fever. Sometimes there is a discharge from the incision. By the fourth or fifth day the edges of the wound separate.

MANAGEMENT OF DISRUPTION

Supportive Management The area is kept clean and free from irritating discharge and debris by warm sitz baths twice daily for 20 minutes. Following this the perineum is lamped for 30 minutes. The wound granulates in and heals from the deep layers up. The patient may go home at the usual time and continue the treatment there. Unless there has been damage to the rectum, this management has always been successful in our experience. The wound heals well, no aftereffects are noted, and prolonged hospitalization is avoided.

Secondary Repair Supportive treatment is carried on until the area is clean. This takes 5 to 6 days. Then the patient is anesthetized, the devitalized tissue debrided, and the episiotomy repaired.

In our experience supportive therapy alone has given the best results and is the simplest to carry out.

A late complication of an infected episiotomy is a rectovaginal fistula. This results from an unrecognized tear of the rectum or from a suture being passed through the rectal wall and left there.

LACERATIONS OF THE PERINEUM

Many women suffer tears of the perineum at birth of the first child. In about half the cases these tears are extensive. Lacerations must be repaired carefully.

Maternal causes include:

1. Precipitate, uncontrolled, or unattended delivery (the most frequent cause)
2. The patient's inability to stop bearing down
3. Hastening the delivery by excessive fundal pressure
4. Edema and friability of the perineum
5. Vulvar varicosities weakening the tissue
6. Narrow pubic arch with outlet contraction, forcing the head posteriorly
7. Extension of episiotomy

Fetal factors are:

1. Large baby
2. Abnormal positions of the head—e.g., occipitoposterior and face presentations

3. Breech deliveries
4. Difficult forceps extractions
5. Shoulder dystocia
6. Congenital anomalies, such as hydrocephaly

Classification of Perineal Lacerations

FIRST DEGREE TEAR

First degree tear involves the vaginal mucosa, the fourchette, and the skin of the perineum just below it.

Repair These tears are small and are repaired as simply as possible. The aim is reapproximation of the divided tissue and hemostasis. In the average case a few interrupted sutures through the vaginal mucosa, the fourchette, and the skin of the perineum are enough. If bleeding is profuse, figure-8 stitches may be used. Interrupted sutures, loosely tied, are best for the skin because they cause less tension and less discomfort to the patient.

SECOND DEGREE TEAR

Second degree lacerations are deeper. They are mainly in the midline and extend through the perineal body. Often the transverse perineal muscle is torn, and the rent may go down to but not through the rectal sphincter. Usually the tear extends upward along the vaginal mucosa and the submucosal tissue. This gives the laceration a doubly triangular appearance with the base at the fourchette, one apex in the vagina, and the other near the rectum.

Repair Repair of second degree lacerations is in layers:

1. Interrupted, continuous, or lock stitches are used to approximate the edges of the vaginal mucosa and submucosa (Fig. 4A).
2. The deep muscles of the perineal body are sewn together with interrupted sutures (Fig. 4B).
3. A running subcuticular suture or interrupted sutures, loosely tied, bring together the skin edges (Fig. 4C).

THIRD DEGREE TEAR

Third degree tears extend through the perineal body, the transverse perineal muscle, and the rectal sphincter. In partial third degree tears only the rectal sphincter is torn; in complete tears the rectal sphincter is severed, and the laceration extends up the anterior rectal wall for a variable distance. Some authors refer to this as a fourth degree tear.

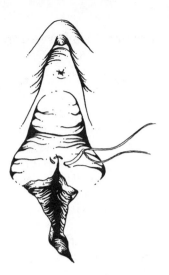

A. Closure of the rent in the vaginal mucosa with a continuous suture.

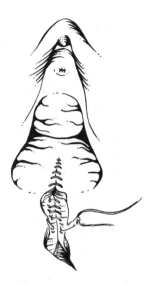

B. Drawing together the perineal muscles and fascia with interrupted sutures.

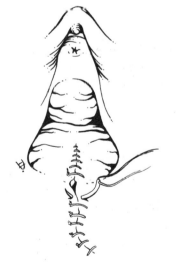

C. Closure of the skin edges with interrupted sutures tied loosely.

FIG. 4. Repair of a second degree perineal laceration.

471

Repair of Complete Tear Complete third degree tear (Fig. 5A) is repaired in layers:

1. The anterior wall of the rectum is repaired with fine 000 or 0000 chromic catgut on a fused needle. Starting at the apex, interrupted sutures are placed submucosally so that the serosa, muscularis, and submucosa of the rectum are apposed (Fig. 5B). Some authors advise that the knot be tied in the lumen of the bowel. Others approximate the edges of the rectum with a continuous suture going through all layers. This part of the repair must be performed meticulously.
2. The line of repair is oversewn by bringing together the perirectal fascia and the fascia of the rectovaginal septum. Interrupted or continuous sutures are used.
3. The torn ends of the rectal sphincter (which have retracted) are identified, grasped with Allis forceps, and approximated with interrupted sutures or two figure-8 sutures (Figs. 5C and D).
4. The vaginal mucosa is then repaired as in a midline episiotomy, with continuous or interrupted sutures
5. The perineal muscles are sewn together with interrupted stitches.
6. The skin edges are sewn together with a continuous subcuticular suture or loosely tied interrupted sutures.

Repair of Partial Tear Repair of partial third degree tear is similar to that of the complete variety, except that the rectal wall is intact and the repair starts with reapproximation of the torn ends of the rectal sphincter.

Aftercare Aftercare of third degree tears includes:

1. General perineal asepsis
2. Low-residue diet
3. Encouragement of soft bowel movements with mild laxatives
4. Suppository or carefully given enema on the fifth or sixth day

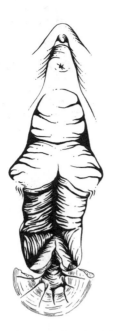

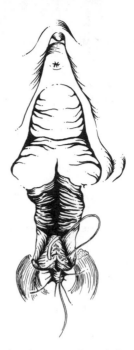

A. Torn and retracted ends of the rectal sphincter, laceration of the anterior wall of the rectum, and the torn vagina and perineum.

B. Closing the tear in the anterior wall of the rectum with interrupted sutures tied in the lumen.

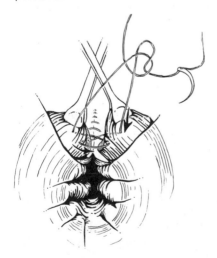

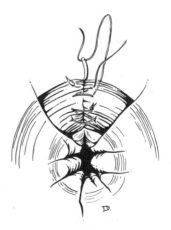

C. Retracted ends of the rectal sphincter are grasped with Allis forceps, and the first figure-eight suture is being placed.

D. Reunion of torn rectal sphincter completed with two figure-eight sutures.

FIG. 5. Repair of a third degree laceration (complete tear).

LACERATIONS OF ANTERIOR VULVA AND LOWER ANTERIOR VAGINAL WALL

Various areas may be involved. Superficial tears are not serious, but with deep tears the bleeding may be profuse.

Locations of Lacerations

1. Tissue on either side of the urethra.
2. Labia minora.
3. Lateral walls of the vagina.
4. Area of the clitoris: With deep tears the corpora cavernosa may be torn. Because of the general vascularity of this structure, as well as the presence of the deep and dorsal blood vessels of the clitoris, these lacerations are accompanied by severe bleeding.
5. Urethra, under the pubic arch.
6. Bladder: The bladder is close to the anterior vaginal wall and may be damaged. Vesicovaginal fistula can occur. The main causes of fistula are prolonged labor with pressure necrosis of the wall of the bladder and instrumental damage during difficult deliveries.

Repair of Lacerations

Superficial small lacerations do not need repair in many cases. When the legs are brought together the torn edges are approximated and heal spontaneously. Larger tears should have the edges brought together with interrupted sutures to promote healing.

Deep lacerations must be repaired. Profuse bleeding is controlled best by figure-8 sutures placed to include and shut off the torn and bleeding vessels. Unfortunately in many cases the lacerated area is the site of varicosities, and passage of the needle through the tissue provokes fresh bleeding. If sutures do not stop the bleeding, a firm pack should be applied against the bleeding site and the hemorrhage controlled by tamponade.

Often the area of bleeding is near the urethra, and when the periclitoral region is involved the hemorrhage can be excessive. Repair is difficult because of the proximity of the urethra. To prevent damaging the urethra a catheter should be inserted to guide the needle away from it.

Tears of the urethra and bladder are repaired in three layers to approximate the bladder mucosa, bladder wall, and anterior wall of the

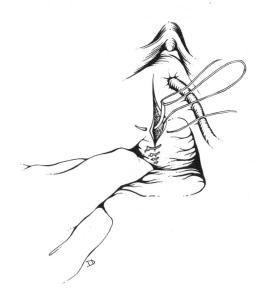

FIG. 6. Anterior paraurethral laceration: placing of fine interrupted sutures. A catheter is in the urethra.

vagina (Fig. 6). An indwelling catheter should be inserted into the bladder for drainage.

LACERATIONS OF UPPER VAGINA

These lacerations may take place during spontaneous delivery but are more common with operative deliveries and are associated with a variety of conditions. Predisposing factors include congenital anomalies of the vagina, a small or infantile vagina, loss of tissue elasticity in elderly primigravidas, scar tissue following the use of caustic substances in attempting to induce abortions, and unhealthy tissues, which tear like wet blotting paper.

Forceps rotation and extractions following deep transverse arrest, persistent occipitoposteriors, or face presentations often cause vaginal tears. The fact that these malpositions are frequently associated with small or male type pelves aggravates the situation and increases the incidence and extent of the lacerations. During rotation the edge of the blades may shear off the vaginal mucosa. Improper traction tends to overstretch the tissues and may result in a large tear. A large infant increases the danger of extensive lacerations.

The majority of vaginal tears are longitudinal and extend in the

sulci along the columns of the vagina. In many cases the lacerations are
bilateral.

Technique of Repair

Lacerations of the upper vagina bleed profusely; the bleeding must
be controlled as soon as possible. As the tear is often high and out of
sight, good exposure, good light, and good assistance are essential. Bleeding from the uterus may obscure the field. The placenta should be removed and oxytocics given before the repair is begun. The operator must
be certain that the apex of the tear is included in the suture, or hemorrhage may take place from a vessel that has retracted. If the apex cannot
be reached, several sutures are placed below it, and traction on these then
expose the apex of the laceration (Fig. 7). Figure-8 sutures are preferable

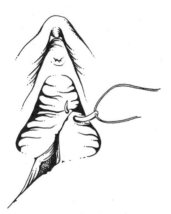

A. Introduction of first suture at highest
point visible.

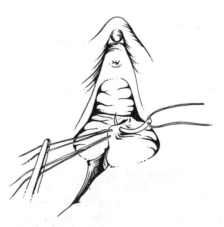

B. Traction on first suture exposes apex
of the laceration and enables top suture
to be placed. The remainder of the vaginal laceration is closed with continuous
or interrupted sutures.

FIG. 7. Right mediolateral episiotomy with high left vaginal sulcus tear.

if bleeding is profuse, or a continuous lock stitch may be employed.

In some instances the sutures do not control the bleeding adequately. The vagina should be packed tightly with a 5-yard gauze. This reduces the oozing and helps prevent the formation of hematomas. The pack is removed in 24 hours.

VESICOVAGINAL FISTULA

A fistula is an abnormal communication between two or more organs. One variety is formed between the vagina and the urinary tract—the urethra, bladder, or ureter. Urine passes into the vagina, and there is an uncontrollable vaginal discharge.

Fistulas occur: (1) at childbirth, (2) during surgery, or (3) as a complication of cancer and radiation therapy. Although, because of improved obstetrics, most fistulas are associated with surgery, they do occur in association with parturition in the following ways:

1. During prolonged and obstructed labor the bladder is trapped between the fetal head and the maternal pubic symphysis. The resulting ischemic necrosis and slough results in fistulas of varying sizes. The proximal urethra, vesical neck, and trigone are involved.
2. Direct injury can occur during a difficult forceps delivery. Usually the trigone and urethra are damaged.
3. At cesarean section the bladder and ureter may be cut or torn.

Management

If the injury is recognized, an immediate two- or three-layer repair should be performed, followed by continuous bladder drainage for 10 days. When the damage is not recognized or if repair is not possible, continuous bladder drainage is instituted. Sometimes spontaneous closure of the fistula takes place. Should the fistula persist, active treatment is delayed for 2 to 3 months to allow the edema to subside, the slough to separate, and a new circulation to be established. Repair of the fistula is then carried out.

RECTOVAGINAL FISTULA

This is an opening between the rectum and the vagina. The patient notices the passage of air from the vagina and an irritating vaginal discharge.

Most of these occur as the result of an unsuccessful repair of a third degree laceration. The sphincter, or part of it, heals, while the area above the sphincter breaks down. A low rectovaginal fistula is the result. Occasionally a stitch in the apex of the episiotomy enters the rectum. Most of these cause no trouble. Once in a while healing does not take place and a fistula develops.

Treatment is by surgical repair.

HEMATOMAS

Vulva and Vagina

PUERPERAL HEMATOMA

1. Vulvar: The bleeding is limited to the vulvar tissue and is readily apparent.
2. Vulvovaginal: The hematoma involves the paravaginal tissue and the vulva, perineum, or ischiorectal fossa. The extent of the bleeding is only partially revealed on inspection of the vulva.
3. Vaginal or concealed: The hematoma is confined to the paravaginal tissue and is not visible externally.
4. Supravaginal or subperitoneal: The bleeding occurs above the pelvic fascia and is retroperitoneal or intraligamentous.

These result from rupture of the blood vessels, especially veins, under the skin of the external genitals and beneath the vaginal mucosa. The causal trauma occurs during delivery or repair. In rare cases the accident takes place during pregnancy or very early labor, in which case a large hematoma can obstruct progress. Damage to a blood vessel may lead to its necrosis, and the hematoma may not become manifest for several days.

Most hematomas are small and are located just beneath the skin of the perineum. While they cause pain and skin discoloration, they are not important. Since the blood is absorbed spontaneously no treatment is required beyond ordinary perineal care.

Rupture of the vessels under the vaginal mucosa is serious, since large amounts of blood can collect in the loose submucosal tissues. Many vaginal hematomas contain over half a liter of blood by the time the diagnosis is made. The mass may be so large that it occludes the lumen of the vagina, and pressure on the rectum is intense. When bleeding occurs at the base of the ligament the blood may extend in the retroperitoneal space even as far as the kidneys.

Many hematomas occur after easy spontaneous deliveries as well as in association with traumatic deliveries. The hematoma often is located on the side opposite the episiotomy. Stretching of the deep tissues can result in rupture of a deep vessel without visible external bleeding. Varicosities play a predisposing role. The possibility of a coagulation defect must be considered. Failure to achieve perfect hemostasis is an important etiologic factor.

DIAGNOSIS

The diagnosis is made within 12 hours of delivery. Classically, the patient's complaints of pain are dismissed as being part of the usual postpartum perineal discomfort. After a time it is realized that the pain is out of proportion to that associated with the ordinary trauma of delivery. Sedatives and analgesics do not alleviate the pain. Careful examination of the vulva and vagina reveals the swelling, discoloration, extreme tenderness, rectal pressure, and large fluctuant mass palpable per rectum or vaginam. Where large amounts of blood have been lost from the general circulation there is pallor, tachycardia, hypotension, and even shock. If the hematoma is high and ruptures into the peritoneal cavity, sudden extreme shock may occur and the patient may die.

TREATMENT

Active treatment is not needed for small hematomas and those which are not getting larger. The area should be kept clean; and since tissue necrosis may be followed by infection, antimicrobial agents are prescribed.

Big hematomas and those which are enlarging require surgical therapy. The wound is opened, the blood clots are evacuated, and if bleeding points can be found these are ligated. The area is packed with sterile gauze and a counter pack is placed in the vagina. This is left in situ for 24 to 48 hours. Antibiotics are given, blood transfusion is used as needed, and the patient is observed carefully for fresh bleeding. An indwelling catheter should be placed.

Since there is a tendency for the bleeding to recur and the hematoma to re-form, careful observation is necessary. Most cases do well, but several weeks pass before the wound heals and the perineum looks normal.

Broad Ligament

The danger of broad ligament hematomas is that they can rupture into the general peritoneal cavity and cause sudden and extreme shock.

DIAGNOSIS

Diagnosis is made by vaginal examination. Rupture of the lower uterine segment must be ruled out. If the hematoma is large the uterus is pushed to the opposite side.

TREATMENT

Treatment depends on the degree of bleeding. Conservative therapy consists of bed rest, antibiotics, blood transfusion, and observation. Serial blood counts are done.

In the event of continued bleeding or progressive anemia, surgical intervention is carried out. The abdomen is opened, and the blood clots are evacuated. Where possible the bleeding points are tied off, care being taken to avoid the ureter. An extraperitoneal drain may be inserted. In older women hysterectomy is considered, and this operation may be necessary in young women to control the situation.

LACERATIONS OF THE CERVIX

As a result of its dilatation, superficial lacerations of the cervix occur during almost every confinement. They are partly responsible for the bloody show. These small tears heal spontaneously and require no treatment.

Deep lacerations, on the other hand, can cause severe hemorrhage and shock to the extent of endangering the life of the patient. This is particularly so when the laceration extends into the lower uterine segment where the large uterine vessels may be involved. The lacerations may be unilateral or bilateral. The most common sites are at the sides of the cervix, at 3 or 9 o'clock.

Etiology

The etiology of deep lacerations includes precipitate labor, a rigid or scarred cervix, the forceful delivery of the child through an undilated cervix, breech extraction, and a large baby.

Diagnosis

Diagnosis is by careful inspection. Some obstetricians inspect the cervix after every delivery. It must be done after all difficult confinements and whenever there is continuous bleeding, especially if the blood is bright red. Ring forceps are used to grasp the lips of the cervix so that the whole circumference can be examined.

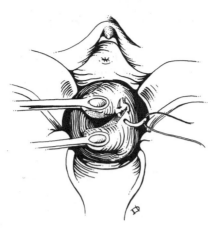

FIG. 8. Laceration of cervix on the left side. Uppermost suture is placed just above the apex of the tear. The laceration is being closed with interrupted sutures. Figure-eight sutures may be used.

Repair

Repair of cervical tears is important. The cervix is exposed with a vaginal speculum or with retractors. An assistant is invaluable. Ring forceps are placed on each side of the laceration. Interrupted or figure-8 sutures are placed starting at the apex and are tied just tightly enough to control the bleeding and to approximate the tissues. Care must be taken not to include the ring of the forceps in the stitch. It is important that the first stitch be placed a little above the apex (Fig. 8) to catch any vessel that may have retracted. If the tear is high there is danger of injury to the ureter. When the tear has extended into the lower uterine segment or into the broad ligament, repair from below may be impossible and laparotomy necessary.

Careful repair of the torn cervix is important, not only to control bleeding but as prophylaxis against scarring, erosions, and chronic ascending infections. Lacerations more than a centimeter in length warrant treatment.

DÜHRSSEN'S CERVICAL INCISIONS

Incisions of the cervix are used to facilitate immediate delivery when the cervix is fully effaced but not completely dilated. This procedure is used rarely today, the incidence being under 1 percent and being needed more often in primigravidas.

Reasons why this procedure is used so seldom today include the following:

1. The employment of the intravenous oxytocin drip has reduced the incidence of failure of cervical dilatation.
2. The increased safety of cesarean section has steered obstetricians away from incising the cervix.
3. It is realized that nondilatation of the cervix may be an indication of disproportion.
4. In the presence of fetal distress cervical incisions and midforceps may be more than the baby can stand.

Indications

This operation may be employed in the presence of fetal distress or arrest of progress when it is considered that vaginal delivery would be relatively easy if the cervix were fully dilated. The obstetrician must beware of diagnosing cervical dystocia when fetopelvic disproportion is the real problem.

Prerequisites

1. There must be no cephalopelvic disproportion.
2. The cervix must be completely effaced.
3. The cervix must be at least half dilated.
4. The station of the fetal skull is at +1 or +2.
5. The patient must have been in good labor for 6 to 8 hours with ruptured membranes.

Technique

The cervix is grasped with ring forceps, and the incisions are made between them at 2, 6, and 10 o'clock (Fig. 9). These are extended to the junction of the cervix and vaginal wall. When the three incisions have been made, the diameter of the cervix is equivalent to full dilatation.

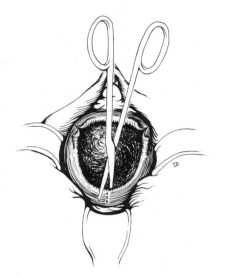

FIG. 9. Dührssen's cervical incisions at 2, 6, and 10 o'clock.

Because the bladder is pulled upward as effacement takes place, its dissection from the anterior vaginal wall is not required.

Appropriate measures for delivery of the child are then carried out. The incisions are repaired with continuous, interrupted, or figure-8 sutures. While there is rarely much bleeding, preparations to treat hemorrhage should be at hand. Most cervices heal well, and future pregnancies deliver normally.

ANNULAR DETACHMENT OF THE CERVIX

The anterior lip of the cervix may be compressed between the fetal head and the pubic symphysis. If this situation continues for a long time, edema, local anemia, anoxia, and even necrosis may develop. Rarely, an entire ring of cervix undergoes anoxic necrosis, and a section of the vaginal part of the cervix comes away. This is known as annular detachment of the cervix. Because the prolonged pressure has caused the blood vessels to thrombose, excessive bleeding from the cervix is unusual.

Etiology

1. Seventy-five percent of cases occur in primigravidas.
2. Prolonged labor is almost always the rule.
3. There is often a history of early rupture of the membranes.

4. The fetal head is low in the pelvis.
5. The cervix is well effaced and often quite thin. It is the external os that does not dilate. Several observers have reported that the cervix feels rigid to palpation during the first stage of labor.
6. The uterine contractions are strong and efficient.

Mechanism

The myometrial contractions press the presenting part against the thinned out, rigid external os; in addition, the retracting upper segment of the uterus pulls the cervix upward. This double action leads to poor circulation in the cervix, anoxia, and necrosis. A tear starts at the cervico-vaginal junction, and a line of cleavage develops and continues until the separation is complete. The characteristic doughnut-shaped ring of tissue becomes detached when the cervix is about 3 to 5 cm dilated. Gross histologic examinations have revealed these cervices to be no different from the normal term organ.

Clinical Picture

The clinical picture is one of good labor obstructed by an unyielding external os. In almost every case the fetus is delivered without difficulty once the cervical obstruction is overcome. Annular detachment is the result of true cervical dystocia.

Treatment

Because the vessels are thrombosed, serious bleeding from the stump is rare. No active treatment is needed. The rare maternal death occurs either from sepsis or from uterine bleeding associated with prolonged labor and postpartum uterine atony. Any hemorrhage that originates in the cervix must be controlled by figure-8 sutures.

Prevention

Prevention is achieved by recognizing the situation before the actual detachment takes place. When the cervix is effaced and thin, cervical incisions are indicated; delivery usually follows. If the situation is not right for the cervical incisions, cesarean section must be done.

Prognosis

Many women avoid future pregnancy. Stenosis and hematometra have been recorded. Several subsequent gestations have been delivered vaginally with no difficulty and there has been one elective cesarean section and one abortion from an incompetent os reported.

RUPTURE OF THE UTERUS

Rupture of the uterus is a dangerous complication of pregnancy. It is responsible for 5 percent of maternal deaths in the United States and Canada, and is an even greater hazard in the underdeveloped countries.

Incidence

The reported incidence varies from 1:93 confinements to 1:8,741, depending on the source of the material. The average incidence is around 1:2,000. Recent publications suggest that the number of uterine ruptures is increasing and blame this fact on (1) more frequent use of cesarean section, (2) careless administration of oxytocic drugs, (3) inadequate professional care during labor, and (4) lackadaisical and poor management of labor and delivery.

Types of Rupture

1. The rupture is complete when all the layers of the uterus are involved and there is a direct communication between the uterine and abdominal cavities. This is the common variety.
2. The incomplete rupture includes the whole myometrium; the peritoneum covering the uterus remains intact.
3. A third variety may occur. In this instance the serosa and part of the external myometrium are torn, but the laceration does not extend into the cavity. A severe intraperitoneal hemorrhage may take place without the condition being diagnosed. This situation should be suspected when there are signs of an intraabdominal catastrophe during or after labor, but no uterine defect is detectable on manual exploration of the uterine cavity.

Site and Time of Rupture

Tears that take place during pregnancy are more often in the upper segment of the uterus, at the site of previous operation or injury. During labor the rupture is usually in the lower segment. The longer the labor, the more thinned out the lower segment and the greater the danger of rupture. The tear may extend into the uterine vessels and cause profuse hemorrhage. Tears in the anterior or posterior walls of the uterus usually extend transversely or obliquely. In the region of the broad ligament the laceration runs longitudinally up the sides of the uterus.

It may occur during pregnancy, normal labor, or difficult labor, or it may follow labor. Most ruptures take place at or near term. Those happening before the onset of labor are usually dehiscences of cesarean section scars.

Classification

SPONTANEOUS RUPTURE OF THE NORMAL UTERUS

These accidents occur during labor, are more common in the lower segment of the uterus, and are the result of mismanagement and neglect. Etiologic factors include:

1. Multiparity
2. Disproportion
3. Abnormal presentation (brow, breech, transverse lie)
4. Improper use of oxytocin

TRAUMATIC RUPTURE

This is caused by ill-advised and poorly executed operative vaginal deliveries. The incidence is decreasing. Etiologic factors include:

1. Version and extraction
2. Difficult forceps operations
3. Forceful breech extraction
4. Craniotomy
5. Excessive fundal pressure
6. Manual dilatation of the cervix

POSTCESAREAN RUPTURE

This is the most common variety seen today. It may occur before or during labor. Upper segment scars rupture more often than lower segment incisions. While hysterograms done 3 months after operation may give an indication as to whether good healing has taken place, there is no accurate way of predicting the behavior of a uterine scar. All cesarean section scars present a hazard. Hence many clinicians follow the rule of "once a cesarean, always a cesarean."

RUPTURE FOLLOWING TRAUMA OTHER THAN CESAREAN

The danger is that often the damage is not recognized, and the accident comes as a surprise. Included in this group are:

1. Previous myomectomy
2. Too vigorous curettage
3. Perforation during curettage
4. Cervical laceration
5. Manual removal of an adherent placenta
6. Placenta percreta
7. Endometritis and myometritis
8. Hydatidiform mole
9. Cornual resection for ectopic pregnancy
10. Hysterotomy

SILENT BLOODLESS DEHISCENCE OF A PREVIOUS CESAREAN SCAR

This is a complication of lower segment cesarean sections. Part or all of the incision may be involved. Usually the peritoneum over the scar is intact. Many of these windows are areas not of current rupture but of failure of the original incision to heal. This complication is in no way as serious as true uterine rupture. Features of this complication include:

1. Usually diagnosed during repeat cesarean section, being unsuspected before operation
2. No hemorrhage at site of dehiscence
3. No shock
4. Hysterectomy not necessary
5. No fetal death
6. No maternal mortality

Clinical Picture

The clinical picture of uterine rupture is variable in that it depends on many factors:

1. Time of occurrence (pregnancy, early or late labor)
2. Cause of the rupture
3. Degree of the rupture (complete or incomplete)
4. Position of the rupture
5. Extent of the rupture
6. Amount of intraperitoneal spill
7. Size of the blood vessels involved and the amount of bleeding
8. Complete or partial extrusion of the fetus and placenta from the uterus
9. Degree of retraction of the myometrium
10. General condition of the patient

On a clinical basis rupture of the uterus may be divided into four groups.

1. Silent or quiet rupture: The accident occurs without (initially) the usual signs and symptoms. Diagnosis is difficult and often delayed. Nothing dramatic happens, but the observant attendant notices a rising pulse rate, pallor, and perhaps slight vaginal bleeding. The patient complains of some pain. The contractions may go on, but the cervix fails to dilate. This type is usually associated with the scar of a previous cesarean section.
2. Usual variety: The picture develops over a period of a few hours. The signs and symptoms include abdominal pain, vomiting, faintness, vaginal bleeding, rapid pulse rate, pallor, tenderness on palpation, and absence of the fetal heart. These features may have arisen during pregnancy or labor. If the diagnosis is not made, hypotension and shock supervene.
3. Violent rupture: It is apparent almost immediately that a serious accident has taken place. Usually a hard uterine contraction is followed by the sensation of something having given way and a sharp pain in the lower abdomen. Often the contractions cease, there is a change in the character of the pain, and the patient becomes anxious. The fetus can be palpated easily and feels close to the examining fingers. The presenting part is no longer at the pelvic brim and can be moved freely. Sometimes the uterus and fetus can be palpated in different parts of the abdomen. Fetal movements cease, and the fetal heart is not heard. The symptoms and signs of shock appear soon, and complete collapse may occur.
4. Rupture with delayed diagnosis: Here the condition is not diagnosed until the patient is in a process of gradual deterioration,

unexplained anemia leads to careful investigation, a palpable hematoma develops in the broad ligament, signs of peritoneal irritation appear, or the patient goes into shock (either gradually or suddenly as when a hematoma in the broad ligament ruptures). Sometimes the diagnosis is made only at autopsy.

Diagnosis

The diagnosis is made easily when the classic picture is present or when the rupture is catastrophic. In atypical cases the diagnosis may be difficult. A high index of suspicion is important. If routine exploration of the uterus is not carried out after every birth, then at least following all difficult deliveries whenever there is unexplained shock or postpartum bleeding the interior of the cavity should be explored manually and the lower segment searched for tears.

Palpatory findings, as described in the previous section, may be pathognomonic. The fetal heart beat is absent in most cases. An x-ray of the abdomen may demonstrate the fetus lying in the peritoneal cavity surrounded by the intestines, with the shadow of the uterus to one side.

Treatment

Treatment must be prompt and in keeping with the patient's condition. Laparotomy is performed, and the bleeding is controlled as quickly as possible. Aortic compression (by the hand or by using a special instrument) is useful in reducing the bleeding until the situation can be evaluated. Most patients are critically ill and are unable to stand prolonged surgery.

In most cases total hysterectomy is the procedure of choice. If the patient is in poor condition rapid, subtotal hysterectomy may be performed. If, however, the tear has extended into the cervix, the bleeding will not be controlled by subtotal hysterectomy. In such cases, if it cannot be removed, the cervix must be sutured carefully to tie off all bleeding points.

In young women and in those who desire more children, treatment may be limited to repair of the tear. This should be done only when the uterine musculature can be so reconstituted as to assure a reasonable degree of success and safety for a future pregnancy. As supportive treatment, blood must be replaced quickly in the amount lost.

Maternal Mortality

The reported maternal death rate ranges from 3 to 40 percent. Spontaneous rupture of the uterus is responsible for the largest number of deaths, followed by the traumatic variety. The amount of hemorrhage is greatest in these types. The lowest death rate is associated with postcesarean ruptures, probably because these patients are observed so carefully during labor.

The main causes of death are shock and blood loss (usually over 1,000 ml). Sepsis and paralytic ileus are contributory factors.

The prognosis for the mother depends on (1) prompt diagnosis and treatment, the interval between rupture and surgery being important; (2) the amount of hemorrhage and the availability of blood; (3) whether infection sets in; and (4) the type and site of the rupture.

The mortality rate is lower today because of:

1. Early diagnosis
2. Immediate laparotomy
3. Blood transfusion
4. Antibiotics
5. Reduction or elimination of traumatic vaginal operative deliveries
6. Better management of prolonged or obstructed labor

Fetal Mortality

Fetal mortality is high, ranging from 30 to 85 percent. Most fetuses die from separation of the placenta. There is a reduction of blood supply available to the fetus after the uterus has ruptured. Probably the prolonged labor before rupture plays a part in causing fetal hypoxia. Many of these babies are premature. The highest mortality is associated with fundal rupture where the fetus has been extruded into the abdominal cavity.

Pregnancy after Rupture of the Uterus

Ritchie reported 28 patients who had 36 pregnancies following repair of a ruptured uterus. Repeat rupture occurred in 13 percent with two maternal deaths. The risk of repeat rupture is:

1. Least when the scar is confined to the lower segment
2. Greater if the scar extends into the upper segment

3. Greatest in women whose original rupture occurred following classic cesarean section

MANAGEMENT
Cesarean section should be performed before the scar is subjected to stress.

1. Scar in lower segment: cesarean section at 38 weeks
2. Scar in upper segment: cesarean section at 36 weeks

INVERSION OF THE UTERUS

Uterine inversion is a turning inside out of the uterus. In the extreme case the doctor may see the purplish endometrium, with the placenta often still attached. In the severe situation the patient may be bleeding profusely, hypotensive, and sometimes pulseless. The reported incidence ranges from 1:100,000 to 1:5,000 deliveries. It is seen rarely in the nongravid uterus with a pedunculated myoma.

Etiology

The disorder's mechanism is not understood completely. It is believed to be related to an abnormality of the myometrium. Some inversions are spontaneous and tend to recur at subsequent deliveries; however, it occurs more often in primigravidas.

Many are caused by improper obstetric manipulations, but they may take place after normal or abnormal labor. Most often inversion is a catastrophe of the third stage of labor.

PREDISPOSING FACTORS

1. Abnormalities of the uterus and its contents
   a. Adherent placenta
   b. Short umbilical cord
   c. Congenital anomalies
   d. Weakness of uterine wall at the placental site
   e. Fundal implantation of the placenta
   f. Neoplasm of the uterus
2. Functional conditions of the uterus
   a. Relaxation of the myometrium
   b. Disturbance of the contractile mechanism

EXCITING CAUSES

1. Manual removal of the placenta
2. Increase in abdominal pressure
   a. Coughing
   b. Sneezing
3. Mismanagement of third stage of labor
   a. Improper fundal pressure
   b. Traction on the cord
   c. Injudicious use of oxytocics

Classification

Classification on the basis of stage is as follows:

1. Acute, occurring immediately after birth of the baby or placenta, before there is contraction of the cervical ring
2. Subacute, beginning when contraction of the cervix becomes established
3. Chronic, present for more than 4 weeks

Classification on the basis of degree includes three types:

1. Incomplete, when the fundus is not beyond the internal os of the cervix
2. Complete, when the fundus protrudes through the external os of the cervix
3. Prolapse, in which the fundus protrudes through the vulva

Pathology

The following stages have been described:

1. Acute inversion
2. Contraction of the cervical ring and lower segment of the uterus around the encircled portion of the uterus
3. Edema
4. Reduction of blood supply
5. Gangrene and necrosis
6. Sloughing

Clinical Picture

Sometimes the symptoms are minor so the diagnosis is not made, or the condition is recognized but treatment is not carried out at the time. These are the chronic inversions. Those that cause shock and require immediate therapy are the acute ones.

When the inversion is complete the diagnosis is easy. Partial inversions may fool the observer. Classically, shock is greater than expected for the amount of bleeding. The extreme shock is probably caused by tension on the nerves of the broad ligament, which are drawn through the cervical ring, and by irritation of the peritoneum. In any situation where shock is out of proportion to hemorrhage the accoucheur should think of uterine inversion. The placenta may have separated or may remain attached. The hemorrhage may be excessive or minimal.

Diagnosis

1. High index of suspicion
2. Absence of uterine fundus on abdominal examination
3. Vaginal examination
4. Uterine rupture must be excluded

Treatment of Acute Inversion

The aim of treatment is to replace the uterus as soon as possible. Blood transfusion is instituted and the patient is anesthetized. In most cases the placenta will have been delivered. If it is still attached it can be removed manually or replaced with the fundus, whichever is easier. In some cases attempts to remove the placenta prior to uterine replacement may lead to profuse bleeding.

The method of replacement described by Johnson is effective (Fig. 10). The entire hand of the operator is placed in the vagina with the tips of the fingers at the uterocervical junction and the fundus of the uterus in the palm of the hand. The uterus is then lifted out of the pelvis and held in the abdominal cavity above the level of the umbilicus. This results in the uterine ligaments becoming stretched and tense. When the ligaments are placed under tension, pressure is exerted first to widen the cervical ring and, second, to pull the fundus through it. In this way the uterus is replaced to its normal position. To accomplish this effect it is

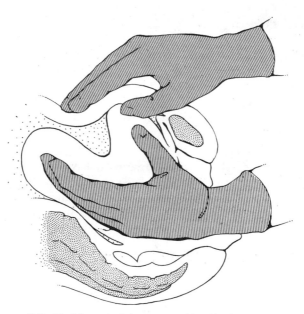

FIG. 10. Manual replacement of inverted uterus.

necessary to hold the uterus in this position for 3 to 5 minutes until the fundus recedes from the palm of the hand.

Treatment of Subacute Inversion

Once the cervix has contracted, immediate replacement of the uterus is no longer feasible.

1. The vagina is packed with 2-inch gauze, without replacing the uterus, pushing the cervix into the abdominal cavity. A Foley catheter is inserted into the bladder.
2. The patient is treated for shock, and blood transfusion is given in the amount lost.
3. Antibiotics may be used.
4. During the next 48 hours fluids and electrolytes are infused in an attempt at restoring the patient to a condition suitable for surgery. At the same time it is hoped that some uterine involution will take place.
5. Laparotomy is carried out and the inversion corrected by a combined abdominovaginal operation, as for chronic inversion.

Treatment of Chronic Inversion

Spinelli Procedure Using the vaginal approach, the contracted cervical ring is incised anteriorly, so that the fundus of the uterus can be pushed back into place.

Haultain Procedure Laparotomy is performed. The cervical ring is incised posteriorly and the uterine fundus is drawn up.

Huntington Procedure The approach is per abdominal incision. The surface of the uterus inside the crater is grasped with Allis forceps about 2 cm below the inversion cup on each side and upward traction exerted. As the uterus comes up through the ring additional forceps are placed below the original ones and further traction is exerted. This procedure is continued until the inversion is completely reversed. Simultaneous pressure on the fundus through the vagina by an assistant may make the procedure easier.

Prognosis

The exact incidence of recurrence is not known, but it is high. Some authorities believe that further pregnancy should be avoided. It is probable that subsequent delivery should be by cesarean section. However, this does not obviate the problem entirely as inversion can occur even at cesarean section.

SEPARATION OF SYMPHYSIS PUBIS

During pregnancy there is relaxation and weakening of the pelvic joints. This begins during the first half of pregnancy and reaches a maximum in the seventh month. Return to normal begins after delivery and is complete by the sixth month.

Incidence and Etiology

This varies from 1:250 to 1:30,000 confinements. Minor degrees of separation take place, but since the symptoms are minimal the diagnosis is not made and spontaneous correction follows. This accident may occur during labor or in the second half of pregnancy.

Rupture of the pubic symphysis occurs in patients with excessive relaxation of the pelvic joints. Precipitating factors include:

1. Tumultuous labor
2. Difficult forceps extractions
3. Cephalopelvic disproportion
4. Excessive abduction of the thighs at delivery
5. Any condition that might place sudden and excessive pressure on the pubic symphysis

Many cases occur following spontaneous delivery.

Pathology

There is an actual tear of the ligaments connecting the pubic bones. The rupture is usually incomplete, and a fibrocartilagenous bridge remains. Hemorrhage and edema are present. Arthritis or osteomyelitis are possible complications.

Clinical Picture and Diagnosis

The onset of symptoms is usually sudden but may not be noted until the patient tries to walk. At the time of rupture the patient may experience a bursting feeling, or a cracking noise may be heard.

Motion of the symphysis (as by moving the legs) causes great pain. If the patient can walk, she does so with a waddling gait.

There is a marked tenderness of the pubic symphysis. Edema and ecchymosis are present frequently. A gaping defect in the joint is often palpable. Walking or pressure causes motion of the loose joint.

Diagnosis is made by the symptoms and signs. X-ray helps, but the degree of separation seen on radiologic study may not be proportional to the clinical manifestations. To be considered pathologic the separation seen on x-ray should be greater than 1 cm.

Management of symptomatic separation must be directed at relieving the patient's discomfort and compensating for her disability. Treatment is governed by the severity of the condition. Analgesia is essential.

Some patients require prolonged bed rest, with a tight corset or peritrochanteric belt to keep the separated bones as nearly apposed as possible. The local injection of Novocain may help. While in hospital the patient should sleep with a bed board under the mattress; she should also use a trapeze to pull herself to a sitting position so as not to strain the pelvis.

When the rupture is minor early ambulation is permissible. When the problem is more severe crutches should be used. Support is needed for 6 weeks. The patient must limit her use of stairs.

Surgical intervention is indicated rarely. When necessary, fusions may be carried out, often supplemented by bone grafts, bolts, and crossed wires.

BIBLIOGRAPHY

Borenstein R, Katz Z, Lancet M: External rupture of the uterus. Obstet Gynecol 40:211, 1972

Cibils L: Rupture of the symphysis pubis. Obstet Gynecol 38:407, 1971

Groen GP: Uterine rupture in Nigeria. Obstet Gynecol 44:682, 1974

Johnson AB: A new concept in the replacement of the inverted uterus and a report of nine cases. Am J Obstet Gynecol 57:557, 1949

Kitchin JD, Thiagarajah S, May HV, Thornton WN: Puerperal inversion of the uterus. Am J Obstet Gynecol 123:51, 1975

Lee WK, Baggish MS, Lashgari M: Acute inversion of the uterus. Obstet Gynecol 51:144, 1978

Ritchie EA: Pregnancy after rupture of the pregnant uterus. J Obstet Gynaecol Br Commonw 78:642, 1971

Schrinksy DC, Benson RC: Rupture of the pregnant uterus: a review. Obstet Gynecol Surv 33:217, 1978

35.

The Placenta, Retained Placenta, Amniotic Fluid Embolism

THE PLACENTA

Normal Placenta

Size and Shape   The placenta is a round or oval disk, 20 × 15 cm in size and 1.5 to 2.0 cm thick. The weight, usually 20 percent of that of the fetus, is between 425 and 550 g.

Organization   On the uterine side there are eight or more maternal cotyledons separated by fissures. The term fetal cotyledon refers to that part of the placenta that is supplied by a main stem villus and its branches. The maternal surface is covered by a layer of decidua and fibrin, which comes away with the placenta at delivery. The fetal side is covered by membranes.

Location   Normally the placenta is implanted in the upper part of the uterus. Occasionally it is placed in the lower segment, and sometimes it lies over the cervix. The latter condition is termed placenta previa and is a cause of bleeding in the third trimester. Ultrasonic examinations in early pregnancy have demonstrated the placenta to be in the lower segment, suggesting placenta previa. At reexamination late in pregnancy the placenta is found in the upper segment. Probably the normal growth of the placenta is away from the cervix. In addition, the uterus enlarges faster than the placenta and, as pregnancy progresses, a proportionately smaller area of the wall of the uterus is occupied by placenta. No cases of downward migration of the placenta have been reported.

Abnormalities of the Placenta

Succenturiate Lobe   This is an accessory lobe that is placed at some distance from the main placenta. The blood vessels that supply this lobe run over the intervening membranes and may be torn when the latter rupture or during delivery. A succenturiate lobe may be retained after birth and cause postpartum hemorrhage.

Circumvallate Placenta   The membranes are folded back on the fetal surface and insert inward on themselves. The placenta is situated outside of the chorion.

Amnion Nodosum   This is a yellow nodule, 3 to 4 cm in diameter, situated on the fetal surface of the amnion. It contains vernix, fibrin, desquamated cells, and lanugo hairs. It may form a cyst. This condition is associated with oligohydramnios.

Infarcts   Localized infarcts are common. The clinical significance is not known, although if the condition is excessive, the functional capacity of the placenta may be reduced.

Discoloration   Red staining is associated with hemorrhage. Green color is caused by meconium and may be an indication of fetal hypoxia.

Twin Placenta   In monochorionic twins the placenta forms one mass, whereas in dichorionic twins the placentas may be fused or separate.

Weight   Placentas weighing over 600 g or under 400 g are usually associated with abnormal pregnancy.

The Placenta in Various Conditions

Prematurity   The placenta is small and often pale.

Postmaturity   The size and weight are usually normal. There may be meconium staining. If there is excessive fibrosis or infarction, the placental function may be reduced.

Intrauterine Growth Retardation   The placenta tends to be small, the decrease in weight being proportional to the weight of the infant.

Diabetes Mellitus   The placenta is usually larger than normal, but in severe cases, when the mother's circulation is affected, the placenta may be small.

Toxemia of Pregnancy No specific changes are seen. Often the placenta appears normal.

Erythroblastosis The placenta is boggy, is pale pink to yellow in color, and may weigh as much as 2,000 g.

Congenital Syphilis The placenta is large, thick, and pale.

Amnionitis The membranes are opaque and have yellow discoloration. The placenta may be foul smelling.

RETAINED PLACENTA

Retention of the placenta in utero falls into four groups:

1. Separated but retained: Here there is failure of the forces that normally expel the placenta.
2. Separated but incarcerated: An hourglass constriction of the uterus, or cervical spasm, traps the placenta in the upper segment.
3. Adherent but separable: In this situation the placenta fails to separate from the uterine wall. The causes include failure of the normal contraction and retraction of the third stage, an anatomic defect in the uterus, and an abnormality of the decidua which prevents formation of the normal decidual plane of cleavage.
4. Adherent and inseparable: Here are the varying degrees of placenta accreta. The normal decidua is absent, and the chorionic villi are attached directly to and through the myometrium.

Technique of Manual Removal

Manual removal of the retained placenta is not considered to be as dangerous as it once was. Many of the bad outcomes of this procedure were the result of too long a delay in treatment until hemorrhage had put the patient in a precarious state. When bleeding is present the placenta must be removed immediately. If there is no associated hemorrhage and the patient is in good condition, a delay of 30 minutes is permissible.

If the patient has been bleeding actively, an intravenous infusion is set up and blood is made available. Anesthesia is necessary. The procedure is carried out under aseptic conditions.

The uterus is steadied by one hand holding the fundus through the maternal abdomen (Fig. 1). The other hand is inserted into the vagina and through the cervix into the uterine cavity. The placenta is reached

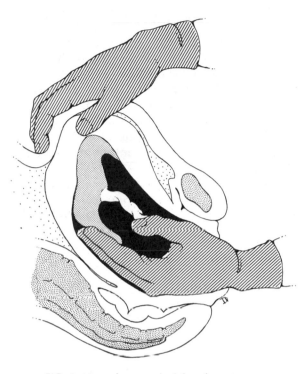

FIG. 1. Manual removal of the placenta.

by following the umbilical cord. If the placenta has separated it is grasped and removed. The uterus is then explored to be sure that nothing has been left.

If the placenta is still adherent to the uterine wall it must be separated. First some part of the margin of attachment is identified and the fingers inserted between the placenta and the wall of the uterus. The back of the hand is kept in contact with the uterine wall. The fingers are forced gently between the placenta and uterus, and as progress is made they are spread apart. In this way the line of cleavage is extended, the placenta is separated from the uterine wall, and it is then extracted. Oxytocics are given to ensure good uterine contraction and retraction.

PLACENTA ACCRETA

Placenta accreta is defined as the abnormal adherence, either in whole or in part, of the afterbirth to the underlying uterine wall. The placental villi adhere to, invade into, or penetrate through the myometrium.

Pathology

Normally the decidua basalis lies between the myometrium and the placenta (Fig. 2A). The plane of cleavage for placental separation is in the spongy layer of the decidua basalis. In placenta accreta the decidua basalis is partially or completely absent (Fig. 2B), so that the placenta is attached directly to the myometrium. The villi may remain superficial to the uterine muscle or may penetrate it deeply. This condition is caused by a defect in the decidua rather than by any abnormal invasive properties of the trophoblast.

In the superficial area of the myometrium a large number of venous channels develop just beneath the placenta. Rupture of these sinuses by forceful extraction of the placenta is the source of the profuse hemorrhage that occurs.

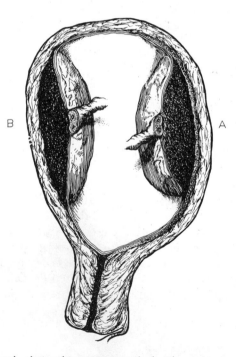

FIG. 2. Utero-placental relationships. **A.** Normal: decidua separates placenta from myometrium. **B.** Placenta accreta: absence of decidua.

Classification

1. By extent
   a. Complete: The whole placenta is adherent to the myometrium.
   b. Partial: One or more cotyledons or part of a cotyledon is adherent.
2. By depth
   a. Accreta: The placenta is adherent to the myometrium. There is no line of cleavage.
   b. Increta: The villi penetrate the uterine muscle but not its full thickness (Fig. 2C).
   c. Percreta: The villi penetrate the wall of the uterus (Fig. 2D) and may perforate the serosa. Rupture of the uterus may occur. A case has been reported in which the villi grew through the wall of the bladder, causing gross hematuria.

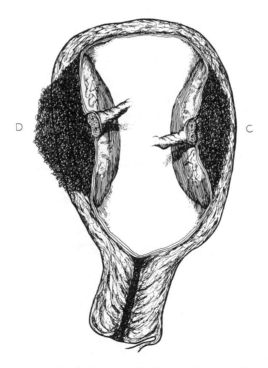

FIG. 2. (cont.) Utero-placental relationships. **C.** Placenta increta: villi penetrate the myometrium. **D.** Placenta percreta: villi extend through the uterine wall.

Incidence

The true incidence is impossible to determine. The reported range varies from 1:540 to 1:93,000 deliveries.

Etiology

1. Maternal factors
   a. Older gravidas.
   b. Multiparity. Placenta accreta is rare in primigravidas.
2. Uterine factors
   a. Previous cesarean section. Often the placenta is implanted over the uterine scar.
   b. Previous uterine surgery.
   c. Previous uterine curettage, mainly following a pregnancy or abortion.
   d. Previous manual removal of placenta.
   e. Previous endometritis.
3. Placental factors
   a. Placenta previa
   b. Cornual implantation.

The significance of most of the etiologic factors is uncertain. The two most frequent predisposing factors are placenta previa and previous cesarean section.

The underlying condition that appears to be common to all causal conditions is a deficiency of the endometrium and the decidua:

1. The decidua overlying the scar of a previous cesarean section is often deficient.
2. In women who have placenta previa the decidua of the lower uterine segment is relatively poorly developed.
3. The decidua of the uterine cornu is usually hypoplastic.
4. With increasing age and parity there is, in many women, a progressive inadequacy of decidua.
5. Previous curettage or manual removal of placenta is probably not an etiologic factor but an indication that an abnormal adherence of the placenta was the reason for the procedure's being necessary.

Clinical Picture

PREGNANCY

1. Most patients have a normal pregnancy.
2. The incidence of antepartum bleeding is increased, but this is usually associated with placenta previa.
3. Premature labor occurs, but only when precipitated by bleeding.
4. Rarely, rupture of the uterus takes place.

LABOR: FIRST AND SECOND STAGES
These are normal in almost all cases.

THIRD STAGE OF LABOR
1. Retained placenta is the main feature.
2. Postpartum hemorrhage. The amount of bleeding depends on the degree of placental attachment. In complete placenta accreta there is no bleeding. In the partial variety bleeding takes place from the uterine vessels underlying the detached area, while the adherent portion prevents the uterus from retracting properly. Often the bleeding is precipitated by the obstetrician as he attempts manual removal of the placenta.
3. A rare but serious complication is uterine inversion. This may occur spontaneously but is usually the result of attempts to remove the placenta.
4. Rupture of the uterus may occur during attempts to extract the afterbirth.

Diagnosis

The gross diagnosis is provisional and is made in two ways. (1) Direct intrauterine palpation. No line of cleavage can be found between the placenta and uterus. The examining fingers slide over the fetal side of the placenta. (2) Study of the uterus and placenta following hysterectomy.

Microscopic examination establishes the diagnosis by demonstrating chorionic villi in the myometrium.

The differential diagnosis includes:

1. Incomplete abortion
2. Retained incarcerated placenta

3. Adherent placenta, where there is a line of cleavage
4. Retained placental fragments
5. Subinvolution of the placental site
6. Choriocarcinoma

Management

The safest treatment is hysterectomy. Since this puts an end to child-bearing, a conservative method of therapy has evolved based on the availability of blood and antibiotics. When placenta accreta is suspected, the following plan of management is useful.

These steps are taken to establish the diagnosis:

1. An intravenous infusion is started with a wide-bore needle.
2. Blood is cross-matched.
3. Expert anesthesia should be available.
4. The operating room must be ready for an emergency.
5. Intrauterine exploration is performed to see whether placenta accreta is present, and if so whether it is complete or partial.
6. In making the diagnosis an attempt is made to remove the placenta. In most instances placenta accreta is not present. Over-zealous attempts to extract the placenta must be avoided since the uterus can be ruptured.

Indications for hysterectomy are:

1. Further pregnancy is not desired
2. Uncontrollable hemorrhage
3. Failure of conservative management
4. Intrauterine suppuration
5. Placenta previa accreta

Conservative management of total placenta accreta includes the following:

1. There is no bleeding unless attempts are made to remove the placenta.
2. The cord is cut short and the blood drained from the placenta.
3. The placenta is left in the uterus.
4. Broad-spectrum antibiotics are given.
5. The placenta becomes organized and partially absorbed, and the superficial portion sloughs off.

6. In some cases suppuration takes place and generalized infection may set in.

Conservative management of partial or focal placenta accreta is as follows:

1. All separated placenta is manually removed. The part of the placenta that is abnormally attached is left.
2. An intravenous oxytocin infusion is maintained for 48 hours.
3. The patient is observed carefully and constantly.
4. Broad-spectrum antibiotics are given.
5. If there is no bleeding after 48 hours, the first stage of conservative management has been successful.

Placenta Previa Accreta

Because the decidua of the lower segment is less abundant than that in the fundus, a placenta implanted near the cervix may be abnormally adherent. The treatment is total hysterectomy.

Maternal Mortality

Before 1937 the reported maternal mortality rate was 37 percent. This figure has decreased steadily because of (1) a greater awareness of the problem, (2) the availability of blood, (3) the effectiveness of antibiotics in combating infection, and (4) the relative safety of timely hysterectomy.

In a recent report the maternal mortality, mainly the result of hemorrhage, was reported as 9.5 percent. Treatment by immediate hysterectomy had a mortality rate of 6.1 percent. Conservative therapy carried a death rate of 25.6 percent. When hysterectomy was performed after conservative therapy had failed, 14.75 percent of patients died. The highest mortality rate was in women delivered per vaginam and treated by conservative methods.

Fetal Results

An incidence of intrauterine fetal death of 9.6 percent indicates that a risk to the fetus exists. Fetal death is associated with antepartum bleeding, uterine rupture, and no discernible cause in equal proportions.

AMNIOTIC FLUID EMBOLISM

Amniotic fluid embolism is a syndrome in which, following the infusion of a large amount of amniotic fluid into the maternal circulation, there is the sudden development of acute respiratory distress and shock. Twenty-five percent of these women die within 1 hour. The condition is rare. Probably many cases are unrecognized, the diagnosis being obstetric shock, postpartum hemorrhage, or acute pulmonary edema.

Amniotic fluid embolism was discovered by Meyer in 1926 at postmortem examination. In 1947 the clinical syndrome was described by Steiner and Lusbaugh. They showed that the sudden infusion of amniotic fluid of sufficient quantity into the maternal circulation is fatal.

Etiology

Predisposing Factors

1. Multiparity
2. Age over 30
3. Large fetus
4. Intrauterine fetal death
5. Meconium in the amniotic fluid
6. Strong uterine contractions
7. High incidence of operative delivery

Clinical Picture

Steiner and Lusbaugh wrote:

Profound shock coming on suddenly and unexpectedly in a woman who is in unusually severe labor or has just finished such a labor, especially if she is an elderly multipara with an excessively large, perhaps dead, fetus, and with meconium in the amniotic fluid, should lead to a suspicion of this possibility [amniotic fluid embolism]. If also the shock is introduced by a chill, which is followed by dyspnea, cyanosis, vomiting, restlessness and the like, and accompanied by a profound fall in blood pressure and a rapid weak pulse, the picture is more complete. If pulmonary edema now develops quickly in the known absence of previously existing heart disease, the diagnosis is reasonably certain.

Nothing has been added to this description except the recognition that there may be an associated failure of coagulation of the patient's blood, and hemorrhage from the placental site.

Diagnosis

The picture includes the following:

1. Respiratory distress.
2. Cyanosis.
3. Cardiovascular collapse.
4. Failure of coagulation and hemorrhage.
5. Coma.
6. Death.
7. In nonfatal cases scan of the lungs using macroaggregated I^{131} albumin may reveal the embolization and establish the diagnosis.

DIFFERENTIAL DIAGNOSIS

1. Thrombotic pulmonary embolism
2. Air embolism
3. Fat embolism
4. Aspiration of vomitus
5. Eclampsia
6. Anesthetic drug reaction
7. Cerebrovascular accident
8. Congestive heart failure
9. Hemorrhagic shock
10. Ruptured uterus
11. Inverted uterus

Clinicopathologic Findings

MODE OF INFUSION

The two major sites of entry into the maternal circulation are the endocervical veins (which may be torn even in normal labor) and the uteroplacental area. Rupture of the uterus increases the chance of amniotic fluid infusion. Abruption of the placenta is a frequent occurrence, this accident preceding or coinciding with the embolic episode.

PATHOGENESIS

The exact mechanism is unknown. Two theories have been advanced: (1) There is an overwhelming mechanical blockade of the pulmonary vessels by emboli of the particulate material in the amniotic fluid, especially meconium. (2) An anaphylactoid reaction to the particulate matter occurs.

The three major aspects of the syndrome are produced probably by a combination of mechanical and spastic processes.

1. The sudden reduction of the amount of blood returning to the left heart and the decreased left ventricular output lead to peripheral vascular collapse.
2. The acute pulmonary hypertension, cor pulmonale, and failure of the right heart produce peripheral edema.
3. The uneven capillary blood flow with derangement of the ventilation/perfusion ratio leads to anoxemia and tissue hypoxia. This can explain the cyanosis, restlessness, convulsions, and coma.

LUNGS
The significant findings are:

1. Edema
2. Alveolar hemorrhage
3. Emboli composed of the particulate material of amniotic fluid (squames, amorphous debris, mucin, vernix, and lanugo)
4. Dilated pulmonary vessels at the area of embolization

HEART
The right side is often dilated. Blood aspirated from the right side reveals amniotic fluid elements.

COAGULATION DEFECTS
The hemorrhage that ensues is the result of a failure of blood coagulation and diminished tonus of the uterus. The probable cause of the failed coagulation process is the release of thromboplastin into the circulation leading to disseminated intravascular coagulation and followed by hypofibrinogenemia and fibrin degradation products. Uterine atony is common, but the exact reason is not known.

Management

While in severe cases nothing does any good, the aims of treatment include reduction of pulmonary hypertension, increased tissue perfusion, relief of bronchospasm, control of hemorrhage, and general supportive measures.

1. Oxygen is given under pressure to increase oxygenation.
2. Antispasmodics and vasodilators such as papaverine, amino-

phylline, and trinitroglycerine may help. Isoproterenol increases pulmonary ventilation and reduces bronchospasm.

3. Coagulation defects must be corrected using heparin or fibrinogen.

4. Fresh blood is given to combat deficits, care being taken not to overload the circulation.

5. Digitalis is useful when cardiac failure is present.

6. Manual exploration of the uterus is performed to rule out rupture or retained placenta.

7. Hydrocortisone is prescribed both to help combat the overwhelming stress and for its inotropic action.

Mortality

While maternal mortality is high, amniotic fluid embolism is not fatal in every instance. Sublethal cases do occur. About 75 percent die as a direct result of the embolism. The rest perish from uncontrollable hemorrhage. Fetal mortality is high, 50 percent of the deaths occurring in utero.

BIBLIOGRAPHY

Breen JL, Neubecker, R, Gregori CA, Franklin JE: Placenta accreta, increta, and percreta. Obstet Gynecol 49:43, 1977
Courtney LD: Amniotic fluid embolism. Obstet Gynecol Surv 29:169, 1974
Fox H: Placenta accreta 1945–1969. Obstet Gynecol Surv 27:475, 1972
Gregory MG, Clayton EM: Amniotic fluid embolism. Obstet Gynecol 42:236, 1973
Teteris NJ, Lina AA, Holaday WJ: Placenta percreta. Obstet Gynecol 47:155, 1976

36.

Assessment of the Fetus in Utero

There are many situations in which it is important to ascertain the health and maturity of the fetus while it is still in utero. In this group are patients with a previous intrauterine fetal death, suspected retarded fetal growth, prolonged pregnancy, toxemia of pregnancy, diabetes, and Rh sensitization. A decision must be made whether to terminate the pregnancy or to let it continue.

There are methods of determining the condition of the fetus while it is still in the uterus. No one test is 100 percent accurate, so several types of examinations are performed and the results collated to help reach a conclusion. Sometimes information is needed to decide whether a fetus is sick and should be delivered immediately. In other cases we want to know about the maturity of the infant and its chances for survival should it be born at that time.

I. During pregnancy, before the onset of labor
   A. Fetal maturity in general
      1. Clinical
         a. Abdominal palpation
         b. Height of fundus and girth of abdomen
      2. X-ray
         a. Ossification of epiphysis of distal femur and proximal tibia
         b. Amniography
      3. Amniocentesis: These data indicate a gestation of 36 weeks or more:
         a. Creatinine level of 2 mg/100 ml amniotic fluid (or higher)
         b. Fat cell concentration over 20 percent
         c. Absence of bilirubin peak at 450 mμ
      4. Ultrasound
         a. Biparietal diameter of 8.5 cm or more: 36 weeks

        b. Serial examinations demonstrating growth or lack of growth of biparietal diameter

B. Maturity of fetal lung: These amniotic fluid test results indicate a gestation of 35 weeks:

    1. Lecithin/sphingomyelin ratio of 2 or more

    2. Positive "shake" test for surfactant

C. Fetal health

    1. Maternal estriol

    2. Amnioscopy: transcervical

    3. Amnioscopy: transabdominal

    4. Examination of fetal heart

        a. Auscultation

        b. Nonstress test

        c. Contraction stress test (oxytocin challenge test)

II. During labor: health of fetus

A. Monitoring the fetal heart rate

B. Microanalysis of fetal blood for pH (acidosis)

The most reliable group of tests to determine that the fetus has reached the stage of maturity of 35 to 36 weeks' gestation are:

1. X-ray

    a. Ossification of the epiphysis of the distal end of the femur

2. Amniotic fluid examination

    a. Creatinine of 2 mg/100 ml fluid

    b. Fat cell concentration over 20 percent

    c. Absence of bilirubin peak at 450 mμ

    d. Lecithin/sphingomyelin ratio of 2 or more

3. Ultrasound

    a. Biparietal diameter of 8.5 cm or more

CLINICAL METHODS

Clinical history and examination are useful. One cannot rely upon a single finding, but by assembling a number of symptoms and signs a reasonably accurate assessment of fetal maturity can be made. Such symptoms and signs include the following:

1. Date of the onset of the last menstrual period. In most cases this is a valid and important parameter. Sources of error include uncertainty of the last menses, bleeding in the early part of preg-

nancy mistaken for a period, oligomenorrhea, and delay of ovulation after discontinuance of the contraceptive pill.

2. Onset of the symptoms of pregnancy.

3. Well-documented evidence of when conception took place; such as an isolated act of coitus or the induction of ovulation in infertile women.

4. Correlation of date of positive pregnancy test and menstrual history.

5. First fetal movement is noticed at 18 to 20 weeks.

6. The fetal heart is heard at 18 to 20 weeks using a fetal stethoscope. However, by means of the Doppler scanner the fetal heart can be identified consistently at 12 weeks and sometimes as early as 10 weeks.

7. Abdominal palpation. In the hands of experienced observers the accuracy is within 1 pound in 80 percent of cases and within 8 ounces in 55 percent. However, the rate of unacceptable estimates is high at the extremes of 2,300 and 4,300 g. There is a

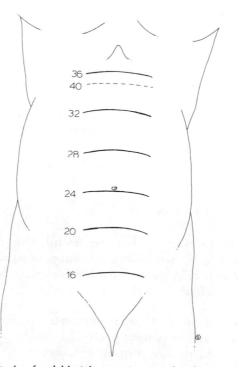

FIG. 1. Uterine fundal height at various weeks of pregnancy.

tendency to overestimate in the lower and underestimate in the higher ranges of birth weight.

8. Measurement of the height of the uterine fundus and the abdominal girth is helpful (Fig. 1).

RADIOLOGIC TECHNIQUES

Flat Plate of Abdomen

A search is made for the epiphyses at the ends of the long bones of the lower limb. The distal (inferior) femoral epiphyseal ossification center is present in 80 percent of fetuses from the 36th week of gestation onward. The proximal (superior) tibial epiphyseal center appears at week 38. Sometimes these centers do not ossify until term. The demonstration of the distal femoral center indicates that the fetus is mature in 90 percent of cases.

Amniography

In performing amniocentesis, 1 ml of amniotic fluid per week of pregnancy is removed and replaced with an equal amount of a radiopaque fluid. Water soluble Hypake-M 75 percent is a good medium. For general diagnostic purposes anteroposterior and lateral x-rays are taken 1 hour after injection. When hydatidiform mole is suspected the films are taken immediately after injection. In the determination of fetal death a delay of 22 to 24 hours is indicated.

Information gained includes the following:

1. The amniotic space can be visualized.
2. The placenta and the umbilical cord are localized.
3. Abnormalities of the uterine cavity are identifiable.
4. Fetal hydrops can be diagnosed.
5. Fetal distress or death can be determined. Normally the fetus swallows the fluid and the gastrointestinal tract is delineated. Total absence of the radiopaque medium in the gut is suggestive of fetal death. Rapid transit through the intestines may indicate fetal distress. Where there is a block of the intestinal tract the level can be established.
6. Since the fluid is excreted via the fetal kidneys, the urinary tract can be outlined.
7. Congenital anomalies of the fetus can be seen.
8. Polyhydramnios is demonstrable.

9. Neural tube defects can be visualized. An elevated level of alpha fetoprotein in the amniotic fluid is suggestive of the presence of an open neural tube defect in the fetus. In order to make a definite diagnosis, demonstration of the lesion is attempted by ultrasonic methods. When this method fails angiography is a useful tool. After injection of the contrast medium into the amniotic sac, the patient is allowed several minutes of normal activity to facilitate dispersion of the contrast material. Under fluoroscopy the mother is rotated until the fetus is seen in the lateral position. A spot film is then taken of the fetal head and spinal region and this is studied to demonstrate the defect.

10. The sex of the fetus can be diagnosed.

AMNIOCENTESIS

Technique

Ultrasonic scanning performed immediately prior to the amniocentesis will provide information as to the location of the placenta, the fetal position, and the area where the amniotic fluid is most accessible. In this way both the site and the depth of the tap can be determined accurately. This is followed by a careful abdominal examination and assessment of the fetal position.

There are two commonly used sites for amniocentesis (Fig. 2): (1) In advanced pregnancy when the head is in the pelvis, the fetal position can be palpated, and the placenta is posterior, the favored site of puncture is in the upper segment of the uterus, in the area of the fetal small parts (Fig. 2A). (2) When the placenta is anterior and in the upper segment of the uterus, and the fetal head can be elevated away from the pelvis, the needle can be inserted easily between the pubic symphysis and the presenting part (Fig. 2B).

The selected area is cleaned with an antiseptic solution and draped. The site of puncture is infiltrated with a local anesthetic. A stylet-containing 18- to 22-gauge needle is used. Entry into the amniotic cavity produces an abrupt loss of resistance.

The return of blood through the needle indicates that the needle is either in the wall of the uterus or in the placenta. If the placenta has been localized by ultrasound one may assume that the needle is in the myometrium and it should be advanced into the amnion. If the placental site is unknown and the depth of the puncture is judged to be adequate, the needle should be removed and another site selected.

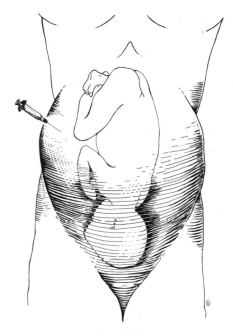

A. Fundal site.

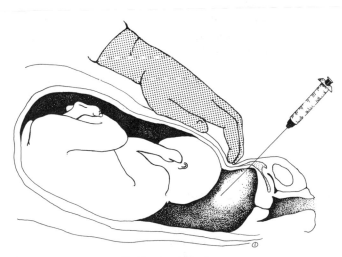

B. Supra pubic site.

FIG. 2. Amniocentesis.

Ten milliliters of amniotic fluid are aspirated and sent to the laboratory for testing. Occasionally no fluid is obtained. This is more common in term or postterm pregnancy in which the volume of amniotic fluid is reduced. In such cases an attempt is made in a different area. However, the procedure may have to be abandoned.

Postamniocentesis care consists of a 20 to 30 minute period of observation with frequent auscultation of the fetal heart. Acceleration of the FHR is the normal response to amniocentesis and is on the order of 20 to 60 beats per minute, lasting for 2 to 3 minutes. The absence of this tachycardia may indicate that the fetus is not in good condition.

Complications of Amniocentesis

Diagnostic amniocentesis is an important procedure. The rate of complications is less than 1 percent. However, they do occur and, as with any invasive technique, amniocentesis should be used only when necessary.

MATERNAL COMPLICATIONS

1. Infection, chorioamnionitis.
2. Puncture of uterine vessels leading to hemorrhage, hemoperitoneum, and formation of hematoma.
3. Vaginal bleeding.
4. Premature rupture of membranes. Leakage of fluid from the site of puncture may track down through the cervix and vagina. This is an occasional and benign event. Rarely, the membranes actually rupture.
5. Premature labor. It is common for patients to experience a few contractions following amniocentesis, but actual labor is rare.
6. Supine hypotension may occur.

FETAL COMPLICATIONS

1. Fetal death is rare.
2. Abortion occurs in less than 1 percent of cases.
3. Infection is rare.
4. Hemorrhage can occur as the result of direct puncture of fetal vessels on the placenta, the cord, or the fetus itself.
5. Fetal injury. In most cases needle trauma is in noncritical areas and no permanent damage results. Occasionally serious injury does take place. The danger is greater in postterm pregnancy, when the volume of fluid is small.

6. Feto-placental-maternal bleeding and potential isoimmuniza-
tion. This occurrence is especially serious when the mother is
Rh negative and the fetus Rh positive. This complication can
be reduced by ultrasonic localization of the placenta preceding
amniocentesis. In any case, Rh immunoglobulin should be administered to Rh negative women following amniocentesis.

Significant Parameters in Amniotic Fluid

No single finding is absolute, but in combination a significant and
reliable estimation of fetal maturity is possible.

CREATININE

Presumably creatinine is a product of fetal urine. It is not established whether the rise in creatinine in the amniotic fluid represents (1)
maturing fetal renal function, (2) a decrease in the volume of amniotic
fluid as term approaches, or (3) an increase in the fetal mass of muscle.
A level of 2.0 mg per 100 ml amniotic fluid (or higher) indicates that the
gestation is over 35 weeks.

BILIRUBIN

The progressive dilution of the amniotic fluid and maturation of
the fetal liver leads to a gradual fall in the concentration of bilirubin. The
spectrophotometric reading of bilirubin at 450 mμ should be zero at 36
weeks. A reading of over 0.01 suggests a gestational age of less than 35
weeks.

In the amniotic fluid there is a normal zone of spectrophotometric
absorbence of bilirubin from 375 to 525 mμ, with a bulge at 450. This
convexity probably represents unconjugated (indirect) bilirubin bound
to albumin. Indirect bilirubin normally circulates in the blood, is insol-
uble in aqueous solutions, and is unable to pass into the urine or bile. It
can cross the placenta into the maternal circulation for elimination. Once
bilirubin is conjugated it becomes water soluble and unable to cross the
membranes of brain or placenta; it cannot return to the blood stream once
it has been excreted into urine or bile. The fetal liver cannot conjugate
bilirubin, so that most fetal serum bilirubin escapes through the placenta in the unconjugated state. It is not known how the unconjugated
bilirubin gets to the amniotic fluid.

FAT CELLS

A drop of amniotic fluid is stained with Nile Blue. Three types of
cells are seen.

1. The immature fetal cell is large and polygonal, with light blue granular cytoplasm and a pyknotic nucleus.
2. The mature fetal cell is an anucleate polygonal cell of intermediate size, with clear cytoplasm and irregular edges. It contains orange "positive fat-staining" granules.
3. The third type of cell is small and round with vacuolated cytoplasm and a small vacuolated nucleus. It probably arises from the amnion or the urinary tract.

When over 20 percent of the cells are mature, orange staining "fat cells," the gestational age is at least 36 weeks.

LECITHIN/SPHINGOMYELIN RATIO: PULMONARY MATURITY

Since the survival of an infant depends on its ability to breathe efficiently, methods to measure this function are of inestimable value. Among other substances, phospholipids increase in the amniotic fluid as the fetus approaches maturity. It has been shown that a decreased concentration of lecithin is associated with respiratory distress. The phospholipids (especially lecithin) that appear in the amniotic fluid originate principally from the fetal lung. Lecithin biosynthesis reflects the status of alveolar stability.

From weeks 20 to 30 of normal pregnancy the amount of sphingomyelin in amniotic fluid is higher than that of surface-active lecithin. By week 30 the concentrations are equal. From this point the amount of lecithin rises above that of sphingomyelin, until at 35 weeks there is a sharp increase in lecithin. The sphingomyelin levels off at week 32 and then declines progressively until at term it is at a low level. At 35 weeks a lecithin/sphingomyelin (L/S) ratio of 2 or more indicates that the lungs are mature and able to sustain extrauterine life.

The accuracy of this test depends on the interval between amniocentesis and birth of the child. Within 24 hours it is close to 100 percent. Since the lungs can mature rapidly, too great a period between testing and delivery makes the significance of the test less precise.

In normal pregnancy the L/S ratio correlates well with gestational age. In high risk pregnancy an L/S ratio of over 2 suggests not only that the lungs are mature but that adequate hepatic and neurologic development has taken place.

In certain situations the achievement of a mature L/S ratio does not occur at the expected time:

Maturational Delay Delay can be caused by:

1. Diabetes, classes A, B, C. Women in these categories tend to have

big babies and large placentas. The L/S ratio usually matures at 36 weeks or later instead of 35 weeks.

2. Hydrops fetalis.
3. Chronic renal disease without hypertension.
4. The smaller of identical twins.

Maturational Acceleration   Acceleration can be caused by:

1. Diabetes, classes D, E, F. Infants in these groups are often small with small placentas; the L/S ratio may mature as early as 33 weeks.
2. Rental disease with hypertension.
3. Hypertension associated with preeclampsia or cardiovascular disease.
4. Retroplacental bleeding.
5. Hemoglobinopathies.
6. Rupture of membranes leads to maturation of the lungs, but only after 24 to 48 hours.
7. Hyperthyroidism.
8. Drugs administered to the mother, such as corticosteroids and isoxsuprine.
9. Heroin and morphine addiction.

L/S Ratio in Diabetes   Although there is evidence that the L/S ratio matures early in some classes of diabetes (D, E, F) and late in others (A, B, C), the L/S ratio is a reliable guide to fetal pulmonary maturity in diabetics. The pregnancy of a diabetic patient should not be terminated until an L/S ratio of 2 or more indicates that the fetal lungs are mature unless complications force early intervention. Falling estriol values, severe preeclampsia, or a positive contraction stress test may indicate that delivery is necessary in spite of an L/S ratio of less than 2.

ULTRASONOGRAPHY

A beam of ultrasound passing through fetal tissue is partially reflected at any physical interface. A given echo returns along the path of the ultrasonic beam and may be recorded on an oscilloscope or on a photographic plate. So far no ill effects have been reported. While ultrasound has many uses and while many structures can be visualized, the technique is discussed here only in terms of determining fetal maturity and size.

The biparietal diameter of the fetal head can be measured with reasonable accuracy starting at 13 weeks. The following information has been noted:

1. The biparietal diameter increases by 1.6 to 1.8 mm per week.
2. Failure of this diameter to grow by 1.5 mm over a 2-week period indicates growth retardation.
3. In 90 percent of cases a biparietal diameter of 8.5 cm denotes a gestation of 36 weeks and a weight of over 2,500 g.
4. In situations of disproportion, measurement of the biparietal diameter offers a good estimate of fetal size.

MATERNAL URINARY ESTRIOL EXCRETION

During pregnancy large amounts of estrogens are excreted in maternal urine. During late pregnancy 90 percent of total estrogen is estriol, which can be measured also in the blood and amniotic fluid.

The fetal adrenal gland secretes dehydroepiandrosterone (DHEA) and 16-hydroxyepiandrosterone (16-OH-DHEA) as sulfates. In the fetal liver some DHEA is converted to 16-OH DHEA. The mixture is desulfated and aromatized by placental enzymes, 16-OH DHEA into estriol and DHEA into estrone. About 10 percent of DHEA comes from maternal sources. The estriol and estrone pass to the maternal liver, which conjugates estriol mainly with glucuronic acid and also metabolizes estrone. The majority of the estriol is excreted in the urine. A small quantity passes into the stool and a little into the amniotic fluid. The major end product of DHEA and 16-OH DHEA is estriol glucuronide. Several organs are involved in the production and excretion of estriol; malfunction of any one of them will affect the level of the hormones.

There is a relationship between the amount of estriol in the mother's urine and the welfare of the fetus. As an index to the status of the fetoplacental complex, the estriol levels are meaningful only after 16 weeks' gestation. Fetal death results in a significant drop in the estriol level within 24 hours.

The assay is performed on 24-hour collections of maternal urine. (It can be done on blood also.) In normal pregnancies the amount increases progressively from a level of 0.1 mg per 24 hours at 6 weeks to values ranging from 12 to 50 mg at term. Variation in any normal patient is great, up to 50 or 60 percent. In problem cases serial assays, as often as every 1 or 2 days, are necessary. Decreasing levels are of great significance.

Serial estriol determinations are essential; a single value should never be used for the evaluation of the patient. Abnormal patterns of estriol excretion include the following:

1. A progressive downward trend is observed.
2. A rapid fall takes place.

3. The estriol values remain persistently below the lower level of normal excretion.

Indices of Trouble

1. Serial values
   a. Progressive decline.
   b. A drop of 50 percent in successive measurements at any level.
2. Absolute values (during last 6 weeks of gestation)
   a. Over 12.0 mg: The fetus is in no immediate danger.
   b. Under 12.0 mg: The fetus is at risk. The lower the levels of estriol, the greater the risk.

Management of the Patient with Low or Falling Estriol Excretion

Depending on the severity of the clinical condition and the level of the estriol values, the test is repeated, daily when indicated. If the abnormal results persist a nonstress test and/or a contraction stress test (oxytocin challenge test) is performed. If these show abnormal findings termination of the pregnancy is considered, especially if the L/S ratio is 2 or more.

Causes of Low Estriol Values

FETUS: REDUCED PRODUCTION OF PRECURSORS

1. Adrenal abnormalities
   a. Anencephaly with hypoplastic adrenals
   b. Primary adrenal hypoplasia
   c. Small adrenals secondary to intrauterine growth retardation
   d. Suppression of maternal and fetal adrenals by exogenous administration of corticosteroids
2. Abnormalities of the hypothalamus and pituitary glands
3. Dysfunction of liver
4. Comprised fetus
5. Abnormal enzymatic systems
6. Down's syndrome

PLACENTA

1. Sulfatase deficiency
2. Acquired placental pathology

MOTHER

1. Impairment of enterohepatic circulation.
2. Reduced renal function.
3. Ampicillin kills the bacteria that hydrolyze the sulfate moiety of estriol to allow its resorption from the wall of the bowel. This leads to an increased excretion of estriol in the feces and lower levels in the urine.
4. Betamethasone given for the purpose of stimulating maturity of the fetal lungs.
5. Glycosuria.
6. Mandelamine. The latter two situations produce aldehydes with acid hydrolysis of the urine leading to the destruction of estriol.
7. Abdominal pregnancy.

Causes of High Estriol Values

1. Multiple pregnancy
2. Oversized fetus

Correlation with Clinical Conditions

The exact value of maternal estriol levels in conditions in which the fetus is at risk is not known. By itself this test may lead to erroneous conclusions and ill-advised interference. It is useful only as one of several clinical and laboratory examinations. Fetal death in utero is unusual when the estriol excretion is normal. Dropping titers are a warning that the fetus may be in danger.

There seems to be reasonable correlation between the levels of maternal estriol and fetal outcome in the following situations:

1. Diabetes mellitus. The value of estriol analyses is controversial. However, daily determinations do provide an index of fetal status and, if normal, can enable the clinician to prolong the pregnancy until fetal maturity has been achieved. Intrauterine death is rare when estriol values are normal. A decrease of more than 35 percent may be ominous.

2. Intrauterine fetal death: Such death is followed by a rapid drop in estriol. Values under 1.0 mg are diagnostic. Impending death may be suspected on the basis of falling levels.
3. Prolonged pregnancy. Estriol studies help differentiate between simple postterm pregnancy and fetal postmaturity, and point out when labor should be induced.
4. Retarded intrauterine growth. Serial studies must be done. Estriols are useful in diagnosing that the problem exists and then deciding when the baby should be delivered.
5. Essential hypertension.
6. Preeclampsia.
7. Patients with a poor obstetrical history.

The correlation between estriol levels and the severity of Rh sensitization is not accurate.

Estriol in Blood

Urinary estriol measurements have certain drawbacks: the inconvenience of a 24-hour collection, errors in collection that often occur, abnormal urinary function that may vitiate the results, and considerable delay in obtaining the results. Hence, many centers now measure the level of estriol in plasma. The normal range is between 5 and 55 g per 100 ml. The accuracy of plasma estriols correlates well with the urinary values.

HUMAN PLACENTAL LACTOGEN

This hormone is synthesized by the placenta and transferred into the maternal circulation. It is related immunologically to growth hormone and has the biologic activity of growth hormone and prolactin. Its function is not known.

HPL can be detected in the maternal blood by the fifth week of pregnancy using radioimmune assay. It rises progressively until the last month of pregnancy, increasing to 500 to 1,000 times the levels of early pregnancy.

Because HPL is of solely trophoblastic origin, it was hoped that it would be an index of placental function. Normal values have not been standardized, the results are controversial, and at present it is believed that HPL levels are of no clinical importance in managing complicated pregnancies.

MECONIUM

Meconium, or fetal stool, is thick, viscous, and green. It consists of bile pigment, bile salts, fetal hair, squamous cells, mucopolysaccharides, and cholesterol. The incidence of meconium staining of the placenta and/or fetal body is between 5 and 10 percent. Once meconium has been passed it takes 4 to 6 hours for the placenta and the fetus to become discolored.

Suggested explanations for the passage of meconium include two extremes. On the one hand it may be a normal physiologic function, no more than a sign of increasing fetal maturity. On the other hand the sequence of events may be that fetal hypoxia leads to hyperperistalsis, sphincteric relaxation, and expulsion of intestinal contents.

Meconium is not prominent in acute emergencies such as prolapse of the umbilical cord, placenta previa, or abruptio placentae. Rather, it is seen in chronic stresses including toxemia of pregnancy, prolonged gestation, intrauterine growth retardation, and chorioamnionitis.

The presence of meconium-stained amniotic fluid is not an absolute sign of severe hypoxia, acidosis, or acute fetal distress. It probably indicates a previous episode of intrauterine hypoxia or a state of compensated fetal distress. It is possible that repeated or prolonged episodes of stress could produce intrauterine or neonatal death.

The exact seriousness of this symptom is not known. Marked fetal distress occurs frequently in the absence of meconium, and meconium is often present in the amniotic fluid with no evidence of fetal distress or asphyxia. However, the neonatal mortality rate is higher and the 1- and 5-minute Apgar scores are lower in infants who have passed meconium than in controls. Yet the fetal heart rate patterns and the incidence of acidosis in infants who passed meconium are not markedly different from those who did not. The presence of meconium in the amniotic fluid does enhance the potential for aspiration.

While the passage of meconium is not a reason for panic, it alerts the physician. These patients should be monitored closely so that any further signs of trouble can be noted immediately.

AMNIOSCOPY

Transcervical Technique

An amnioscope (endoscope) is a tube with a source of light that is inserted into the cervical canal to the internal os so that the amniotic fluid can be inspected. Abundant and clear liquor suggests that the fetus is in good condition. Scanty amniotic fluid or meconium indicates that the fetus is at risk and that the pregnancy should be terminated. The membranes are ruptured, and if labor does not ensue within 24 hours cesarean section is considered.

In suspect pregnancies amnioscopy is performed every second day during the late weeks. Indications include (1) the elderly primigravida, (2) postterm pregnancy, (3) intrauterine growth retardation, and (4) toxemia of pregnancy.

Occasionally the amnioscope cannot be passed. Complications include (1) accidental rupture of membranes, (2) onset of labor, and (3) pyrexia.

Transabdominal Technique

A new instrument (fetoscope) has been devised which can be passed into the amniotic sac through the abdomen and the fetus examined under direct vision.

BIOELECTRONIC MONITORING

Techniques

FETAL STETHOSCOPE

Intermittent auscultation of the fetal heart rate using a fetal stethoscope is a valuable and satisfactory method in normal situations. It has certain drawbacks:

1. It is not continuous.
2. The fetal heart is not heard clearly during a uterine contraction.
3. The relationship of the fetal heart rate to the uterine contractions cannot be shown.
4. Only gross abnormalities are observed; subtle clues are missed.
5. There is no permanent record.
6. There is an inherent error in counting.

CONTINUOUS MONITORING OF THE FETAL HEART RATE

FETAL ELECTRODE The most accurate technique is by the application of an electrode to the fetal scalp or buttocks. A fetal electrocardiographic signal is obtained which is filtered, amplified, fed into a cardiotachometer, and recorded as the FHR on one channel of a recorder. The electrode can be applied only after the membranes have ruptured.

PER MATERNAL ABDOMEN The fetal cardiac signal may be obtained by a technique that uses an ultrasonic type of fetal heart detector applied to the mother's abdomen. The signal is less clear than with the direct method, but it has the advantage of being noninvasive, with no need to rupture the membranes.

UTERINE ACTIVITY RECORDING

INTRAUTERINE CATHETER Direct pressure measurements are obtained via a transcervical intrauterine catheter connected to a strain-gauge transducer whose output is registered on the second channel of the recorder.

EXTERNAL TOKODYNAMOMETER This is placed on the abdominal wall. Only semiquantitative recordings are obtained, and these are not as accurate as with the intrauterine method. However, they do indicate when the contractions begin and end, and the method is noninvasive.

Baseline Fetal Heart Rate

This is the pattern that obtains when the patient is not in labor or is between uterine contractions. Four groups are recognized (Fig. 3A).

NORMAL The FHR is 120 to 160 beats per minute. There is a beat-to-beat variation of 5 to 15 per minute. A minor baseline irregularity is normal and indicates that the central nervous system is functioning and is capable of controlling the FHR. Gross irregularity is a bad sign.

TACHYCARDIA The basal rate is above 160 beats per minute, persisting for 10 minutes or more. This situation is seen with maternal fever and hyperthyroidism, fetal immaturity, or the administration of parasympatholytic drugs. In the absence of the above factors, persistent and severe tachycardia indicates the possibilty of fetal hypoxia.

BRADYCARDIA This is a rate of less than 120 beats per minute, lasting for at least 10 minutes. Temporary bradycardia in the absence of marked deceleration patterns is, in most cases, not associated with depressed newborn infants. However, when severe (under 100 beats per minute) and prolonged it may indicate fetal hypoxia.

SILENT PATTERN This refers to a loss of the normal baseline variability, with fluctuations of less than 5 beats per minute. It is a bad sign, suggesting that the fetus cannot respond to normal physiologic and biochemical changes and that the central nervous system is immature or depressed. If the mother has not been administered drugs that account for this pattern, the prognosis for the fetus is grave. Fetal death may be imminent.

Fetal Heart Rate During Labor

Each uterine contraction exerts stress on the fetus in one of three ways: (1) Pressure is applied to the fetal head and body. (2) The circulation in the intervillous spaces is impeded. (3) There is occlusion, partial or complete, of the blood vessels in the umbilical cord.

The main response of the FHR to stress is bradycardia. Deceleration is classified:

1. *Uniform:* When the FHR relates to the intrauterine pressure curve
   a. Early deceleration
   b. Late deceleration
2. *Variable:* When there is no relation between the uterine contraction and the FHR

In interpreting the FHR patterns (Fig. 3) the following features are significant:

1. The baseline FHR
2. The increase or decrease of the FHR in response to a uterine contraction
3. Whether the curve of the FHR is uniform or variable
4. The time relationship between the onset of the contraction and the start of the deceleration of the FHR
5. The lag time, i.e., the interval between the peak of the intrauterine pressure curve and the lowest level of the FHR
6. The recovery time, i.e., the interval from the nadir of the FHR until its return to the baseline

EARLY DECELERATION OF FHR

1. The curve is of uniform shape and appears the same from one contraction to the next (Fig. 3B).
2. The FHR pattern mirrors that of the uterine contraction.
3. The deceleration of the FHR begins early in the uterine contraction.
4. The FHR returns to the baseline by the time the uterine pressure has done so.
5. The FHR stays within the normal range of 120 to 160 beats per minute.
6. Baseline beat-to-beat variation is maintained.

ASSESSMENT OF THE FETUS IN UTERO

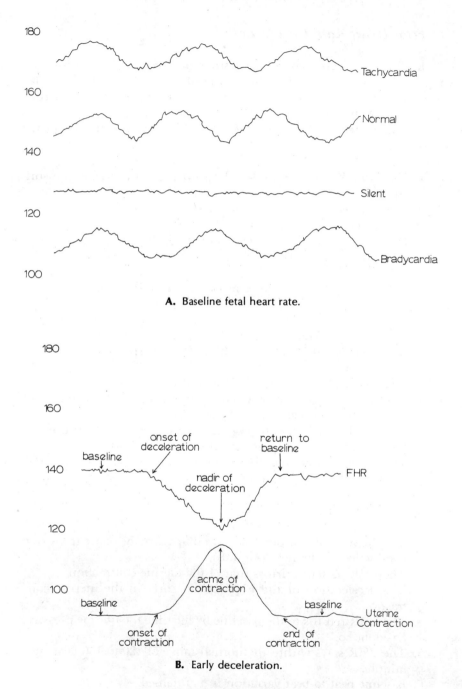

A. Baseline fetal heart rate.

B. Early deceleration.

FIG. 3. Fetal heart patterns

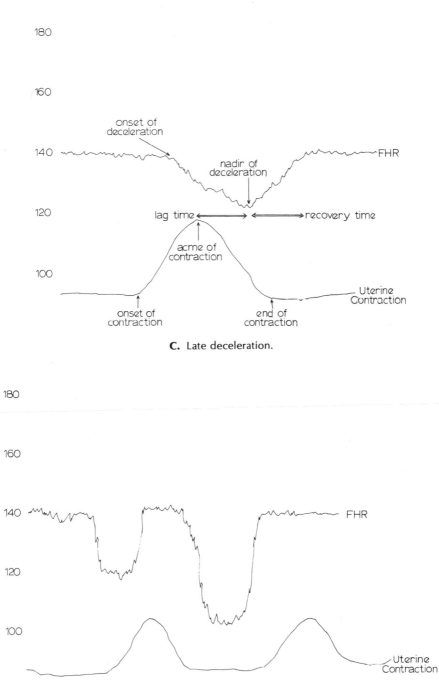

C. Late deceleration.

D. Variable deceleration.

7. The lag time is less than 20 seconds and the recovery time is less than 15 seconds.
8. Administration of oxygen to the mother or a change in her position has no effect on the FHR pattern.

Early deceleration is believed to be the result of compression of the fetal head and is mediated by a vagal reflex. It is a normal pattern. Apgar scores are good and there is no fetal acidosis.

LATE DECELERATION OF FHR

1. The pattern is of uniform shape, one similar to the next. The deceleration begins and returns to the baseline gradually (Fig. 3C).
2. The depth of the deceleration mirrors the intrauterine pressure curve.
3. The onset of the deceleration occurs late in the uterine contraction, 20 to 30 seconds after the onset.
4. The deceleration exceeds 20 beats per minute.
5. The FHR does not return to baseline until after the uterine pressure is back to normal. The deceleration may persist for 30 to 60 seconds after the end of the contraction.
6. The baseline FHR may show signs of irregularity and tachycardia.
7. The lag time is greater than 20 seconds and/or the recovery time is greater than 15 seconds.
8. A pattern exists when 5 or more late decelerations occur consecutively.

Late deceleration is the most ominous of the FHR patterns. Hypoxia is a major cause. The probable mechanism is:

uterine contraction $\longrightarrow$ reduction of intervillous flow of blood $\longrightarrow$
uteroplacental insufficiency $\longrightarrow$ reduced fetal oxygenation (hypoxia or anoxia) $\longrightarrow$
late deceleration of FHR

The infant is often depressed and asphyxiated at birth. Apgar scores are low and acidosis may be present. The normal fetus is able to tolerate reduced oxygenation; the fetus who is already compromised cannot. Late deceleration is seen in patients with high-risk pregnancies, intrauterine growth retardation, postterm pregnancy, maternal hypotension, uterine hyperactivity, excessive stimulation by oxytocin, and other conditions.

Corrective measures include: (1) relief of maternal hypotension by turning the patient on her side, (2) reduction of uterine overactivity by discontinuing the administration of oxytocin, and (3) breathing of high concentrations of oxygen by the mother.

Should the abnormal patterns persist after treatment has been in effect for 10 minutes, preparations must be made for early delivery. If fetal scalp blood sampling techniques are available, this should be done, and if the pH is normal delivery may be delayed.

It must be noted that, while late deceleration patterns increase the likelihood of a depressed infant being born, a number of babies showing this pattern are born with no evidence of hypoxia.

VARIABLE DECELERATION OF FHR

1. The curve is not uniform and varies from one contraction to the next (Fig. 3D).
2. The depth of the deceleration is not related to intrauterine pressure.
3. The onset of deceleration is not related to that of the uterine contraction.
4. The drop in the FHR to 100 beats per minute or lower is dramatic. The return to the baseline is also often abrupt.
5. If the fetus is developing hypoxia, the return of the FHR to the baseline may be slow, the beat-to-beat variation may be decreased, and the baseline FHR may rise.

Variable deceleration is thought to result from compression of the umbilical cord. The pattern of the FHR can be altered by changes in the position of the mother, manipulative or spontaneous movements of the fetus, and the administration of atropine. This pattern may be associated with transient fetal respiratory acidosis.

Variable decelerations lasting less than 30 seconds without slow return to baseline, without loss of baseline irregularity, and without an increase in the baseline FHR do not require intervention. If the decelerations drop to less than 60 beats per minute for longer than 30 to 40 seconds or are associated with a slow return to baseline, loss of baseline variability, and marked fetal tachycardia and are not corrected by changes in maternal position, immediate delivery must be considered.

Intrauterine Death: False Recording of FHR

The fetus acts as a conductor for the low voltage maternal electrocardiogram. When the fetus is alive the maternal signal is overridden by the higher voltage fetal signal. If the fetus is dead the automatic gain control at the monitor amplifies the maternal ECG until it is as large as the usual fetal signal, and then the maternal heart rate is recorded by the monitor. This occurs even when the scalp electrode is in use. It can lead to an erroneous impression that the fetus is alive, and unnecessary emergency cesarean section may be performed.

Indications for Continuous FHR Monitoring

1. Clinically detected abnormalities of the FHR
2. Meconium in the amniotic fluid
3. Oxytocin stimulation of labor
4. Premature labor
5. Slow progress in labor
6. Patients at risk for uteroplacental insufficiency:
   a. Previous stillbirth
   b. Hypertension and preeclampsia
   c. Intrauterine growth retardation
   d. Postterm pregnancy
   e. Abnormal presentation
   f. Rh affected infant
   g. Diabetes
   h. Premature rupture of membranes
   i. Multiple gestation

The Role of Continuous FHR Monitoring

The achievements of electronic monitoring of the fetal heart, both as an adjuvant in the management of difficult labor and as a tool in the extension of knowledge, have been impressive. Success depends upon the availability of proper equipment maintained in good working order, upon the correct use of the monitors, and upon the accurate interpretation of the tracings. The last is not yet an exact science.

It is unfortunate that, too often, excessive reliance is placed on the machinery while clinical acumen is denigrated. The total picture of the high-risk gravida must be kept in mind. Good clinical evaluation encompassing all factors and data must be the final arbiter in selecting the optimal management for the particular patient.

It has been shown that for almost all normal cases and even for many high-risk pregnancies intermittent human auscultation of the fetal heart is as effective as continual monitoring. To achieve this degree of excellence, an almost one-to-one relationship is necessary between the patient and nurse, the auscultator must be an experienced person, and the fetal heart must be evaluated rigidly every 15 minutes in the first stage and every 5 minutes in the second stage of labor. Auscultation of the fetal heart every 1 to 2 hours, not infrequently seen on a busy obstetrical service, is inadequate observation of the laboring patient.

Nonstress Test (NST)

This test is performed on the patient who is not in labor. The external FHR and uterine monitors are applied to the mother's abdomen. The recording is carried on for 20 minutes when the pattern is normal, and for 40 minutes when abnormalities are present or the recording is unsatisfactory. The nonstress test is judged on two features: (1) baseline beat-to-beat variation, and (2) reaction of the FHR to Braxton Hicks contractions and fetal movements.

INDICATIONS

1. Intrauterine growth retardation
2. Prolonged gestation, over 42 weeks
3. Diabetes mellitus
4. Chronic hypertension
5. Preeclampsia
6. Unexplained previous stillbirth
7. Low excretion of estriol

This test has certain advantages over the contraction stress test. The CST is time consuming and expensive, requiring careful and continuous supervision. It may induce premature labor. It may cause tetanic uterine contractions and fetal distress.

Abnormal NST may result from maternal sedation, congenital anomaly of the fetus, and intrauterine growth retardation.

CLASSIFICATION
1. Normal NST (reactive pattern)
   a. Basal FHR of 120 to 160 beats per minute
   b. Baseline variability of 5 to 20 beats per minute
   c. Acceleration of FHR by 15 beats per minute in response to fetal movement or Braxton Hicks contractions (at least four such responses in 20 minutes)
   d. No deceleration of FHR
2. Abnormal NST (nonreactive pattern)
   a. Basal FHR of less than 120 or more than 160 beats per minute
   b. Baseline variability of less than 5 beats per minute
   c. Acceleration of FHR in response to fetal movement or Braxton Hicks contractions of less than 15 beats per minute

    d. Any deceleration lasting over 30 seconds or of an amplitude of over 30 beats per minute

    e. Repeated late deceleration in response to Braxton Hicks contractions

The nonreactive NST may be subdivided in order of increasing severity:

1. Those showing no accelerations in response to fetal movements, or an absence of fetal movements
2. Flat tracings, without baseline variability
3. Late decelerations

INTERPRETATION AND MANAGEMENT

Normal Reactive Nonstress Test   The normal reactive NST indicates that the fetus is in good condition on that day and will survive for 1 week at least. Fetal death almost never occurs within a week of a normal non-stress test. However, the test should be repeated weekly. No further action is necessary unless there is a deterioration in the clinical condition.

Abnormal Nonreactive Nonstress Test   A nonreactive tracing is not an absolute indicator of a poor outcome, but it suggests the presence of fetal hypoxia and does provide a serious warning. Perinatal mortality, fetal distress in labor, cesarean section for fetal distress, and low Apgar scores are all significantly increased in the nonreactive group. The NST is af-fected by sedative drugs, such as diazepam, and in these patients abnormal tracings should be repeated after the drug has been withdrawn.

1. When a nonstress test produces a nonreactive tracing one of two courses are indicated:
    a. Some workers advise that the test be repeated in 24 to 48 hours.
    b. Probably, it is better to proceed to a contraction stress test and to base further management on the combined results.
2. If the pregnancy is near term, the L/S ratio is 2 or more, and the levels of estriol are low or falling, delivery of the baby is consid-ered. Induction of labor under continual fetal monitoring is satisfactory.
3. In preterm pregnancies when the L/S ratio is under 2 the ad-vantages of delay are weighed against giving the patient gluco-corticoids and delivering the baby after 24 hours.
4. When the nonstress test shows a complete loss of beat-to-beat variation and late decelerations in response to fetal movement

or Braxton Hicks contractions, the fetus is in trouble and immediate delivery by cesarean section is indicated.

Contraction Stress Test (Oxytocin Challenge Test)

This test is based on the principle that, in late pregnancy, the response of the fetal heart rate to oxytocin-induced contractions is a useful method of evaluating the status of the fetoplacental unit and of predicting the capacity of the fetus to withstand the stress of labor. It is rarely indicated before 28 weeks of gestation, a time when the fetus would not be viable if delivery were necessary.

INDICATIONS

1. Intrauterine growth retardation
2. Prolonged gestation, over 42 weeks
3. Diabetes mellitus
4. Chronic hypertension
5. Preeclampsia
6. History of unexplained previous stillbirth
7. Low excretion of estriol

CONTRAINDICATIONS

1. Ripe cervix—because of danger of accidental induction of labor
2. Ruptured membranes
3. Polyhydramnios
4. Multiple pregnancy
5. Placenta previa
6. Previous cesarean section

TECHNIQUE

The patient is placed in a 30 degrees semi-Fowler's position, with a slight lateral tilt to reduce the impact of pressure of the uterus on the inferior vena cava, which can cause subsequent supine hypotension. The maternal blood pressure is measured every 10 minutes. The baseline fetal heart rate and uterine contractions are recorded for 15 minutes.

Oxytocin is given by pump, starting with a dose of 0.5 mU per minute. The dose is increased incrementally every 15 minutes until at least three uterine contractions, each lasting 60 to 90 seconds, occur per 10-minute interval. To avoid uterine hypertonus the maximum safe dose is 20 mU per minute. If no contractions occur by 30 minutes the procedure is discontinued. The test should not be performed when the cervix is ripe because an accidental and undesirable induction of labor may occur.

RESULTS

1. POSITIVE TEST The occurrence of six consecutive late deceleration patterns of the FHR, or late deceleration patterns in over 50 percent of all contractions.
2. SUSPICIOUS TEST Late onset deceleration patterns that occur less frequently than defined for the positive test.
3. NEGATIVE TEST Absence of any late deceleration patterns of the fetal heart rate.
4. UNSATISFACTORY TEST
   a. The quality of the recording is poor so that interpretation is not possible.
   b. Uterine contractions are less than 3 per 10 minutes
   c. Hyperstimulation: The frequency of uterine contractions is greater than 5 per 10 minutes or the contractions last longer than 90 seconds. In these situations the OCT should be repeated on another day.

SIGNIFICANCE OF THE CONTRACTION STRESS TEST

It is believed that the CST is a sensitive indicator of uteroplacental function and fetal condition and is effective in detecting the fetus in jeopardy in utero. The CST and other tests of fetus state have two main benefits: (1) A negative test is a reliable indicator of fetal well-being and suggests that the placenta can sustain the fetus for at least 1 week. This helps the clinician avoid unnecessary early delivery and exposure of the neonate to the hazards of prematurity. It is rare for a stillbirth to occur when the CST is negative. (2) A positive test alerts the physician to the possibility of fetal distress so that intervention can be carried out before the fetus succumbs to inadequate placental exchange. Yet the limitations of a positive CST must be kept in mind. Certainly the test indicates a group of patients who are at increased risk, but false-positive tests are frequent. A positive test is not an indication for cesarean section. Each patient should be evaluated carefully. Many of these women can have a successful vaginal delivery of an healthy infant. Intrapartum monitoring is mandatory in these cases.

MANAGEMENT

1. Negative test: Repeat weekly until labor begins.
2. Suspicious test: Repeat in 72 hours.
3. Positive CST:

a. If the L/S ratio is greater than 2.0 intervention is considered, especially if the estriol excretion is low or falling.
b. If the L/S ratio is less than 2.0 and the daily 24-hour urinary estriol excretion is normal, intervention is avoided.
c. If the L/S ratio is less than 2.0 and the estriol is low and/or falling, intervention is considered after consultation with the neonatologist.
d. The method of delivery depends on the status of the cervix and the likelihood of easy induction.

Combined Stress and Nonstress Test

Because the nonstress test is easier and perhaps safer than the stress test (CST), some centers perform the nonstress test first and carry on with the CST only when the nonstress test does not provide the necessary information.

Psychologic Response to Fetal Monitoring

Valuable as the fetal monitor is, it transforms the labor room into an intensive care environment, and some patients manifest strong reactions.

Positive Response Many women find that their state of anxiety is relieved, the machine providing valuable information that is otherwise unavailable. The clicking of the monitor confirms that the baby is alive. Both patient and husband can tell when the next contraction is coming and are able to prepare for it. Women who have had a fetal loss in a previous pregnancy are strongly in favor of fetal monitoring.

Negative Response The patients complain about the discomfort from the abdominal transducers and from the wires of the intravaginal electrode, which hangs between their thighs. They are unhappy with their enforced immobility, the loss of privacy, and their loss of control of the labor. Some are concerned that the electrode may damage the baby or that fetal monitoring is carried on only in dangerous situations and become anxious by variations in the FHR. A few resent the doctor and the husband paying more attention to the equipment than to the patient and feel that they are being used as guinea pigs.

The solution to these problems lies in educating the patient in the antepartum period. A description and demonstration of the apparatus, correction of erroneous impressions as to the purposes of and indications for fetal monitoring, reference to the scalp electrode as a small clip attached to the skin, and reassurance that the procedure is not part of a research project will make electronic monitoring more acceptable.

During labor the working and purposes of the monitor should be explained, the patient should be allowed as much mobility as possible, her comfort must be a paramount consideration, and her privacy maintained.

BIOCHEMICAL ANALYSES

Hypoxia produces bradycardia as a symptom and acidosis as a metabolic result. The pH of fetal blood will be lowered when lactic acid increases as a result of anoxia and anaerobic metabolism of glucose.

Saling developed a method of testing fetal blood for acidosis before birth. After the membranes are ruptured an endoscope is placed through scalp or buttocks. Microanalysis is performed mainly to determine the pH, but other parameters can be measured as well. These include hemoglobin, PO_2, glucose, electrolytes, blood type, and Coombs' test.

During labor there is a gradual shift toward acidity in the fetal blood. The pH decreases from 7.33 to 7.25. In normal cases this change does not represent significant anoxia. Apgar scores are normal.

An arbitrary setting of 7.20 as the lower level of normal has been established. A pH of less than 7.20 is indicative of fetal acidosis and distress. When the pH is under 7.10 shortly before delivery there will be significant fetal depression in 90 percent of cases. On the other hand, a pH above 7.25 predicts that 90 to 95 percent of fetuses will be born healthy and nondepressed.

A scheme of management was proposed by Saling:

1. An abnormal FHR is an indication for analysis of the fetal blood.
2. If the pH is over 7.25 labor is allowed to go on, and the analysis is repeated only if the FHR remains abnormal.
3. When the pH is 7.20 to 7.25 another sampling is performed in 30 minutes.
4. With the pH under 7.20, another sample is collected immediately and preparations are made for operative delivery. If the second analysis confirms the first one, delivery is carried out immediately.

Many workers have been unable to establish a consistent relationship between actual pH during the second stage of labor and the condition of the newborn. They cannot assign a pH value below which the fetus is at unquestionable risk and surgical intervention is mandatory. The main use of the technique may be in the avoidance of cesarean section, when the diagnosis of fetal distress is made on invalid criteria.

Nonetheless, there is good correlation with the Apgar scores. A pH of over 7.25 is associated with an Apgar score of over 7 in 90 percent of cases.

Falsely normal results (pH over 7.20, low Apgar score) occur in association with sedative drugs, anesthesia, obstruction of the airway, congenital anomalies, prematurity, hypoxia subsequent to the sampling, trauma of delivery, or a previous episode of asphyxia (the acid-base balance returns to normal, but the central nervous system does not).

Falsely abnormal results (pH under 7.20, good Apgar score) may occur in the presence of maternal acidosis. Hence, it is important to measure the maternal pH when low values are obtained in the fetus before definitive action is taken.

BIBLIOGRAPHY

Brinsmead MW: Complications of amniocentesis. Med J Aust 1:379, 1976

Caterini H, Sama J, Iffy L, et al: Reevaluation of amniography. Obstet & Gynecol 47:373, 1976

Doran, TA, Benzie RJ, Harkins JL, et al: Amniotic fluid tests for fetal maturity. Am J Obstet Gynecol 119:829, 1974

Flynn AM, Kelly J: Evaluation of fetal well being by antepartum fetal heart monitoring. Br Med J 1:936, 1977

Freeman RK: Intrapartum fetal evaluation. Clin Obstet Gynecol 17:83, 1974

Freeman RK, Goebelsman U, Nochimson D, Cetrulo C: An Evaluation of the significance of a positive oxytocin challenge test. Obstet Gynecol 47:8, 1976

Garite TJ, Freeman RK, Hochleutner I, Linzey EM: Oxytocin challenge test. Obstet Gynecol 51:614, 1978

Gluck L, Kulovich MV: Lecithin/sphyngomyelin ratios in amniotic fluid in normal and abnormal pregnancy. Am J Obstet Gynecol 115:539, 1973

Harbert GM: Evaluation of fetal maturity. Clin Obstet Gynecol 16:171, 1973

Haverkamp AD, Thompson HE, McFee JG, Cetrulo C: The evaluation of continuous fetal heart rate monitoring in high-risk pregnancy. Am J Obstet Gynecol 125:310, 1976

Ostergard DR: Estriol in pregnancy. Obstet Gynecol Surv 28:215, 1973

Ott WJ: The current status of intrapartum fetal monitoring. Obstet Gynecol Surv 31:339, 1976

Patrick JE, Perry TB, Kinch RAH: Fetoscopy and fetal blood sampling: A percutaneous approach. Am J Obstet Gynecol 119:539, 1974

Perkins RF: Antenatal assessment of fetal maturity. Obstet Gynecol Surv 29:369, 1974

Starkman MN: Fetal monitoring. Psychological consequences and management recommendations. Obstet Gynecol 50:500, 1977

Visser GHA, Huisjes HJ: Diagnostic value of the unstressed antepartum cardiotocogram. Br J Obstet Gynaecol 84:321, 1977

Ylikorkala O: Maternal serum HPL levels in normal and complicated pregnancy as an index of placental function. Acta Obstet Gynecol Scand Suppl 26, 1973

37.

Radiography and Ultrasonography

As a diagnostic aid the x-ray has a wide range of uses in obstetrics. Because the exact effects of the rays on the maternal ovaries and on the fetus are not known, radiography should be employed in pregnancy only when there is a clear and definite indication. The first trimester is considered to be the most dangerous time.

USES OF RADIOGRAPHY IN OBSTETRICS

Fetus

The following information regarding the fetus can be determined by radiography:

HYDATIDIFORM MOLE
In cases where hydatidiform mole or chorionepithelioma is suspected and clinical examinations and hormonal tests are inconclusive, a flat plate of the abdomen can demonstrate the presence or absence of a fetus.

MULTIPLE PREGNANCY
The presence of multiple pregnancy can be proved and the positions of the babies in utero shown.

FETAL MATURITY
Sometimes fetal maturity can be determined. From 36 weeks onward, well developed bony structure is seen in all major parts of the skeleton. The distal (lower) femoral epiphyseal ossification center is present in over 80 percent of infants from week 36 onward. The proximal (upper) tibial epiphyseal ossification center appears at about week 38. It is ill-defined at this time but becomes clearly visible at 40 weeks. Between

weeks 40 and 43 the proximal tibial epiphyseal ossification center becomes as large as the distal femoral center. The demonstration by films of the maternal abdomen of the distal femoral center indicates that the fetus is mature in 96 percent of cases.

POSITION AND STATION

When manual examination is inconclusive, x-ray can be used where it is necessary to establish the lie, presentation, position, and attitude of the fetus. Engagement and descent of the presenting part can also be demonstrated.

ABNORMALITIES

Fetal abnormalities such as hydrocephaly, anencephaly, and spina bifida may be demonstrated. In hydrops fetalis the fetus sometimes assumes the Buddha position.

INTRAUTERINE DEATH

Loss of Fetal Tone   When the fetus dies the muscles become flaccid and there is loss of flexion. The uterus becomes reduced in size as it tends to become more spherical. This loss of height is accentuated by resorption of amniotic fluid. The fetus appears rolled up and the term ball sign has been used. This sign takes several days to become apparent, but it is fully established by 1 week after fetal death.

Spalding's Sign (1922)   The overlapping and angulation of the cranial bones is consequent to the shrinkage of the brain and the collapse of the skull. In late pregnancy, before the onset of labor or rupture of the membranes, disalignment of more than 4 mm is indicative of fetal death. Spalding's sign may be present as early as 7 days after death and can be identified without difficulty by 10 days.

Gas in the Fetus   Gas has been demonstrated in intra- and extravascular areas after death in utero. The common sites for accumulation of gas are the heart, the aorta, and the portal veins. The pattern may be confused with gas in the maternal bowel. In the umbilical vessels, however, the finding of gas is pathognomonic. In the umbilical arteries the gas assumes the pattern of a coil or helix; in the vein it has the appearance of a kinked piece of string. The nature and origin of the gas are uncertain; it is probably carbon dioxide. This sign may be seen as early as 12 hours after death. It is present within 10 days in 84 percent of cases.

Halo Sign (Devel 1947)   The fetal skull is covered by the scalp. The layers from the deepest to the most superficial are as follows:

1. The periosteum is closely adherent to the bony skull.
2. The galea (an aponeurotic layer) is attached loosely to the periosteum.
3. The subcutis is attached firmly to the galea. During the last months of pregnancy the subcutis is densely infiltrated by fat cells and is the thickest soft tissue layer of the scalp.
4. Outside the subcutis is the cutis.

The fat-containing subcutaneous layer has a lower density than the other soft tissue and appears on the x-ray of the fetus in utero as a dark line.

When there is edema of the scalp the fluid lies mainly between the periosteum and the galea and to a lesser degree between the galea and the subcutis. The edema fluid elevates the fat-containing subcutis from the skull. On x-ray the fat layer is seen as a dark line apart from the skull and more or less parallel to it. This sign appears no sooner than 3 days after fetal death. Severe erythroblastosis with hydrops fetalis is the only condition in which the halo sign is seen in a live fetus.

Mother

The following conditions of the mother can be determined by radiography:

1. Abdominal pregnancy. The fetus may be seen to lie outside of the uterus.
2. Congenital anomalies of the pelvis.
3. Bony injury to the pelvis, e.g., after an accident.
4. Pelvimetry: investigation of fetopelvic disproportion.

AMNIOGRAPHY

Amniocentesis is performed. Some 30 ml of amniotic fluid are removed and an equal amount of radiopaque fluid is injected into the amniotic cavity. The opaque fluid is dispersed quickly through the amniotic fluid. For the diagnosis of fetal abnormalities the x-ray films are taken within 15 minutes. The fetus swallows the fluid, which is identifiable by 3 hours, and reaches its highest density by 12 to 24 hours after injection. The fluid is excreted via the kidneys. By use of amniography:

1. The amniotic cavity can be visualized.
2. The placenta is localizable.

3. Abnormalities of the uterine cavity can be identified.
4. Fetal hydrops can be diagnosed.
5. Absence of radiopaque medium from the intestines suggests a blockage.
6. The urinary tract can be outlined.
7. Fetal anomalies can be seen.

X-RAY PELVIMETRY

X-ray pelvimetry is the most frequently used method of radiography in obstetrics. It is a valuable aid to mensuration of the pelvis, but only when used in conjunction with clinical examination and judgment. Information is obtained concerning (1) the shape and inclination of the pelvis, (2) the length of the diameters, and (3) the relationship and fit of the fetus to the pelvis.

X-ray pelvimetry not only provides greater precision of mensuration but makes possible the measurement of many important diameters that cannot be obtained manually, e.g., the transverse diameter of the inlet and the distance between the ischial spines. Moreover, it affords a better understanding of the configuration of the pelvis. This has enabled the female pelvis to be classified according to shape, permitting a more accurate clinical prognosis to be made of the outcome of labor.

The distortion produced by divergence of the x-rays because of the distances between the tube, the patient, and the film can be a problem (Fig. 1). This factor must be taken into consideration when measurements are calculated.

FIG. 1. Principle of divergent distortion. Size of the image depends on object-film distance (d) and tube-film distance (D). (From Eastman and Hellman. *Williams Obstetrics*, 14 ed, 1971. Courtesy of Appleton-Century-Crofts.)

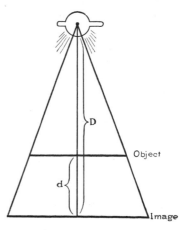

Abdominal View

An anteroposterior view is taken of the abdomen with the patient positioned on her back. This view gives a good picture of the entire fetus.

INFORMATION GAINED

1. Attitude of the fetus
2. Lie, presentation, and position
3. Rough estimate of the size of the baby
4. Presence of more than one fetus
5. Ossification centers that may provide an estimate of fetal maturity
6. Fetal abnormalities or death

Standing Lateral View

A lateral view of the pelvis is taken with the patient erect. A metal ruler with notches or perforations 1 cm apart is placed in the gluteal folds between the buttocks. The ruler has the same degree of distortion as the pelvis and the desired diameters can be measured.

INFORMATION GAINED

1. Inclination, curve, and length of the sacrum
2. Depth of the pelvis
3. Relationship of the promontory of the sacrum to the inlet
4. Sacrosciatic notch—whether it is wide or narrow
5. Anteroposterior diameters of the inlet, the obstetric conjugate; midpelvis; the plane of least dimensions; and the outlet
6. Posterior sagittal diameter of the midpelvis and the outlet
7. Size and shape of the ischial spines. Are they small or large? Are they prominent and posterior? Do they shorten the posterior sagittal diameter and narrow the sacrosciatic notch?
8. Length and inclination of the symphysis
9. Station of the fetal presenting part
10. In cephalic presentations, the presence of synclitism or asynclitism
11. Attitude of the fetus: flexion or extension
12. Relationship or fit of the head to the pelvis

Anteroposterior View

The anteroposterior film is taken with the patient positioned in a semirecumbent position so that the x-ray tube is aimed at the inlet, looking into the midpelvis. A special grid is used for making measurements.

INFORMATION GAINED

1. Shape of the inlet, the posterior and anterior segments. Is the posterior segment well rounded or heart-shaped? Is the anterior segment round or wedge-shaped?
2. Widest transverse diameter of the inlet.
3. Distance between the ischial spines, the transverse diameter of the plane of least dimensions.
4. Anterior and posterior sagittal diameters of the inlet.
5. Size and shape of the ischial spines.
6. Slope of the sidewalls. Are they straight, convergent, or divergent?
7. Classification of the pelvis.

Indications for X-ray Pelvimetry

1. Nonpregnant state
   a. History of difficult delivery
   b. Grossly abnormal pelvis e.g., fracture
   c. Previous cesarean section; vaginal delivery being considered
2. During pregnancy, before labor
   a. Breech presentation
3. During active labor
   a. Breech, undiagnosed antepartum
   b. Cephalic presentation; arrest in second stage; station, attitude, position unclear; decision to be made: forceps or cesarean section.

Once an important tool in the diagnosis and management of obstetric problems, x-ray pelvimetry plays a reduced role today. Clearer understanding of uterine dysfunction, the realization that most disproportion is relative and its seriousness can be assessed properly only by a trial of labor, acceptance of the use of oxytocin stimulation in trials of labor, elimination of the fear of doing a cesarean section after the patient has been in labor for some time, and the knowledge that radiation may be harmful have all helped narrow the indications for pelvimetry.

X-ray pelvimetry is needed rarely in modern times because:

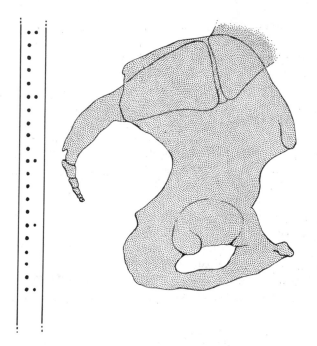

A. Relation of the centimeter scale image to the lateral view of the pelvis.

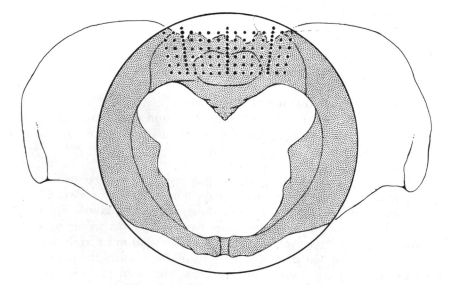

B. Relation of the centimeter scale image to the anteroposterior view of the pelvis.

FIG. 2. Thoms' technique.

1. In most cases the decision can be made on clinical examination and a trial of labor.
2. Often the reason for failure of progress is not demonstrated by x-ray.
3. In cases of disproportion the cause is a large baby more often than a contracted pelvis.
4. Inefficient labor is a frequent factor when progress ceases, and this is not shown by x-ray.
5. Most cesarean sections are performed in women with normal pelves.
6. If the cervix does not dilate, vaginal delivery is impossible.

PLACENTOGRAPHY

The main purpose of these techniques is to localize the placenta when placenta previa is suspected.

METHODS THAT DEPEND ON FETAL DISPLACEMENT

1. Anteroposterior and lateral films are taken with the patient erect. If the presenting part lies within 2 cm of the sacral promontory or the symphysis pubis it is unlikely that placenta previa exists.
2. The bladder is filled with radiopaque fluid and standing anteroposterior and lateral films are taken. If the fetal presenting part lies close to the bladder, placenta previa is unlikely.

SOFT TISSUE PLACENTOGRAPHY

By the use of an aluminum filter the margins of the uterus and the fetal subcutaneous layer of fat can be demarcated. The tissues between the fetus and the uterine wall are of equal density, and the placental site is deduced from variation in the thickness of this intervening area.

RADIOISOTOPES

A radioactive isotope is injected into the maternal circulation. The extensive vascularity of the placenta leads to a high degree of radioactivity in this area, which is detectable by an external counter. The total dose of radiation to the fetus is small and safe, less than with an x-ray film. The isotope is attached to a high-molecular-weight carrier such as radioiodinated serum albumin or Technetium, and it does not cross the placenta.

ULTRASOUND

Ultrasonic localization of the placenta is accurate, safe, and the preferred method.

DANGER OF RADIATION

The possible deleterious effects of x-ray on the embryo and fetus can be grouped in the following way:

1. DEVELOPMENTAL EFFECTS A disturbance of growth during organogenesis may result in hypoplasia, absence, or gross distortion of part or all of an organ. If the effect is of major proportions death and abortion will occur.
2. MUTATION This refers to an unusual and permanent change in the structure of the genetic material or the chromosome. In such cases the infant may appear normal at birth, the abnormalities appearing only later in life.
3. EFFECTS ON THE CENTRAL NERVOUS SYSTEM The CNS is unique in being susceptible to radiation-induced damage through the entire period of gestation.
4. LATE EFFECTS There may be a higher incidence of neoplasia (especially leukemia) in children who were exposed to radiation in utero.

The degree of risk to the fetus in utero engendered by radiologic examination of the mother is not known and may, indeed, prove to be minimal. However, until the final truth is established, diagnostic x-ray should be used only when there is a clear and necessary indication and avoided whenever possible.

ULTRASOUND

Ultrasonics are vibrational waves of a frequency above the hearing range of the normal human ear and include waves with a frequency of more than 20,000 cycles per second. For purposes of medical diagnosis wave frequencies of 1 million to 15 million vibrations per second are used.

Since 1880 it has been known that when a force is applied to a piezoelectric crystal an electrical current is generated. Conversely, when an electrical current is passed across the surface of such a crystal a high frequency vibrational wave is produced. The transducer that sends out the waves also receives the echoes when they return. In medicine the pulsed ultrasonic system is used; the transducer is sending out signals less than 1 percent of the time and is listening for their return the rest of the time. The sonar systems use a high-powered burst of sound referred to as a pulse.

The transducer is coupled to the body by a fluid such as water, mineral oil, or olive oil, enabling the ultrasonic beam to penetrate the body. At the time when the beam crosses an interface, an echo is reflected. This is picked up by the transducer, which converts the returning vibrations into electrical energy, amplifies them, converts them into audible sounds, and/or records them on an oscilloscope screen. Objects of differing densities vary in the amount of energy they reflect back to the receiver, accounting for the pictures produced and enabling diagnoses to be made.

The purposes for which diagnostic ultrasound is used depend on the ability it offers: (1) to determine the distance of an object from a known point on the surface, (2) to determine its angular position from a known point on the surface, and (3) to detect movement.

Systems measuring only movement depend on the Doppler effect. The closer the object is, the higher is the frequency of the arrival of waves at the observer. These systems use a continuous wave transmission and detect the change in the frequency of returned signals as a result of movement of the target being investigated. An example is the use of signals corresponding to cardiac movements to provide a heart rate sound for monitoring purposes.

The A-scan is a simple, inexpensive mechanism with a limited field of usefulness. Providing linear measurements, it can demonstrate the extent of movement but does not show the character of the motion. The A-scope gives a one-dimensional view, measuring the space between two interfaces. It can determine the biparietal diameter of the fetal head.

The B-scan is more complicated and has a wide range of diagnostic capabilities. This sonar system provides a noninvasive technique of producing cross-sectional pictures (B-scan) of internal organs and structures which enable size and position to be determined. The B-scan shows what would be seen if the subject were cut through along the plane defined by the beam and the cut surface surveyed. It can outline the fetal skull, the thorax, the extremities, and the placenta. The machine measures the time interval between two echoes, and this is converted to distance on the basis of assumed speed of transmission through the tissues.

There are no contraindications to the use of ultrasound. No evidence of tissue damage has been demonstrated.

Use of Ultrasound in Obstetrics

EARLY DETECTION OF PREGNANCY

In the first trimester the patient's bladder should be full during use of ultrasound because sound waves pass through fluid more easily and reach the deeper structures. The amniotic sac can be seen by 6 weeks. Fetal echoes are obtainable from the 9th to 10th week. After 39 days the diagnosis is 95 percent accurate. If the sac is not visible by 6 weeks it is doubtful that a normal pregnancy exists. After the 12th week the gestational sac is no longer seen.

FETAL HEART ACTIVITY
This has been noted as early as 45 days. It is accurate after 8 weeks. By the use of real-time imaging, fetal movement can be detected at 6 to 7 weeks by observing the patient for 5 minutes.

ABORTION
Ultrasonic examination can distinguish between a normally developing pregnancy and a missed abortion. Serial scans may be necessary. Signs of early failure of pregnancy include:

1. A poorly formed gestational sac with fragmentation
2. An empty sac
3. Absence of fetal heart action
4. A gestational sac over 2 weeks behind the dates, with no growth in the next week

The diagnosis can be made early and appropriate therapy instituted, saving time and hospital stay and obviating uncertainty.

ECTOPIC PREGNANCY
The finding of an intrauterine sac rules out ectopic pregnancy in most cases. In some cases an adnexal mass can be seen.

HYDATIDIFORM MOLE
The appearance is that of a diffuse intrauterine "snowflake" pattern, which is finer than that of the normal placenta. Theca-lutein cysts with septa can be detected. Following evacuation of the mole the regression in the size of these cysts can be observed by serial ultrasonic scans.

FETAL CEPHALOMETRY
The head of the fetus may be visible as early as the 11th week of pregnancy. Actual measurement of the biparietal diameter (BPD) is feasible by the 13th week in 75 percent of cases, by the 14th week in 95 percent, and in the 15th week in 100 percent. The accuracy is greatest between the 20th and 30th weeks of gestation. In 95 percent of fetuses the measurement of the BPD is reliable to ± 3 mm on serial examinations. A single BPD estimation gives an accuracy of 84 percent with an error of ±9 days. The reliability is less in the third trimester. In the first half of pregnancy the mean weekly growth of the BPD is 0.3 cm.

INTRAUTERINE GROWTH RETARDATION

Serial scans are helpful in following suspected cases of intrauterine growth retardation on the basis of actual size and rate of growth. An interval of 3 weeks is necessary for an accurate diagnosis. The biparietal diameter alone is not always conclusive, and the ratio between the size of the body and that of the head is more significant in this area. Up to 32 to 36 weeks the circumference of the head is greater than that of the body. At 32 to 36 weeks the measurements are the same. After 36 weeks the circumference of the body becomes larger than that of the head. In many cases of IUGR this reversal of the ratio does not take place, and is a point in favor of the diagnosis.

MULTIPLE PREGNANCY

This can be diagnosed as early as the 10th week and easily by the 16th week.

DETECTION OF FETAL ANOMALIES

1. Anencephaly. A single screening can confirm the presence or absence of the fetal head. Two examinations at a weekly interval are advised in suspicious cases at 14 to 15 weeks' gestation.
2. Hydrocephaly may be identified when the BPD is over 11.0 cm.
3. Microcephaly may be suspected but is difficult to diagnose.
4. Meningocele can be recognized sometimes by the double-ring outline produced by the double sac of the meningomyelocele.

FETAL PRESENTATION

The lie of the fetus and whether the head or the breech is presenting can be ascertained easily.

POLYHYDRAMNIOS

The diagnosis is based on the impression that there is a larger amount of amniotic fluid than expected relative to the size of the fetus and the duration of the pregnancy.

INTRAUTERINE FETAL DEATH

The fetal heart is unobtainable by Doppler technique or echocardiography. The B-scan evidence of fetal death, seen within 24 to 48 hours, consists of the development of a fluffy fetal contour and a double skeletal outline. The latter is indicative of gross edema. Subsequently the loss of fetal structure is seen in the collapsed thorax and the misshapen skull. Multiple intercranial echoes appear with the loss of the midline echo complex of the head. The double skull is seen also in severe maternal diabetes and advanced Rh disease.

LOCALIZATION OF THE PLACENTA

Ultrasound is the safest and most reliable method of placentography. By the use of gray scaling, the texture, quality, margins, and thickness of the placenta can be noted. In the first part of pregnancy sonograms have shown placentas that were low lying and even over the cervix. Later in pregnancy the placenta was found to be in the upper segment. Probably the normal growth of the placenta is away from the cervix. In addition the uterus enlarges faster than the placenta and, as pregnancy progresses, a proportionately smaller area of the uterus is covered by placenta. The finding of a low-lying placenta in early pregnancy is an indication for reexamination later—nothing more. No cases have been reported of a placenta moving downward once it has located itself in the upper segment.

PUERPERAL OR POSTABORTAL UTERUS

This organ can be scanned to see if there are any retained products of conception. Blood clot may confuse the picture.

Limitations of Ultrasound

1. The picture obtained is a cross-sectional, two-dimensional view, and only those structures directly in the line of the beam can be seen. Those in a different plane cannot be seen at the same time.
2. In early pregnancy twins may be missed if the heads are at different poles and are not seen at the same time and especially if the diagnosis is not suspected on clinical grounds.
3. Cephalometry is tricky as the correct angle must be located. Deep engagement of the head in the pelvis makes measurement of the BPD difficult or impossible.
4. The time needed to determine growth with reasonable confidence is not less than 3 weeks.
5. Considerable experience is needed. Sources of error include those of the apparatus and those of the observer:
   a. The reading error in measuring the BPD on a given occasion.
   b. The error involved in measuring the BPD on different occasions.
   c. The limitations of the physical properties of the apparatus.

BIBLIOGRAPHY

Campbell S, Johnstone FD, Holt EM, May P: Anencephaly: Early ultrasonic diagnosis and active management. Lancet 9 Dec 72:1226

Davidson JM, Lind T, Farr V, Whittingham TA: The limitations of ultrasonic cephalometry. J Obstet Gynaecol Br Commonw 80:769, 1973

Gaulden ME: Possible effects of diagnostic x-rays on the human embryo and fetus. J Arkansas Med Soc 70:424, 1974

Hellman LM, Kobayashi M, Cromb E: Ultrasonic diagnosis of embryonic malformations. Am J Obstet Gynecol 115:615, 1973

King DL: Placental migration demonstrated by ultrasonography. Radiology 109:167, 1973

Malvern J, Campbell S, May P: Ultrasonic scanning of the puerperal uterus following secondary post partum hemorrhage. J Obstet Gynaecol Br Commonw 80:320, 1973

Piiroinen O: Studies in diagnostic ultrasound. Acta Obstet Gynaecol Scand Suppl 46, 1975

Shaff MI: An evaluation of the radiological signs of the fetal death. South African Med J 49:736, 1975

38.

Normal and Abnormal Uterine Action

DEFINITIONS

CONTRACTION   Contraction is the shortening of a muscle in response to stimulus, with return to its original length after the contraction has worn off.

RETRACTION   The muscle shortens in response to a stimulus but does not return to its original length when the contraction has passed. The muscle becomes fixed at a relatively shorter length, but the tension remains the same. In this way the slack is taken up and the walls of the uterus maintain contact with the contents. Retraction is responsible for descent. Without this property the fetus would move down with the contraction, only to return to the original level once the contraction had ceased. With retraction, on the other hand, the fetus remains at a slightly lower level each time. During contraction it is as though three steps are taken forward and then three backward. With retraction, three steps are taken forward and then two backward. In this way a little ground is gained each time. In the control of postpartum bleeding retraction is essential. Without it many patients might bleed to death.

PHYSIOLOGIC RETRACTION RING   As labor and retraction proceed, the upper part of the uterus becomes progressively shorter and thicker, while the lower portion gets longer and thinner. The boundary between the two segments is the physiologic retraction ring (Fig. 1).

PATHOLOGIC RETRACTION RING   In cases of obstructed labor the physiologic ring becomes extreme and is known as the pathologic retraction (Bandl's) ring.

CONSTRICTION RING   This is a localized segment of myometrial spasm which grips the fetus tightly and prevents descent.

556

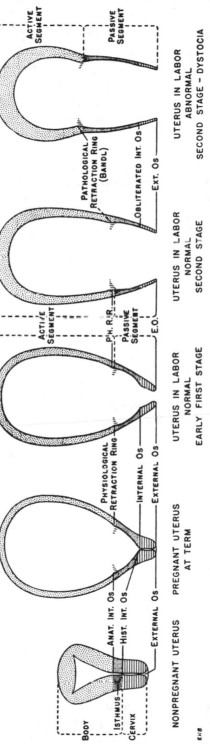

FIG. 1. Progressive development of the segments and rings of the uterus at term. Note comparison between the nonpregnant uterus, uterus at term, and uterus in labor. The passive segment is derived from the lower uterine segment (isthmus) and cervix; the physiologic retraction ring from the anatomic internal os. The pathologic ring which forms under abnormal conditions develops from the physiologic ring. (From Hellman and Pritchard. *Williams Obstetrics*, 14th ed, 1971. Courtesy of Appleton-Century-Crofts.)

TONUS Tonus is the lowest intrauterine (intraamniotic) pressure between contractions. It is expressed in millimeters of mercury (mm Hg). The normal resting tension is 8 to 12 mm Hg.

INTENSITY Intensity or amplitude is the rise in intrauterine pressure brought about by each contraction. The normal is 30 to 50 mm Hg.

FREQUENCY Caldeyro-Barcia defined this as the number of contractions per 10 minutes. For the patient to be in good labor the frequency must be at least two per 10 minutes.

UTERINE ACTIVITY Uterine activity is described by Caldeyro-Barcia as the intensity multiplied by the frequency and is expressed in Montevideo units (millimeters of mercury per 10 minutes).

POLARITY OF THE UTERUS When the upper segment contracts, the lower segment relaxes. Actually the lower part does contract, but much less than the upper part. The effect is as though the lower portion did relax.

PAIN OF LABOR

Pain during labor is related to contractions of the uterus. In normal labor the pain is intermittent. It starts as the uterus contracts, becomes more severe as the contraction reaches its peak, and disappears when the uterus relaxes. The degree of pain varies in different patients, in the same patient during succeeding labors, and at different stages in the same labor. In some cases the contractions are painless.

Causes

1. Distention of the lower pole of the uterus.
2. Stretching of the ligaments adjacent to the uterus.
3. Pressure on or stretching of the nerve ganglia around the uterus.
4. Contractions of the muscle while it is in a relatively ischemic state (similar to angina pectoris). This occurs especially when the uterine tonus is too high or when the contractions are too frequent and last too long. Adequate amounts of blood do not get to the muscles and they become anoxic.

PAIN IN LOWER ABDOMEN

Pain in the lower abdomen seems to be related to activity in the upper uterine segment and is present during efficient labor.

PAIN IN BACK

Pain in the back is related to tension in the lower uterus segment and the cervix. In normal labor back pain is prominent only at the start of a contraction and in the early stages of cervical dilatation. When the cervix is abnormally resistant the backache is severe. Backache is prominent also in posterior positions. In general, the less the backache the more efficient the uterus.

PAIN IN THE INCOORDINATE UTERUS

1. An excessive amount of pain is felt in the back.
2. Because of persistent high tonus or spasm in some parts of the uterus the pain seems to be present even in the intervals between contractions.
3. The patient complains of pain before the uterus is felt to harden, and the pain persists even after the uterus relaxes and softens.

NORMAL UTERINE CONTRACTIONS

Caldeyro-Barcia has published a logical and understandable description of the normal uterine contraction wave.

Triple Descending Gradient (TDG) of Caldeyro-Barcia

Each contraction wave has three components:

1. The propagation of the wave is from above downward. It starts at the pacemaker and works its way to the lower part of the uterus.
2. The duration of the contraction diminishes progressively as the wave moves away from the pacemaker. During any contraction the upper portion of the uterus is in action for a longer period of time than the lower.
3. The intensity of the contraction diminishes from top to bottom of the uterus. The upper segment of the uterus contracts more strongly than the lower.

In order that normal labor may take place all parts of the triple descending gradient must perform properly. The activity of the upper part dominates and is greater than that of the lower part. All parts of the uterus contract, but the upper segment does so more strongly than the lower segment; in turn, the latter's contractions are stronger than those of the cervix. Were this not so there would be no progress. This is the modern interpretation of uterine polarity.

The normal contractions are regular and intermittent. There is contraction (systole) and relaxation (diastole). The most efficient uterus is one showing moderately low tonus and strong contractions.

PACEMAKERS
Normally there are two, one situated at each uterine end of the fallopian tube. Since one pacemaker is responsible for initiation of a contraction, their activities must be coordinated. In the abnormal uterus new pacemakers may spring up anywhere in the organ, resulting in incoordinate uterine action.

PROPAGATION
The wave begins at the pacemaker and proceeds downward to the rest of the uterus. A small wave goes up to the fundal portion of the uterus above the level of the pacemaker.

COORDINATION
Coordination is such that, while the wave begins earlier in some areas than in others, the contraction attains its maximum in the different parts of the uterus at the same time. The places where the contraction starts later achieve their acme more rapidly. Thus at the peak of the contraction the entire uterus is acting as a unit. Relaxation, on the other hand, starts simultaneously in all parts of the uterus. For normal uterine action there must be good coordination between the two halves of the uterus as well as between the upper and lower segments.

DILATATION OF THE CERVIX
Dilatation of the cervix is caused by two mechanisms:

1. The pressure on the cervix by the presenting part: When this part of the fetus is regular and well fitting—e.g., the flexed head— it favors effective uterine action and smooth cervical dilatation. The bag of waters does not play an important role in helping promote good contractions and rapid cervical opening.
2. The longitudinal traction on the cervix by the upper part of the uterus as it contracts and retracts: After each contraction the upper segment becomes shorter and thicker; the lower uterine segment becomes longer, thinner, and more distended; and the cervix becomes more and more dilated.

Cervical dilatation is the result of a gradient of diminishing activity from the fundus through the lower uterine segment.

ROUND LIGAMENT CONTRACTION
These ligaments contain muscle, and they contract at the same time

as the upper segment of the uterus. This anchors the uterus, prevents its ascending in the abdomen, and so helps force the presenting part down.

Uterine Contractions During Pregnancy

Some uterine activity goes on throughout pregnancy. During the first 30 weeks the frequency and strength of the contractions are low, less than 20 Montevideo units.

After 30 weeks and especially after 35 weeks the contractions become more frequent and may be noticed by the patient. Sometimes they are painful and are called false labor pains. Prelabor, as evidenced in the increasing activity of the uterus during the later weeks of pregnancy, is an integral part of the process of evacuating the human uterus. The contractions of this period are associated with steadily increasing uterine activity, cervical ripening, and general readiness for true labor. Prelabor merges into clinically recognizable labor by such small degrees that the exact point at which so-called true labor begins is difficult to determine.

CLASSIFICATION OF UTERINE ACTION

Clinical Conditions with Normal Contractile Waves

NORMAL LABOR

The intensity or amplitude of the contractions varies from 30 to 50 mm Hg, and frequency is two to five contractions per 10 minutes.

TRUE INERTIA

When the intensity of the contractions is less than 25 and the frequency is under two per 10 minutes, progress is slow and labor prolonged. If the intensity is less than 15, labor does not begin, or if it has started it ceases.

The uterine tonus is normal, the pattern of activity is coordinated, and the relaxation of the lower segment is adequate. The uterus, however, is inactive, and the expulsive efforts are weak, infrequent, or both. There is progress neither in descent of the presenting part nor in dilatation of the cervix. It is often difficult to be sure that the patient is in labor. Pain is mild or even absent entirely.

The force exerted on the fetus is small and no caput succedaneum is formed. No damage is done to either mother or child.

PRECIPITATE LABOR

Precipitate labor lasts less than 3 hours. In some cases an amplitude over 50 is responsible for the rapid labor. In most instances, however, the chief factor enabling the baby to pass easily through the pelvis is the lack of resistance of the maternal tissues.

Conditions that predispose to or contribute to the etiology of precipitate labor include:

1. Multiparity
2. Large pelvis
3. Lax and unresistant soft tissues
4. Strong uterine contractions
5. Small baby in good position
6. Induction of labor by rupture of membranes and oxytocin infusion
7. Previous precipitate labor

The distinction must be made between precipitate labor and precipitate delivery. The latter, being sudden and unexpected, carries with it the dangers of an unattended birth.

While many authors have warned of the dangers of rapid labor, such as maternal lacerations, cerebral hemorrhage, brain damage in the fetus, and asphyxia from interference with the placental circulation, some recent studies suggest that the risk to mother and child is not greater than the average labor.

CERVICAL DYSTOCIA

Cervical dystocia includes two main groups:

1. Primary dystocia
   a. Achalasia of the cervix: The failure or inability of the structurally normal cervix to relax and open
   b. Rigid cervix: An anatomic abnormality of the cervical tissue
   c. Conglutination of the external os: The sticking together of the lips of the cervix
2. Secondary dystocia
   a. Post delivery
   b. Postoperative scarring
   c. Cancer

If the condition is not treated the cervix may rupture or annular detachment may take place. The constant and prolonged pressure on the cervix leads to anoxia and devitalization of the tissue, which eventually separates and comes away as a ring. Usually there is thrombosis in the vessels at the site of separation, so bleeding is rarely a problem.

In some cases the cervix becomes well effaced and the external os very thin, but dilatation does not take place. In this situation incision of the rim of cervix is followed by easy delivery.

OBSTRUCTED LABOR

Etiologic factors range from fetopelvic disproportion through malpresentations to neoplasms blocking the birth canal. As labor proceeds and the uterus tries to overcome the obstruction, the contractions become more frequent and stronger, and the tonus rises. There is progressive retraction of the upper segment with stretching and thinning of the lower part of the uterus. The physiologic retraction ring becomes the pathologic (Bandl's) ring. The round ligaments are tense and may be palpable through the abdomen. The pain is severe and felt in the abdomen.

If the obstruction is not relieved and the contractions go on, rupture of the lower segment is the final outcome. In some cases the myometrium becomes exhausted and inertia sets in before rupture occurs.

While the uterus itself does not impede the descent and birth of the baby, the strong, frequent contractions and high tonus may cut off the placental circulation and kill the baby.

RAPID OVERDISTENTION OF THE UTERUS

Acute polyhydramnios is an example. The rapidly accumulating amniotic fluid leads to a rise in tonus and a fall in the intensity of the contractions.

SLOW DISTENTION OF THE UTERUS

Slow distention of the uterus is seen in multiple pregnancy or in chronic polyhydramnios. The increase in the intrauterine volume is slow and gradual, so there is time for compensatory hypertrophy and hyperplasia of the uterine muscles. For this reason the tonus and intensity of the contractions are normal.

Contractile Waves with Inverted Gradient

Caldeyro-Barcia described the normal contraction wave as having three properties:

1. The propagation of the wave is from above downward.
2. The duration of the contraction diminishes progressively as the wave moves away from the pacemaker.

3. The intensity of the contraction decreases from the top of the uterus to the lower part.

One of the varieties of inefficient uterine action takes place when the gradients of the normal contraction are inverted. The inversion may be total or partial.

1. Total: All three gradients are affected. The uterine contractions are completely ineffective. There is no progress—neither dilatation of the cervix nor descent of the fetus.
2. Partial: One or two of the gradients are involved. Some cervical dilatation may take place, but it is very slow.

Inversion of the propagation gradient means that the contraction begins in the lower segment and moves upward. Normally it goes the other way. Inversion of the duration gradient means that the contraction lasts longer in the lower than in the upper segment. This is the opposite of the normal wave. When there is inversion of the intensity gradient, the lower segment contractions are stronger than those of the upper segment. This is the hypertonic lower segment of Jeffcoate. Normally the opposite is true.

When these conditions are present the polarity of the uterus is reversed. The contractions are of no value in furthering progress as they produce no effacement or dilatation of the cervix. They are the type of contraction seen often in false labor and prelabor.

Clinically, as compared with true inertia, these patients do have pain and it may be severe. Backache is often the main complaint. Typically, the fetus remains high, and the cervix stays thick, uneffaced, and poorly applied to the presenting part.

Incoordination of the Uterus: Localized Contraction Waves

ASYMMETRICAL UTERINE ACTION

The pacemakers do not work in rhythm, and each half of the uterus acts independently. Small contractions alternate with large ones. The minor contractions are entirely ineffective. The major ones do bring about some cervical dilatation but much less effectively than normal waves. Progress is painfully slow.

UTERINE FIBRILLATION: THE COLICKY UTERUS

In this condition new pacemakers appear all over the uterus. The myometrium contracts spasmodically, frequently, irregularly, and purposelessly. The tonus is elevated slightly, but the action is not effectively expulsive. The fetus is not pushed down, and the cervix does not dilate well.

Pain is present all the time—before, during, and after contractions. The pain is out of proportion to the intensity of the contractions.

CONSTRICTION RING

A constriction ring is a localized phenomenon. A ring of myometrium goes into tetanic contraction. The most common site is 7 to 8 cm above the external os of the cervix. A constriction ring can develop rapidly. Causes include:

1. Intrauterine manipulations
2. Failed forceps
3. The use of oxytocin when the uterus is hypertonic
4. Spontaneous constriction ring, which usually occurs in a colicky uterus

The constriction ring grips the fetus tightly and prevents its descent. It is the cause of the obstruction. In the pathologic contraction ring of Bandl, on the other hand, the obstruction to the passage of the fetus comes first and it is the cause of the ring.

The area of spasm is thick, but the lower segment is neither stretched nor thinned out. Constriction rings never lead to uterine rupture. The patient experiences severe pain, and the tenderness of the uterus makes her resist palpation of the abdomen.

While deep surgical anesthesia is needed to relax the major rings, lesser degrees of anesthesia, sedation, or Adrenalin Chloride may be effective in the milder forms.

Diagnosis is made by abdominal, vaginal, and intrauterine examinations:

1. The ring may be felt on abdominal examination.
2. There is no change in the station of the presenting part during a contraction.
3. The fetal head is loose in the pelvic cavity both during and between uterine contraction.
4. The portion of the uterus between the external os and the ring is lax during the contraction.
5. The cervix is floppy and is not well applied to the presenting part.
6. Because of the laxity of the cervix a hand can be passed into the uterine cavity and the ring palpated.
7. By placing a finger between the cervix and the head, the impact

TABLE 1. Differential Diagnosis of Constriction Ring and the Pathologic Retraction Ring

Constriction Ring	Pathologic Retraction Ring
Localized ring of spastic myometrium.	Formed by excessive retraction of upper segment.
May occur in any part of the uterus.	Always at junction of upper and lower segments.
Muscle at the ring is thicker than above or below it.	Myometrium is much thicker above than below the ring.
Uterus below the ring is neither thin nor distended.	Wall below is thin and overdistended.
Uterus never ruptures.	If uncorrected, uterus may rupture.
Uterus above ring is relaxed and not tender.	Uterus above ring is hard.
Round ligaments are not tense.	Round ligaments are tense and stand out.
May occur in any stage of labor.	Usually occurs late in the second stage.
Position of the ring does not change.	The ring gradually rises in the abdomen.
Presenting part is not driven down.	Presenting part is jammed into the pelvis.
Fetus may be wholly or mainly above the ring.	Part of the child must be below the ring.
Patient's general condition is good.	Patient's general condition is poor.
Uterine action is inefficient.	Uterine action is efficient or overefficient.
Abnormal polarity.	Normal polarity.
Results in obstructed labor.	Caused by an obstruction.

on the finger during a strong contraction is found to be quite weak.

The differential diagnosis may be made by studying Table 1.

SPASM OF THE INTERNAL OR EXTERNAL CERVICAL OS

The cervix does not relax and does not dilate. The contractions of the cervix are stronger than those of the lower uterine segment, and no progress is made.

Abnormal Uterine Action: Third Stage of Labor

Separation and expulsion of the placenta and the control of hemorrhage are dependent on normal uterine action. Abnormal uterine contractility can lead to the following complications:

1. Uterine inertia may cause delayed separation of the placenta and postpartum hemorrhage.
2. The colicky uterus interferes with normal separation.
3. A constriction ring prevents normal expulsion.
4. Cervical spasm may trap the placenta in the uterus.
5. Incoordinate uterine action may lead to inversion of the uterus.

INCOORDINATE UTERINE ACTION

Etiology

The quoted incidence varies from 1 to 7 percent, but it is doubtful that the real syndrome occurs in more than 2 percent of labors. Mild disproportion and malpresentations predispose to abnormal uterine action.

AGE AND PARITY

This is mainly a condition of primigravidas. About 95 percent of severe cases occur in first labors, and the uterus is almost always more efficient during the next pregnancy. The incidence in elderly primigravidas is only a little higher than in young women.

CONSTITUTIONAL FACTORS

Especially prone to incoordinate uterine action is the thickset, obese, masculine, relatively infertile woman. There appears to be a familial tendency. It is not associated with general debility or malnutrition.

NERVOUS AND EMOTIONAL CONDITIONS

We do not know how nervous and emotional problems act in causing or aggravating incoordination of the uterus in labor. It has been claimed that fear increases the tension of the lower uterine segment. However, there are placid women who have difficult labors, and highly emotional ones who have easy deliveries. Most grave disorders of the central nervous system do not affect labor adversely.

ERRORS OF THE UTERUS

While some workers believe that overdistention, fibroids, and scars of the uterus predispose to poor uterine contractions, others deny it. Certainly the congenitally abnormal, incompletely fused, or bicornuate uterus does not behave well in labor.

RUPTURE OF THE MEMBRANES

Rupture of the membranes under proper conditions stimulates the uterus to better contractions and speeds progress. However, rupture of the bag of waters when the cervix is unripe—i.e., uneffaced, hard, thick, and closed—does lead to a prolonged and inefficient type of labor.

MECHANICAL ERRORS IN THE RELATION OF FETUS TO BIRTH CANAL

A close and even application of the presenting part to the cervix and lower uterine segment during the first stage of labor and to the vagina and perineum in the second stage results in good reflex stimulation of the myometrium. Anything that prevents this good relationship causes the reflex to fail, and poor contractions may be the result.

The relationship of posterior positions, extended attitudes, and transverse arrest to faulty uterine action is well known. The malposition precedes the uterine disturbance, and if it can be corrected good contractions often return.

Late engagement and incomplete formation of the lower uterine segment may be an early sign of an incoordinate uterus. Mild degrees of cephalopelvic disproportion predispose to incoordinate uterine action.

IRRITATION OF UTERUS
Improper stimulation of the uterus by drugs or intrauterine manipulations may bring about incoordination.

Clinical Picture

LABOR
The clinical picture is of prolonged labor in the absence of feto-pelvic disproportion. There is hypertonus, increased tension, and spasm in some areas of the uterine muscle which persist even between the contractions. The resting intrauterine pressure is increased. The contractions may be frequent and are usually irregular in strength and periodicity. Despite uterine contractions that are often strong and always painful, progress is slow or absent. The cervix dilates slowly, and the presenting part advances little or not at all. This condition occurs in all degrees, from mild to most severe.

Labor may be normal at first or it may be incoordinate from the beginning. Premature rupture of the membranes while the cervix is closed and uneffaced is seen frequently. The patient complains bitterly of pain, and when examination shows no progress the assumption is made that she is making more fuss than the condition warrants. The experienced obstetrician, however, recognizes the condition and orders sedation. After a rest the contractions may resume in a normal pattern, or they may still be incoordinate. As time passes the colicky nature of the pain increases. The patient holds her hands over the sensitive uterus to protect it. Eventually more sedation is needed.

Labor is long, especially the first stage, because with incoordinate uterine action the cervix fails to dilate normally. After a long period: (1) the cervix may dilate fully, and the baby may be born spontaneously or by forceps; (2) some method of promoting cervical dilatation may have to be used before the baby can be extracted; or (3) vaginal delivery may be abandoned and cesarean section performed.

It is characteristic of this condition that the patient complains of the pain before the uterus is felt to harden, and the pain persists after the uterus softens. Sometimes there is continual pain, especially severe in the back. The patient realizes that she is not making progress, and her anxiety and loss of morale aggravate the situation. Eventually she becomes exhausted and dehydrated, and the pulse and temperature rise.

The cervix may be thick or thin, it may be applied tightly to the presenting part or hang loosely in the vagina. It dilates very slowly and may never reach full dilatation. In most cases dilatation stops at 6 to 7 cm. Sometimes a thick, edematous anterior lip is caught between the pubis and the fetal head.

The patient often experiences the acute desire to bear down before the cervix is fully dilated. The attendant must stop the patient from doing this, for it exhausts her without furthering progress. There is a tendency to urinary retention. Vomiting is common and adds to the dehydration.

DIAGNOSIS
Diagnosis is based on the following:

1. The patient's subjective impression of the strength and duration of the pains
2. The physician's objective impression of the duration of the contractions, and his partly objective opinion of their strength
3. Observation of the effectiveness of the contractions in promoting progress, especially cervical dilatation
4. The use of electronic equipment to monitor the uterine contractions and the fetal heart rate

MATERNAL DANGERS
1. Exhaustion
2. Hemorrhage and shock
3. Infection
4. Lacerations of the vagina during difficult deliveries
5. Appular detachment or lacerations of the cervix

After 24 hours the dangers to the mother and fetus rise sharply. Many women suffer so much that they refuse to have more children. Maternal mortality is under 1 percent.

FETAL DANGERS

1. Asphyxia from prolonged labor and from interference with utero-placental circulation during long, hard uterine contractions
2. Injury during traumatic delivery

3. Pulmonary complications from aspiration of infected amniotic fluid

The fetal mortality is under 15 percent. The prognosis used to be bad, especially because of traumatic forceps deliveries performed often before the cervix was fully dilated and with the head not engaged. The improvement in the results are due to:

1. Early diagnosis of ineffective uterine action
2. More timely forceps extractions
3. Increased use of cesarean section
4. Better anesthesia
5. Early diagnosis of fetal hypoxia by electronic monitoring of the fetal heart rate

False Labor

False labor is attended by irregular contractions. There is no progress, no dilatation of the cervix, and no descent of the presenting part. No damage is done to the fetus. The contractions may be painful and prevent the patient from resting. Sometimes they do have an effect in effacing the cervix and are called prelabor contractions. Treatment is sedation and rest.

Secondary Uterine Inertia

Secondary uterine inertia is a condition of myometrial and general fatigue. It is often associated with prolonged obstructed labor. The contractions become feeble, infrequent, and irregular and may stop altogether. Progress ceases. Treatment is hydration and rest.

Management of Incoordinate Uterine Action

INVESTIGATION AND DIAGNOSIS

1. The patient is observed as to her general condition, the amount of pain, and the degree of progress.
2. The uterus is palpated to determine the type and severity of the contractions.
3. Vaginal examination shows the position, station, size of the

caput, condition of the cervix, presence of a constriction ring, and any disproportion.
4. In cases of doubt, x-rays are taken to rule out fetopelvic disproportion or abnormal position.
5. Questions to be answered include:
    Is there disproportion?
    Is the fetus placed badly?
    Is the woman in true labor?
    Is the uterus hypertonic or hypotonic?
    Is the uterine action incoordinate?
    Is the basic problem at the cervix?

PREVENTION

1. Fear is counteracted by good prenatal care.
2. Analgesia is used when necessary to prevent loss of control.
3. Heavy sedation is prescribed for false labor, so that the patient is not exhausted when she goes into true labor.

GENERAL MEASURES

1. The morale of the patient should be maintained.
2. Intravenous infusions are given for hydration. Glucose in water provides nourishment and prevents acidosis.
3. The bladder and bowel should be emptied when necessary.
4. Antibacterial measures are used when indicated.

SEDATION AND ANALGESIA
While an excessive amount of sedation can inhibit uterine contractions, properly used it does not interfere with true labor. The patient needs sedation to relieve her anxiety and analgesia to make the pain less severe. Often sedation and rest change poor labor into a better variety. Continuous lumbar epidural analgesia is frequently effective in improving uterine coordination.

UTERINE STIMULATION
The uterus should be stimulated only in hypotonic conditions. If the uterus is hypertonic, stimulation makes the situation worse. Methods include:

1. Keeping the patient walking around to maintain the presenting part against the cervix
2. Oxytocin, given best as a dilute intravenous infusion
3. Artificial rupture of the membranes

OPERATIVE MEASURES

1. When the head is low and the cervix thin, the cervix may be dilated manually or an anterior rim pushed over the fetal head.
2. Forceps rotation and extraction can be performed when the cervix is fully dilated. The operation should not be delayed until the mother and fetus are in poor condition.
3. Cesarean section is used more often today. It is safer for mother and chlid than a traumatic vaginal delivery.

CONSTRICTION RING

Relaxing drugs and deep anesthesia can be tried. If these succeed in releasing the constriction, the fetus is extracted with forceps. Cesarean section, however, is probably the method of choice.

BANDL'S PATHOLOGIC RETRACTION RING

Since the basic problem here is cephalopelvic disproportion, cesarean section is the proper therapy. If the baby is dead craniotomy may be considered.

CERVICAL DYSTOCIA

1. Cesarean section is the procedure of choice when the cervix does not dilate.
2. Manual dilatation or incisions of the cervix are used rarely.

39.

Uterotonic Agents: Oxytocin, Ergot, Prostaglandin, Sparteine Sulfate

OXYTOCIN, PITUITRIN, PITOCIN, AND PITRESSIN

To fill the need for an agent to stimulate uterine contractions in selected obstetric situations, posterior pituitary extract has been available for 70 years. At first, whole posterior pituitary extract (pituitrin) was used. It contains mainly an oxytocic agent and an antidiuretic hypertensive factor. The extract has been divided into its two main components: an almost pure oxytocic (pitocin) and its hypertensive counterpart (pitressin).

During the early 1950s DuVigneaud and his colleagues succeeded in the purification, chemical identification, and synthesis of oxytocin and vasopressin. The natural and synthetic products are equally efficient in regard to their action on the myometrium. Synthetic oxytocin is a chemically pure substance and is free from the danger of reaction to animal protein. At the present time all commercial preparations of oxytocin used in obstetrics are synthetic.

Oxytocin, an octopeptide, is produced in the supraoptic and paraventricular nuclei of the hypothalamus and is stored in the posterior pituitary gland. Oxytocin-releasing stimuli include: (1) cervical dilatation, (2) coitus, (3) emotional reactions, (4) suckling, and (5) drugs such as acetyline choline, morphine, nicotine, and certain anesthetics.

573

Effects of Oxytocin

UTERUS

In causing the uterus to contract, oxytocin is believed to act on the myometrial cell membrane. It increases the normal excitability of the muscle but adds no new properties. The myometrial sensitivity to oxytocin rises as pregnancy progresses.

CARDIOVASCULAR SYSTEM

Oxytocin has numerous effects on the cardiovascular system.

1. Heart rate: a small to moderate increase.
2. Systemic arterial blood pressure: a decrease results mainly from a lowering of peripheral resistance.
3. Cardiac output: given as a single dose oxytocin causes a rise in cardiac output, followed by a fall; continuous infusion results in an increased cardiac output.
4. Renal blood flow: no significant change.
5. Skin: the blood vessels are sensitive to the vasodilatory action of oxytocin, and flushing of the face, neck, and hands may occur.
6. Uterine flow: the decrease is caused mainly by the extravascular resistance around the uterine blood vessels as the result of the increased uterine contractions.

KIDNEYS

Oxytocin can induce antidiuresis. The human kidney is not damaged, the excretion of electrolytes is not changed, and renal blood flow is not reduced. The antidiuretic action probably occurs by resorption of water from the distal convoluted tubules and the collecting ducts.

Administration

Routes of administration include intramuscular or repeated subcutaneous injections of small or large doses and the placing of a cotton pledget soaked in 5 or 10 units of oxytocin in the nostril, whence the drug is absorbed. However, the intravenous infusion of a dilute solution of oxytocin is so superior to other methods that it is the procedure of choice, to the virtual exclusion of the others.

ADVANTAGES OF THE INTRAVENOUS ROUTE

1. The amount of oxytocin entering the bloodstream can be regulated. With other techniques the amount given to the patient is

known, but there is no control over the rate of absorption. It can be fast or slow, regular or intermittent, and it may accumulate in the tissues to be released later in a large amount and high concentration.

2. Minute amounts are effective.

3. The blood level and the activity of oxytocin are constant as long as the rate of the drip is maintained. It can be speeded up or slowed down with instant changes in effect.

4. The plasma of pregnant women near term contains an enzyme, pitocinase, in such high concentration that half of an intravenously given dosage of pitocin is destroyed in 2 to 3 minutes. Thus, within 3 to 4 minutes of shutting off an intravenous infusion, the oxytocic activity has ceased.

5. The contractions brought on by this technique seem to be mainly of the normal triple descending gradient type.

TECHNIQUE OF INTRAVENOUS ADMINISTRATION

The two methods of intravenous infusion are by the use of a constant infusion pump or by a Murphy drip. Whichever system is employed it is advisable to start the drip at a rate of 1.0 mU per minute to test for untoward reactions. If none occur the speed of the infusion is increased until the desired effect is achieved. The maximum safe dose is 20 mU per minute. In most cases doses of less than 10 mU per minute are adequate.

In high-risk cases, when extreme accuracy and control are essential, the constant rate infusion pump should be used. Changes in the patient's position or movement will not affect the speed at which the solution is being infused.

For the average situation the drip technique is satisfactory. The popular strengths of the solutions are 5 or 10 U. of oxytocin in a liter of 5 percent glucose in water. In most instances a concentration of 2 U. per liter will be effective. The advantages of the dilute solution are that the physiologic dose is being employed, the control is easier, and the danger is reduced. When used for induction or augmentation of labor, it is advisable to maintain the infusion for 1 hour post partum to control uterine atony. To avoid water intoxication the amount of oxytocin and fluid must be controlled carefully; 1 liter per 24 hours is the maximum.

When the drip method is used the two-bottle system is advised. One bottle contains a liter of 5 percent glucose in water. The other contains a liter of 5 percent glucose in water to which the oxytocin has been added; this must be labeled clearly. The two tubes leading from the bottles are connected by a Y adapter, which connects to the needle in the vein. The Y adapter should be as close to the needle as possible so that change from one solution to the other has an immediate effect.

The drip is started with the pure glucose solution; when it is running at 10 to 15 drops a minute the switch is made to the oxytocin solution. Careful observation is made as to the type, strength, and duration of the contractions and to their effect on the fetal heart. If no untoward reactions are noted, the drip is continued. If excessive uterine contractions occur, or if there is fetal bradycardia (under 100), tachycardia (over 160), or irregularity of the heart, the oxytocin is stopped and plain glucose is infused. Oxytocin is one of the most potent drugs known. It may vary a hundredfold in its actions on different people. The dosage is regulated by the effect on the individual receiving it. The speed of the drip is determined by and correlated to the frequency, intensity, and duration of the resulting contractions, rather than by any arbitrary number of drops per minute. The aim is to bring about strong uterine contractions lasting 40 to 50 seconds, and recurring every 2 to 3 minutes. Care must be exercised to avoid tumultuous contractions so frequent and prolonged that there is no interval between them. This carries the danger of uterine rupture, placental separation, and fetal asphyxia.

Indications for Use of Oxytocin

MANAGEMENT OF ABORTIONS
Oxytocin is used during abortions to stimulate the uterus to pass retained tissue and to control bleeding.

Inevitable Abortion   The symptoms are bleeding and cramps. The cervix is partly open, but the products of conception have not been passed. Oxytocin stimulates the uterus to contract and expel its contents after the cervix has been opened widely. Curettage is easier through an open cervix. The oxytocin keeps the uterus firm, makes it easier to avoid perforation of the uterine fundus, and helps control hemorrhage.

Incomplete Abortion   The fetus has been passed, but part or all of the placenta is in situ. Oxytocin helps expel what is left, makes curettage easier, and controls hemorrhage.

Complete Abortion   Oxytocin is used to reduce postabortal bleeding.

Missed Abortion   While most missed abortions terminate spontaneously, in some instances (e.g., danger of hypo- or afibrinogenemia) one can wait only so long and then steps must be taken to empty the uterus. Oxytocin is valuable to soften the cervix, to open it sufficiently so that dilatation and curettage can be performed safely, and to keep the uterine tone high so that bleeding is controlled.

INDUCTION OF LABOR

Elective Induction of Labor   Elective induction of labor is performed for a variety of reasons including the following:

1. Convenience to the mother and doctor
2. Patients with a history of precipitate labors
3. Patients who live a long distance from the hospital

As long as the cervix is ripe (soft, less than 1.3 cm (0.5 inch) long, effaced, open to admit at least one finger, and easily dilatable) and the head is well in the pelvis, induction of labor is feasible. Artificial rupture of the membranes increases the efficiency of inducing labor with oxytocin.

Spontaneous Rupture of the Membranes   If the membranes rupture prematurely, much before term, an attempt is made to prolong the pregnancy to a point where the baby is big enough to survive. On the other hand, most patients who rupture the membranes near or at term go into spontaneous labor. If this does not take place within 24 hours induction of labor is indicated.

Fetal Salvage   In certain instances where the pregnancy has gone past the date of expected confinement by 2 weeks or more, induction is indicated. Rupture of the membranes and an oxytocin drip are the methods of choice, providing the cervix is ripe and the head engaged. In diabetic mothers and in those who are sensitized to the rhesus factor, induction of labor before term may be necessary. If conditions are right this can be done with oxytocin and rupture of the membranes. If the cervix is not ripe and the presenting part is high, cesarean section may be safer.

Maternal Indications   In conditions such as preeclampsia, premature separation of the placenta, and fetal death in utero, the time comes when medical management or watchful expectancy is no longer indicated and the pregnancy must be terminated artificially in the interests of the mother. This is especially true if her condition is deteriorating.

Ripening of the Cervix   As a general rule, induction of labor by artificial rupture of the bag of waters is not attempted unless the cervix is ripe and the head is in the pelvis. Should induction be essential in the presence of an unripe cervix, an attempt is made to ripen it. The patient is given an oxytocin drip several hours daily for a few days. In most instances, this does not institute true labor, but the oxytocin-induced contractions often bring the head down into the pelvis and ripen the cervix so that the membranes can be ruptured and good labor instituted.

TO IMPROVE EFFICIENCY OF UTERINE CONTRACTIONS

Prolonged Labor due to Hypotonic Uterine Inertia In prolonged labor due to hypotonic uterine inertia oxytocin is most valuable. The effect is to increase the type of contraction already present. In true hypotonic inertia the pattern is normal, but the contractions of the upper segment are weak and progress is not made. Before using oxytocin in these conditions one must be sure that there is no disproportion or malpresentation, since these abnormalities signal poor uterine action.

In hypotonic uterine action an oxytocin drip may result in an immediate improvement of the labor, with steady progress to successful delivery of the child. The proper use of pitocin in these cases has resulted in:

1. Successful termination of the labor
2. Reduction in the incidence of midforceps, cervical lacerations, cesarean section, Dührssen's incisions, and traumatic deliveries
3. Shortening of prolonged labor

Treatment of Postpartum Hemorrhage In postpartum hemorrhage caused by uterine atony an oxytocin drip is a good method of treatment. Other causes of the bleeding must of course be ruled out. The drip is effective in improving the tone of the uterus, and it can be kept running as long as necessary.

Prevention of Postpartum Hemorrhage Such conditions as uterine inertia, twin pregnancy, polyhydramnios, difficult delivery, and excessive anesthesia predispose to uterine atony and postpartum hemorrhage. The complication should be anticipated and guarded against by starting an oxytocin drip before the hemorrhage takes place.

Normal Management of the Third Stage To hasten delivery of the placenta and to reduce the bleeding of the placental stage, oxytocin may be given before or after delivery of the placenta.

Prerequisites for the Use of Oxytocin

1. The presenting part should be well engaged.
2. The cervix must be ripe, effaced, soft, and partially dilated.

3. There must be a normal obstetric history and the absence of an abnormal one.
4. There must be no fetopelvic disproportion.
5. The fetus should be in normal position.
6. The fetus should be in good condition with normal fetal heart.
7. Adequate personnel must be available to watch the patient.
8. The patient must be examined carfully before the oxytocin is started.
9. The doctor in charge of the case should:
   a. Examine the patient himself before the drip is set up.
   b. Be present when the infusion is started.
   c. Observe the patient and the fetal heart for the first few contractions. He should then regulate the speed.
   d. Not order the drip by telephone.
   e. Be in hospital and available while the drip is running.
10. The response of the human uterus to intravenous oxytocin increases with the length of pregnancy, reaching a peak during the 36th week. After this the reactiveness changes little. Induction is as successful during weeks 36 to 39 as later. However, in the earlier period the induction takes longer, and more oxytocin is needed.

Contraindications to the Use of Oxytocin

1. Absence of proper indication.
2. Absence of the prerequisites.
3. Disproportion, generally contracted pelvis, and obstruction by tumors.
4. Grand multiparity: There is too great a chance of uterine rupture.
5. Previous cesarean section.
6. Hypertonic or incoordinate uterus. The hypertonic or incoordinate uterus is made worse by oxytocin and may lead to a constriction ring.
7. Maternal exhaustion. This condition should be treated by rest and fluids, not by oxytocin stimulation.
8. Fetal distress. Not only should oxytocin not be given, but the appearance of an irregular or slow heart while the drip is running demands that the drip be stopped.
9. Abnormal presentation and position of all types.
10. Unengaged head.
11. Congenital anomalies of the uterus.
12. Placenta previa.
13. Previous extensive myomectomy.

Dangers of Oxytocin

MATERNAL DANGERS

1. Uterine rupture. If the patient is oversensitive to the drug she may get hard and even tetanic contractions, enough to rupture the uterus, whereas normal contractions would do no harm.
2. Cervical and vaginal lacerations can be caused by too rapid passage of the baby through the pelvis.
3. Uterine atony and postpartum hemorrhage may develop when the oxytocin is discontinued.
4. Abruptio placentae has been reported.
5. Water intoxication is induced by retention in the body of large amounts of water in excess of electrolytes.

WATER INTOXICATION
Oxytocin has an antidiuretic effect that begins when the rate of infusion is 15 mU per minute and is maximal at 45 mU per minute. Single doses have no effect; the antidiuretic activity seems to depend on the maintenance of a constant and critical level. The action is on the distal convoluted tubules and collecting ducts of the kidneys, causing increased resorption of water from the glomerular filtrate. The combination of oxytocin and large amounts of electrolyte-free glucose in water leads to retention of fluid, low serum levels of sodium and chloride, and often progressive oliguria.

The symptoms range from headache, nausea, vomiting, mental confusion, and seizures to coma and death. These have been attributed to edema and swelling of the brain.

Management of Water Intoxication

1. Prevention. Patients receiving an infusion of oxytocin should not receive more than 1 liter of electrolyte-free fluid in 24 hours.
2. Mild cases. Discontinue the oxytocin and withhold all fluids.
3. Severe cases require, in addition, the infusion of hypertonic (3.0 percent) sodium chloride intravenously. This will withdraw fluid from the tissues and bring about a diuresis. The rate of infusion must be slow and should be discontinued when the diuretic phase ends to avoid overcorrection, lest the cerebral effects of hypernatremia be imposed upon those of water intoxication.

FETAL DANGERS FROM OXYTOCIN

1. Anoxia caused by contractions that are too hard, too frequent,

and last too long. The uterus never relaxes enough to maintain adequate circulation. In some cases separation of the placenta has taken place.

2. Damage to the baby from too rapid propulsion through the pelvis.

3. Forcing the fetus through a pelvis too small for it.

In a large series it was shown that the signs of fetal distress are more common in patients receiving an oxytocin drip than in those without stimulation of labor. In almost all instances slowing or stopping the oxytocin infusion resulted in the rapid return to normal of the fetal heart. The incidence of emergency obstetric intervention was no higher, and the final fetal results were comparable.

ERGOT DERIVATIVES

The first pure ergot alkaloid, ergotamine, was isolated in 1920. Later another active alkaloid was discovered and named ergometrine (ergonovine). Only the latter is used in obstetrics. It has no adrenergic blocking action and the emetic and cardiovascular effects are less than those of ergotamine. These are powerful ecbolic agents, exciting a tonic contraction of the myometrium. The maximum effect is during labor and the puerperium. They are never used during the first and second stages of labor.

Undesirable effects include (1) hypertension, (2) tachycardia, (3) headache, and (4) nausea and vomiting. The vasomotor effects are worse in patients delivered under regional anesthesia. The ergot alkaloids should not be used in hypertensive patients, in women with cardiac disease, or in those being delivered under spinal or epidural anesthesia.

PROSTAGLANDIN

Prostaglandins are 20-carbon carboxylic acids that are formed enzymatically from polyunsaturated essential fatty acids. Most organs are capable of synthesizing prostaglandins, as well as metabolizing them to less active compounds.

On the basis of their structure prostaglandins are divided into four groups, namely E, F, A, and B. Three of the E group and three of the F group are primary compounds. The other eight are metabolites of the parent six. Thirteen of the 14 known prostaglandins occur in man.

First isolated from the seminal fluid, these substances are distributed widely in all mammalian tissues. Their exact mode of action is not known, but prostaglandins are thought to be part of the mechanism that controls transmission in the sympathetic nervous system. Two generalized activities are apparent: (1) alteration of smooth muscle contractility and (2) modulation of hormonal activity. How an organ will respond depends upon (1) the specific prostaglandin, (2) the dose, (3) the route of administration, and (4) the hormonal or drug environment. Prostaglandins are metabolized rapidly and their systemic effects are of short duration.

Prostaglandins produce a wide variety of physiologic responses. Both E and F have profoundly stimulating effects on the myometrium. In adequate dosage they can initiate labor at any stage of pregnancy. These drugs have not replaced oxytocin in the induction and augmentation of labor. Response is less predictable and side effects are more pronounced. However, when oxytocin is contraindicated, prostaglandin may have a role in the stimulation of uterine activity at term.

Adverse Reactions and Contraindications

1. Gastrointestinal symptoms, including nausea, vomiting, and diarrhea, occur in half the patients. In most cases these effects are short in duration and not severe.
2. A syndrome of bronchial constriction (asthma attack) with tachycardia, vasovagal effects, and alterations in blood pressure may take place. Should this occur the drug is discontinued and supportive therapy instituted. The vital signs return to normal within a few minutes, probably because the drug is metabolized rapidly.
3. Hyperpyrexia occurs occasionally.
4. Convulsive seizures have been reported, and patients with epilepsy should not be given prostaglandin.
5. Contraindications include asthma, cardiovascular disease, and hypertension.

SPARTEINE SULFATE

Sparteine sulfate is an alkaloid derived from the plant *Cytisus scoparius* (Scotch broom). It has the property of increasing the intensity, frequency, and duration of uterine contractions.

For induction of labor the dosage is 150 mg given intramuscularly every hour to a maximum of three doses or 450 mg. Once labor has started, no more is given. Because some patients react strongly to the drug, it has been suggested that the first dose be only 75 mg.

The original claims that the drug has no side effects, that the margin of safety is wide, that it poses no danger to mother and child, and that constant supervision is not required during its adminstration have not been borne out by further experience. Sparteine sulfate is not a safe oxytocic. The same care must be exercised as with any other oxytocic drug.

Advantages of sparteine sulfate include:

1. Administration to the patient is easy.
2. Induction is successful in many cases.
3. Labor is shortened.
4. It is a simple way of getting labor into the active phase.

Disadvantages and dangers include:

1. Uterine hypertonus and tetanic contractions.
2. Tumultuous labor and delivery.
3. Rupture of uterus and lacerations of the cervix.
4. Separation of the placenta from the uterus.
5. Fetal distress.
6. The intramuscular injection is unpredictable and potentially dangerous.
7. There is great variability in the effect of sparteine, not only in different patients but in the same patient from one injection to the next.

These factors must be noted concerning sparteine sulfate:

1. It is an efficient oxytocic drug.
2. Its use requires the same constant and careful supervision as any other oxytocic drug.
3. The prerequisites and contraindications to its administration are the same as those given for oxytocin.
4. The safest time for its use is during the latent phase when the cervix is effaced and dilated to 3 cm. By giving one injection of 150 mg the labor can be lifted into the active phase in many cases.
5. Sparteine should never be given when the patient is in active labor. Sudden tumultuous contractions may ensue.
6. Sparteine sulfate must not be given concomitantly with oxytocin. At least 2 hours must elapse before a change is made from one agent to the other.
7. There is no advantge in using sparteine rather than oxytocin. On the contrary we have found oxytocin to be more efficient, more reliable, and more predictable.

BIBLIOGRAPHY

Barber HRK, Graber EA, Orlando A: Augmented labor. Obstet Gynecol 39:933, 1972

Gupta DR, Cohen NH: Oxytocin, salting-out, and water intoxication. JAMA 220:681, 1972

Nakano J: Cardiovascular actions of oxytocin. Obstet Gynecol Surv 28:75, 1973

Pauerstein CJ: Use and abuse of oxytocic agents. Clin Obstet Gynecol 16:262, 1973

Sogolow SR: An historical review of the use of oxytocin prior to delivery. Obstet Gynecol Surv 21:155, 1968

40.

Induction of Labor

Induced labor is labor started by artificial methods.

INDICATIONS FOR THE INDUCTION OF LABOR

Maternal Indications

SPONTANEOUS RUPTURE OF MEMBRANES If the pregnancy is within 2 weeks of term and labor does not begin after 24 hours, induction with oxytocin should be considered.

TOXEMIA OF PREGNANCY When medical therapy is unable to control toxemia the pregnancy must be terminated.

POLYHYDRAMNIOS Polyhydramnios is the accumulation of an excessive amount of amniotic fluid. Pressure symptoms and dyspnea may be so severe that the patient is unable to carry on.

ANTEPARTUM BLEEDING Included here are cases of low-lying placenta and mild placental separation, in which the bleeding is not controllable by bed rest, or when the baby is dead.

INTRAUTERINE FETAL DEATH In selected cases labor is induced to relieve the mother of the strain of carrying a dead child and to prevent the development of afibrinogenemia.

CANCER Termination of the pregnancy is for the purpose of permitting surgical, radiation, or chemical treatment of the lesion, or simply to remove a drain on the patient's resources and powers of resistance.

HISTORY OF RAPID LABORS The aim is to avoid birth of the baby at home or en route to hospital.

PATIENTS LIVING FAR FROM HOSPITAL

ELECTIVE Here the procedure is being carried out for the convenience of the patient, the doctor, or both. Because there is no pressing medical reason for the induction, great care must be taken in selecting the patient and no risks should be taken. The labor must be supervised constantly. If there is the least doubt about the procedure it should not be instituted.

585

Fetal Indications

MATERNAL DIABETES The babies tend to be large and often die in utero during the later weeks of pregnancy. Hence the pregnancy should be terminated at around the 37th week.

RHESUS INCOMPATIBILITY When the fetus is being sensitized or when there has been fetal death in utero during previous pregnancies, premature induction of labor is sometimes indicated.

RECURRENT INTRAUTERINE DEATH Intrauterine death near term in past pregnancies is a rational reason for premature induction of labor.

EXCESSIVE SIZE OF THE FETUS

POSTTERM PREGNANCY There is some evidence that there is a progressive decrease in placental function and in the oxygen content of fetal blood as pregnancy proceeds past term. Occasionally there is fetal death in utero, or often the baby is born with poor nutrition and has difficulty during the postnatal period.

Advantages

1. The patient is admitted to hospital the previous night and a hypnotic is prescribed to assure her of sleep.
2. No food is given by mouth; the empty stomach decreases the anesthetic risk.
3. The rush to hospital is avoided.
4. It is a daytime procedure when full staff is available.
5. The doctor chooses a day when he has no other duties and can remain in hospital with the patient.
6. The length of labor is shortened.

PREREQUISITES AND CONDITIONS

PRESENTATION The presentation should be cephalic. Labor is never induced in the presence of attitudes of extension, transverse lies, or compound presentations, and almost never when the breech presents.

STAGE OF THE PREGNANCY The closer the gestation is to term the easier is the induction.

STATION The head must be engaged: the lower the head, the easier and safer the procedure.

CERVICAL RIPENESS The cervix must be effaced, less than 1.3 cm (0.5

inch) in length, soft, dilatable, and open to admit at least one finger and preferably two. The firm ring of the internal os should not be present. It is advantageous for the cervix to be in the center of the birth canal or anterior. When the cervix is posterior conditions for induction are less favorable.

PARITY It is much easier and safer to induce a multipara than a primigravida, and the success rate increases with parity.

FETAL MATURITY In general the nearer the gestation is to 40 weeks the better the fetal results. When preterm termination of pregnancy is necessary, tests for fetal maturity should be performed to establish, as far as possible, that the fetus will be able to survive outside the uterus. These tests include clinical examination, ultrasonic measurement of the biparietal diameter of the head and circumference of the body, and determination of the L/S ratio, creatinine, bilirubin, and fat cells in the amniotic fluid.

DANGERS

1. Prolapse of the umbilical cord may occur if artificial rupture of the membranes is performed when the presenting part is not well engaged.
2. Fetal death, unexplained.
3. Prolonged labor.
4. Prematurity as a result of miscalculating the expected date of confinement.
5. Genital and fetal infection following a long period of ruptured membranes.
6. Failure of induction may be defined as occurring (a) when the uterus does not respond to stimulation at all or (b) when the uterus contracts abnormally and the cervix does not dilate. As long as the prerequisites are observed, the rate of successful labor inductions is over 90 percent. Some 10 percent of women are delivered by cesarean section. It must be kept in mind that in many cases the original indication for the induction and the cesarean are the same—e.g., diabetes or Rh immunization.

METHODS OF INDUCING LABOR

Medical Methods

Castor oil, 2 ounces, followed by soapsuds enema may succeed in inducing labor.

Hormonal Methods

Oxytocin is used to achieve two purposes:

1. To induce labor when conditions are correct.
2. To ripen the cervix: When induction is necessary but the cervix is not ripe, intravenous oxytocin is given for several hours daily until the cervix is ripe, when induction can be carried out. (For details of technique see Chapter 39.)

Artificial Rupture of Membranes

1. The fetal heart is checked carefully.
2. Sterile vaginal examination is made to determine that the necessary conditions and prerequisites are present.
3. With a finger placed between the cervix and the bag of waters, the cervix is rimmed, stripping the membranes away from the lower uterine segment.
4. Pressure is maintained on the uterine fundus through the abdomen to keep the head well down.
5. Using a uterine dressing forceps, an Allis forceps, a Kelly clamp, or a membrane hook, the bag of waters is torn or punctured.
6. A gush of fluid from the vagina or the grasping of fetal hair in the clamp is proof of success.
7. The fetal heart is checked carefully.
8. Although the head may be pushed upward slightly to allow escape of the amniotic fluid, this must be done with caution for there is danger of umbilical cord prolapse.
9. Amnioscope. Artificial rupture of the membranes can be performed through a vaginal amnioscope. Advantages include:
   a. The procedure is carried out under direct vision, which adds to the safety.
   b. The color of the fluid and the presence of meconium can be ascertained before the membranes are ruptured.
   c. The presence of a low-lying umbilical cord or vasa previa can be ruled out.
   d. Amniotic fluid, uncontaminated by vaginal contents, can be collected for biochemical analysis.
   e. The amnioscope provides a sterile pathway to the cervix and reduces the danger of amnionitis.

CONTRAINDICATIONS TO ARTIFICIAL RUPTURE OF THE MEMBRANES

1. High presenting part
2. Presentation other than vertex
3. Unripe cervix
4. Abnormal fetal heart rate

Laminaria Tents

The use of laminaria tents to dilate the uterine cervix during pregnancy, given up many years ago because of the high rate of infection, has been revived as a consequence of the obviation of sepsis by modern methods of sterilization. *Laminaria digitata* is a species of seaweed. The dried stem is hygroscopic: when it comes in contact with moisture it swells to 3 to 5 times its original diameter. In so doing it brings about gradual softening and dilatation of the cervix. The most rapid swelling occurs in the first 4 to 6 hours and the maximal effect is achieved in 24.

INDICATIONS

1. *First trimester abortions:* Precurettage or vacuum aspiration.
2. *Midtrimester abortions:* In association with the intraamniotic injection of ecbolic solutions.
3. *Term or preterm pregnancy:* To ripen the unfavorable cervix prior to induction of labor.

ADVANTAGES

1. The cervix becomes soft and dilated, making amniotomy easier.
2. The length of the first stage of labor is shortened.

TECHNIQUE: PREINDUCTION OF LABOR

1. In the evening before the day of induction two to five laminaria are placed in the cervix. The number depends on the capacity of the cervix. As many as possible are inserted.
2. Care is taken not to rupture the membranes.
3. A sterile gauze is placed against the cervix to hold the laminaria in place.
4. Next morning the laminaria tents are removed.

5. Amniotomy is performed.
6. An infusion of oxytocin may be started immediately. However, some obstetricians prefer to use oxytocin only if labor does not begin after 6 to 8 hours.

Intraamniotic Injection of Ecbolic Solutions

The intraamniotic instillation of various solutions will induce labor. Some exert this effect by virtue of their hypertonicity. Others have a different mode of action. In most cases delivery of the products of conception takes place within 40 hours. Retained placenta, bleeding, and the need for curettage are common. This technique is feasible only after 16 weeks' gestation because of the difficulty of locating the amniotic sac before this time and the inadequate quantity of amniotic fluid.

MECHANISM OF ACTION
Hypotheses as to the mechanism of action include:

1. Normally progesterone blocks the onset of labor. The hypertonic solution disrupts the placenta and releases the local progesterone block; labor then follows.
2. Uterine volume is an important factor in controlling the onset of labor. The body attempts to equilibrate the hypertonic solution, the volume of intraamniotic fluid is increased, and uterine contractions begin.
3. The injected drug has a direct effect on the myometrium, stimulating it to contract.

Indications

This method is used for the induction of labor when the fetus is dead or when the termination of pregnancy is so essential to the interests of the mother that the fetus is being disregarded. This technique is useful in missed abortions. It works even when the cervix is unripe. This procedure is not employed to induce labor in a normal pregnancy or when the fetus is viable.

TECHNIQUE

1. For maximum safety the placenta is localized and the diagnosis of fetal presentation confirmed by ultrasonic scan.

2. While premedication with an analgesic such as Demerol is helpful, general anesthesia must never be used as it would mask untoward reactions.
3. The patient is placed on an operating table in moderate Trendelenburg position.
4. An intravenous infusion of 5 percent glucose in water is instituted.
5. The bladder must be empty.
6. The procedure is performed under aseptic conditions. The abdomen is sterilized as well as possible.
7. Transabdominal amniotomy is performed under local anesthesia, using a 10-cm (4-inch) spinal needle with stylet. The needle is inserted halfway between the symphysis pubis and the umbilicus, 2.5 cm (1-inch) from the midline, toward the side where the fetal small parts are located.
8. The first bit of amniotic fluid removed may be tested to be certain it is not urine. If it is alkaline and positive for glucose and protein, it is probably amniotic fluid and not urine.
9. One of the dangers is that the needle may become displaced and injection made into the wrong area. To avoid this the needle must be fixed in position or, preferably, replaced by a catheter, which is easier to set and has less chance of moving out of the amniotic sac.
10. A three-way stopcock is helpful.
11. Amniotic fluid is removed and replaced with the drug being used. The amount of fluid withdrawn depends on the medication to be instilled. The injection is made slowly, with frequent aspirations to check the position of the needle or catheter and to make certain that it is not in a blood vessel.
12. After a small amount of drug has been injected the patient is observed for untoward effects. If these are absent the total dose is instilled. If abnormal reactions occur the procedure is discontinued.
13. The patient is returned to bed, the intravenous infusion maintained at a slow rate, and the patient kept under close supervision to await the onset of labor.

At the conclusion of the injection two laminaria tents may be inserted into the cervical canal to soften and dilate the cervix gradually so that the danger of cervical trauma may be reduced, including cervicovaginal fistula and cervical incompetence. Often the injection-to-delivery time is reduced. Care must be taken not to rupture the membranes.

The laminaria tents are inserted after the injection is complete so that, if the intraamniotic injecton is unsuccessful, the procedure can be reattempted the following week. Once the laminaria have been inserted the evacuation of the uterus cannot be postponed.

POSTINJECTION COURSE

1. If labor does not begin by 24 hours an oxytocin infusion may be instituted.
2. Some physicians start an oxytocin drip routinely after the intraamniotic injection is made.
3. If induction of labor fails a second intraamniotic injection is made.
4. In rare cases hysterotomy may be necessary. Under these conditions this is a dangerous procedure.
5. Retention of placenta or excessive bleeding requires immediate curettage.

ADVANTAGES
This method is an effective way of inducing labor and obviates the need for hysterotomy when the pregnancy must be terminated after the first trimester.

DANGERS

1. Maternal death may result.
2. Infection may be introduced, especially when glucose is used.
3. Damage to placental vessels during amniotomy may allow fetal erythrocytes to enter the maternal circulation.
4. The bladder or bowel may be injured.
5. Intravascular injection may occur.
6. There may be water intoxication from overabsorption of saline into the maternal tissues.
7. Retained placenta or excessive bleeding occurs in 20 percent of cases.
8. Many patients show some changes in blood clotting, and a few develop a picture of consumption coagulopathy when hypertonic saline is used.

ECBOLIC AGENTS

Hypertonic Glucose Originally a solution of 50 percent glucose was employed with success. However, because of a high rate of infection, its use was discontinued.

Hypertonic Saline A 20 percent solution is effective in inducing labor and is used widely. The amount of amniotic fluid removed ranges from 100 to 300 ml and is replaced with an equal quantity of saline. In the interests of safety no more than 200 ml of hypertonic saline should be injected.

The initial 10 ml of hypertonic saline is administered and the patient observed. Indications for discontinuance of the procedure include burning abdominal pain (myometrial or intraperitoneal injection) and sudden onset of headache, generalized flush, and thirst (suggesting intravascular injection). In the latter case 5 percent glucose in water is infused rapidly. In the absence of untoward symptoms the remainder of the saline is injected slowly.

The mechanism of action is not clear. Intraamniotic injection of saline leads to an increase in the production and release of prostaglandin, a substance known to stimulate the uterus to contract. The saline may also cause suppression of the synthesis of placental progesterone, thereby allowing myometrial activity to begin.

COMPLICATIONS

1. Hypernatremia is common, and, in most cases, it is insignificant. However, this complication accounts for most deaths. These fatalities are associated with rapid transfer of sodium chloride into the vascular system either by direct injection or through a tear in the uterine vessels. Death occurs from excessive dehydration of the brain.
2. Disseminated intravascular coagulation is rare. It may be related to a release of thromboplastin from the amniotic fluid into the maternal circulation. The removal of the products of conception results in rapid correction of the abnormality.
3. Hemorrhage and retained placenta require operative removal of tissue from the uterus.
4. The cervix may be lacerated. Occasionally, failure of the cervix to dilate leads to the fetus and placenta being extruded through the cervical canal, resulting in a cervicovaginal fistula.
5. If oxytocin is used, water intoxication may occur.
6. Hypertonic saline should not be used in women with cardiac disease, hypertension, severe renal abnormalities, or hemolytic processes.

Because of the rapid fetal death after injection of hypertonic saline, there are no live births with this method.

Urea To avoid the dangers of hypertonic saline, urea may be employed. The mode of action is similar to saline in that decreases in circulating progesterone levels and increases in prostaglandin release have been reported. Fetal death and maceration occur in all cases.

TECHNIQUE Amniocentesis is performed in the usual way; 200 ml of amniotic fluid is removed and replaced with 200 ml of 5 percent dextrose in water containing 80 g of urea. The solution is injected slowly. The incidence of retained placenta and bleeding is higher than with saline. Operative evacuation of the uterus is necessary frequently.

COMPLICATIONS

1. Nausea and vomiting.
2. Urea is an osmotic diuretic and dehydration of clinical significance may occur, especially when there is vomiting.
3. If massive diuresis takes place, hyponatremia and hypokalemia may cause problems.
4. Coagulation defects are apparent but are not severe.
5. Infection and cervical laceration may occur.
6. Urea is contraindicated in patients with renal or hepatic impairment.

ADVANTAGES

1. There are no significant complications if inadvertent intravenous injection is made.
2. Intramural injection does not cause myometrial necrosis.

Prostaglandin F_2 *Alpha* Injected intraamniotically, this is an efficient agent in bringing about termination of pregnancy in the second trimester.

TECHNIQUE Amniocentesis is performed in the usual way. At least 1 ml of amniotic fluid is removed. One milliliter (5 mg) of prostaglandin F_2 alpha is injected. The patient is observed for pain, vomiting, or bronchospasm. Then the rest of the 40 mg is injected. The patient may be ambulatory.

ADVANTAGES Advantages of PG over saline include the following:

1. Injection-to-abortion time is shorter.
2. There is no significant change in heart rate, cardiac output, or intravascular volume.
3. There is no alteration in the clotting factors.
4. There is no risk of hypernatremia.
5. Myometrial necrosis does not occur even if the injection is made into the wall of the uterus.

DISADVANTAGES

1. A number of patients will require a second injection.
2. The incidence of nausea, vomiting, diarrhea, dyspnea, flushing, and chest pain is higher than with saline.
3. Heavy bleeding, often necessitating blood transfusion, is more common than when saline is used.
4. Postabortal curettage, both for bleeding and retained secundines, is often necessary.
5. Prostaglandins do not cause fetal death in utero and the fetus may be born alive, leading to potential medical, psychological, and legal problems. This situation may be obviated by combining prostaglandin with urea.

BIBLIOGRAPHY

American College of Obstetrics and Gynecology: Termination of second trimester pregnancy using prostaglandin F_2 alpha. Tech Bull No 27 April 1974

Ballard CA, Ballard FE: Four years' experience with mid trimester abortion by amnio-infusion. Am J Obstet Gynecol 114:575, 1972

Barham K: Amnioscopy amniotomy: A look at surgical induction of labor. Am J Obstet Gynecol 117:35, 1973

Berk H, Ullman J, Berger J: Experience and complications with the use of hypertonic intraamniotic saline solution. Surg Gynecol Obstet 133:955, 1971

Burnett LS, Wentz AC, King TM: Techniques of pregnancy termination. Part II. Obstet Gynecol Surv 29:6, 1974

Cross WG, Pitkin RM: Laminaria as an adjunct in induction of labor. Obstet Gynecol 51:606, 1978

Lauerson, NH, Schulman JD: Oxytocin administration in mid-trimester abortions. Am J Obstet Gynecol 115:420, 1973

Triconi V: Induction of labor. Clin Obstet Gynecol 16:226, 1973

Weinberg PC, Shepard MK: Intraamniotic urea for induction of mid-trimester abortion. Obstet Gynecol 41:451, 1973

41.

Fetal Dysmaturity, Retarded Intrauterine Growth, Prolonged Pregnancy, Term Intrapartum Fetal Death

CLASSIFICATION OF FETAL STATUS

1. According to gestational age
   a. Preterm: less than 37 completed weeks (259 days) from the first day of the last menstrual period
   b. Term: from 37 to less than 42 completed weeks (259 to 293 days)
   c. Postterm: 42 completed weeks (294 days) or more
2. According to pattern of growth
   a. Appropriate for gestational age (AGA): between the 10th and 90th percentiles
   b. Large for gestational age (LGA): above the 90th percentile
   c. Small for gestational age (SGA): below the 10th percentile

FETAL DYSMATURITY

The term fetal dysmaturity refers to the syndrome in which either the infant's stage of development is less than expected for the period of gestation or it shows the regressive changes and signs of intrauterine hypoxia.

Children who demonstrate soft tissue wasting have the following appearance:

1. The weight is low in relation to body length.
2. The limbs are long and lean.
3. The baby looks undernourished and has only a small amount of subcutaneous fat.
4. The vernix is scanty or absent and when present is yellow or green.
5. The hair is abundant.
6. The nails are long.
7. The skin hangs in folds. There is a tendency to desquamation, especially on the palms and soles. The skin dries after birth and becomes parchment-like.
8. The skin, nails, umbilical cord, and amniotic fluid are stained with meconium.
9. In advanced cases the amniotic fluid becomes scanty and thick with meconium. There is a tendency to aspiration of this fluid with subsequent pulmonary complications.

INTRAUTERINE GROWTH RETARDATION

Infants whose intrauterine growth has been retarded are small for gestational age (SGA). The condition has been defined in two ways: (1) infants whose weight is below the tenth percentile for their gestational age, and (2) infants whose weight is two standard deviations below the mean weight for their gestational age. These babies are small, but not premature. They do not have the problems of infants born preterm.

Mechanisms of Growth Retardation

Slow growth of the fetus is utero may be a reflection of chronic intrauterine insufficiency, a fetal anomaly beyond correction, or no more than a normal variation. The two basic mechanisms of intrauterine growth retardation are a reduction in fetal growth potential and a reduction in fetal growth support.

REDUCED FETAL GROWTH POTENTIAL

One-third of clinically recognizable cases of growth retardation are in this group. Most of these infants are small because of constitutional limitations. A few are congenitally abnormal as a result of chromosomal aberrations or damage by noxious agents such as rubella, toxoplasmosis, cytomegalic virus disease, and others. The basic defect is an interference with the hyperplastic phase of development. There is no actual cessation of growth. Rather, beginning in the first trimester, there is a persistently slow rate of growth and reduced absolute size. The total number of cells in the body, including those of the brain, is reduced. Because the brain and body are affected equally, the ratio of the size of the body to that of the head may be normal. There is no association with hypertensive disorders of pregnancy and no increased incidence of fetal distress, meconium aspiration, asphyxia neonatorum, or postpartum hypoglycemia. Clinically these neonates are symmetrically small and appear runted.

REDUCED FETAL GROWTH SUPPORT

This form of slowing or cessation of growth occurs in infants with normal growth potential. The basic defect implies impairment in the transplacental supply of nutrients. This form of growth retardation is associated with hypertensive disorders, with their consequent reduction in uterine blood flow. Chronic maternal malnutrition and poor weight gain in pregnancy appear to play a causal role. There is a high association with fetal distress, meconium aspiration, asphyxia, and postpartum hypoglycemia. This group represents about 60 percent of cases of intrauterine growth retardation. Hypoxia is probably the common denominator in this type of retarded growth. Interference occurs with both hyperplasia and hypertrophy, and these infants appear wasted. Because the brain is spared, the circumference of the head remains greater than that of the body.

Diagnosis

Because of the high perinatal mortality, early diagnosis is important. However, it is difficult, being made in only one-third of cases. There is no reliable screening test. Often the growth-retarded infant is identified only after birth. On the other hand, overdiagnosis is a problem. Only one-third of infants suspected of being growth-retarded turn out to be so. This leads to unnecessary investigation and interference.

The signs of intrauterine growth retardation or placental insufficiency are seldom elicited before 28 weeks of gestation. The clinical features are:

1. Failure of the uterus and fetus to grow at the normal rate over a 4-week period.
2. The uterine fundal height is at least 2 cm less than expected for the length of gestation.
3. Absence of maternal gain in weight.
4. Diminished fetal movements.

5. Often the uterus is irritable.
6. A reduced volume of amniotic fluid.

IUGR is more common:

1. In women with a previous SGA (small-for-gestational-age) baby
2. When there has been a pregnancy loss in a former pregnancy
3. With poor maternal gain in weight
4. With maternal complications, especially those associated with reduced uterine and placental flow of blood
5. With maternal smoking of cigarettes

Antepartum Assessment

1. Menstrual history is important.
2. History of quickening and first auscultation of the fetal heart, around 18 weeks.
3. Clinical estimation of fetal size.
4. Serial ultrasonic measurements of the biparietal diameter of the head and the thoracic and abdominal girth are carried out every 3 weeks. Because of the brain-sparing tendency in some cases, the cephalic measurements may be misleading. The head-to-body ratio is important. Up to 32 to 36 weeks the abdominal circumference at the umbilicus is smaller than that of the head. At 32 to 36 weeks the measurements are the same. After 36 weeks the circumference of the abdomen becomes larger than that of the head. In many cases of IUGR the reversal of this ratio does not take place.

    Campbell described two ultrasonic patterns of biparietal measurements seen with intrauterine growth retardation.
    a. Low profile. This pattern correlates with the group described as having reduced fetal growth potential. A persistently slow rate of growth is evident from early in the second trimester. Growth occurs steadily, but the absolute values are below the mean. These babies have symmetrical growth retardation.
    b. Late flattening pattern. This group correlates with that described under reduced fetal growth support. An abrupt slowing and eventual cessation of growth are seen following a period of normal development.
5. Urinary estriol, on a serial basis, is done twice a week, or more often if indicated. While normal values do not rule out IUGR, it is unlikely that the fetus is in any danger. Subnormal values call for further assessment.

6. Nonstress test of fetal heart rate. This is done weekly. A reactive pattern (Braxton Hicks contractions or fetal movement cause fetal tachycardia) suggests that the baby is safe in utero for at least 1 week. Nonreactive patterns indicate the need for careful observation and repeated tests. Absence of beat-to-beat variation is a bad sign.
7. Contraction stress test. A negative test is significant in that the fetus is safe for 1 week. A positive test is not as meaningful because of a high percentage of false-positives. A positive test is not a contraindication to a monitored vaginal delivery.
8. Some congenital anomalies can be identified by ultrasound and useless intervention avoided.
9. Amniocentesis is used to measure the L/S ratio, fat cells, creatinine, and bilirubin in the amniotic fluid to determine fetal maturity.

Antepartum Management

1. Investigation of placental function and fetal condition is carried out (Fig. 1).
2. In the absence of signs of fetal distress the pregnancy is allowed to continue. One should let the fetus mature as much as possible. The pregnancy is terminated only when serious signs of fetal or maternal distress are present. There is no advantage in being born prematurely.
3. Once the diagnosis of IUGR has been made, delivery should be accomplished by 38 weeks. The baby that is no longer developing in the uterus will grow better in the nursery.
4. An attempt is made to improve the situation by (a) correcting underlying disorders such as hypertension and uncontrolled diabetes and (b) enhancing blood flow to the uterus by the patient's resting a great deal in the lateral recumbent position.
5. Most fetal deaths in utero occur after the 36th week of gestation and before the onset of labor. Intervention may save these infants.

The Delivery

These babies should be born in hospitals with specialized high-risk facilities, both obstetrical and pediatric. A neonatologist should be present at birth.

1. Ripe cervix: Induction, careful monitoring, and vaginal delivery

INTRAUTERINE GROWTH RETARDATION

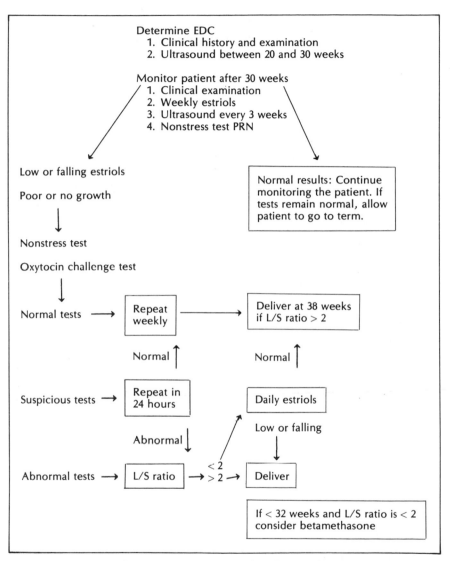

FIG. 1. Management of High-Risk Pregnancy

2. Unripe cervix: Oxytocin drip to ripen the cervix, followed by artificial rupture of membranes.
3. Liberal indications for cesarean section:
   a. Fetal distress
   b. Failed induction
   c. Malpresentation

    d. Disproportion
    e. Unripe cervix in a patient with severe disease such as diabetes or toxemia
    f. Previous cesarean section

Postnatal Problems

1. Asphyxia neonatorum is common.
2. Meconium aspiration is a danger. Meconium acts as a foreign body and may obstruct the flow of air into the alveoli. The nares and nasopharynx should be aspirated as soon as the head is born.
3. The respiratory distress syndrome is rare.
4. Hypoglycemia and hypocalcemia occur frequently.
5. Hypothermia is common.
6. Congenital anomalies occur in 10 percent of IUGR infants. Included in this group are trisomy 18 and 21, neural tube defects, and Potter's syndrome.
7. In the neonatal period most babies who do not have congenital anomalies do well.
8. The congenital infection syndrome must be ruled out.
9. Nutritional management should support growth, but there must be no preoccupation with the attainment of "normal" weight.
10. The perinatal morbidity and mortality are increased, but the long-term prognosis remains unclear.
11. Long-term problems include emotional maladjustment, impaired hearing, decreased coordination and motor skills, poor speech, and reduced reading ability.
12. The neurologic behavior fits the age rather than the size of the newborn infant.
13. The degree of growth retardation is not the same in all organs. There is a tendency for the brain to be spared.

PROLONGED (POSTTERM) PREGNANCY

In calculating the expected date of confinement Naegele's rule is that term is reached 40 weeks after the first day of the last normal menstrual period. This is based on the belief that conception takes place on about the 14th day of the cycle. In most instances the exact date of conception is not known.

By definition postterm pregnancy is one that has lasted 42 weeks (294 days) or more. This includes 12 percent of all pregnancies. The incidence of pregnancy that reaches 43 weeks or more is 4 percent.

Reasons for errors associated with Naegele's rule include these:

1. The menstrual history is unreliable. Many women do not remember when the last menstruation began.
2. Women whose cycle is longer than 28 days or whose ovulation is late may deliver after the expected date.
3. Even under normal conditions the length of pregnancy varies.
4. Women have been known to falsify the menstrual history for social reasons.

Assuming that the expected date of confinement is known accurately, the following questions must be answered:

1. Does postterm pregnancy add any risk to mother and child?
2. At what stage do these dangers play a part?
3. How do they compare with the problems of artificial termination of the pregnancy?

There are two opposite views as to the implications of postterm pregnancy:

1. This is a physiologic variation. In itself it poses no danger to the fetus; hence no routine interference is indicated.
2. Prolongation of gestation carries with it an increased fetal mortality, and termination of the pregnancy should be considered in all cases.

Fetal Size and Condition

1. Most babies are normal.
2. A number keep growing and some weight over 4,000 g. Disproportion and dystocia may result with the attendant danger to the infant.
3. Fetal postmaturity (dysmaturity). A birth some postterm babies are small, undernourished, and asphyxiated as a consequence of reduction in the respiratory and nutritive function of the aging placenta. The incidence of fetal postmaturity in postterm pregnancy is 20 percent. In these infants disadvantages in general health persist for 2 years. After 5 years of age data on growth, intelligence, and health are no different from the findings in children born at term.

Fetal Mortality

Perinatal mortality is increased in prolonged pregnancy, but this occurs almost entirely in dysmature infants. Quoted figures vary, but the probable rates of death at 43 weeks are twice, at 44 weeks thrice, and at 45 weeks five times that of babies born at term. The increased fetal mortality occurs before the onset of labor, during labor and delivery, and in the neonatal period.

It was believed that the postterm fetus had a special intolerance to labor. Recent work has not confirmed this idea. While postterm women in labor should be monitored carefully, there is no justification for over-aggressive intervention in anticipation of problems of intrauterine hypoxia. Fetal death during labor is rare unless signs of danger are ignored.

Therapeutic Rationale

Some authorities advise that, because of the dangers of placental insufficiency, every pregnancy should be terminated at 42 weeks. Others disagree, pointing out that the diagnosis is often uncertain, that the dangers of prolonged pregnancy have been exaggerated, and that the hazards of induction under unfavorable conditions, such as an unripe cervix, are greater than those of delay.

Tests for fetal distress are done as soon as a diagnosis of prolonged pregnancy is made and are repeated as often as necessary until the baby is born.

Investigation: Tests of Fetal Well-being

1. Clinical assessment.
   a. Menstrual history.
   b. Date of quickening and first auscultation of fetal heart.
   c. Size of uterus, height of fundus, abdominal girth.
   d. Ripeness of cervix.
   e. Station of presenting part.
   f. Estimation of fetal size.
2. Estriol levels in maternal urine or blood.
3. Ultrasonic measurement of fetal head and body.
4. Meconium in amniotic fluid: amnioscopy or amniocentesis. By itself the presence of meconium-stained amniotic fluid is not a reliable indicator for termination of the pregnancy, especially when the cervix is not ripe. Amniocentesis is rarely necessary in

the clinical management of prolonged pregnancy. As long as the other tests of fetal well-being are normal, postterm pregnancy is not an indication to terminate the gestation. If these tests are not reassuring, amniocentesis or amnioscopy should be performed. If the fluid is stained with meconium, delivery should occur soon to prevent fetal death from dysmaturity.

5. Nonstress recording of fetal heart rate.
6. Oxytocin challenge test (Contraction stress test).
7. Amniocentesis, in those patients in whom it is uncertain that the pregnancy is really postterm and the fetus seems to be small, to determine:
   a. L/S ratio.
   b. Percentage of fat cells.
   c. Bilirubin.
   d. Creatinine.
8. Continuous monitoring of FHR during labor.
9. Measurement of pH of fetal blood during labor, if indicated.

Management

As a general rule vaginal delivery is preferred. During labor:

1. Careful monitoring of the FHR is essential.
2. An intravenous infusion of glucose should be running.
3. If possible, the patient lies on her side to avoid supine hypotension.
4. Excessive sedation may be harmful.
5. Prolonged labor is dangerous; cesarean section is considered after 12 to 18 hours.
6. Fetal distress calls for delivery by the safest method.

NO SIGNS OF FETAL DISTRESS: NORMAL PREGNANCY

1. Induce labor if the cervix is ripe and the fetal head is in good position.
2. Allow the pregnancy to continue when:
   a. Tests for fetal health are normal.
   b. Estimated fetal weight is under 2,500 g.
   c. The period of gestation is uncertain.
   d. The cervix is unfavorable in young, healthy women.

NO SIGNS OF FETAL DISTRESS: COMPLICATED PREGNANCY
Included here are:

1. Elderly primigravidas.
2. Patients with toxemia or diabetes.
3. Intrauterine growth retardation.
4. Previous unexplained stillbirth or neonatal death.
5. Dystocia in a previous pregnancy.
6. Erythroblastosis.

These patients should not go past term.

1. Ripe cervix: induce.
2. Unripe cervix:
   a. Consider induction after oxytocin to ripen cervix.
   b. Cesarean section may be best.

SIGNS OF FETAL DISTRESS
These include:

1. Low or falling estriol levels
2. Abnormal nonstress FHR patterns
3. Positive oxytocin challenge test

If these signs are present, the pregnancy should be ended as indicated below:

1. Elderly primigravidas and multiparas with a complicated medical history: cesarean section.
2. Young primigravidas and normal multiparas:
   a. Unripe cervix: cesarean section.
   b. Favorable cervix: induction may be attempted under careful FHR monitoring. If induction is not successful or if abnormalities of the FHR supervene, emergency cesarean section must be done.
   c. Breech presentation: cesarean section.

TERM INTRAPARTUM FETAL DEATH

Babies may die during labor. The definition of the term intrapartum fetal death includes the following: (1) documentation of fetal heart tones after the onset of labor, (2) birth weight over 2,500 g, (3) gestation of 37 to 40 weeks, and (4) no sign of life after delivery of the child.

On an etiologic basis two large groups are noted. In half the cases there is a definite and acceptable explanation. In the rest there is no clearly defined cause of the fetal death, but associated conditions are present which may have played a part. The presence of these situations should prewarn the obstetrician to expect trouble.

1. Definite cause of death
    a. Difficult and traumatic delivery
    b. Prolapse of the cord
    c. Abruptio placentae
    d. Congenital anomalies incompatible with life
    e. Rh sensitization
    f. Ruptured uterus
2. Concomitant problems
    a. Highly significant conditions
        Prolonged gestation
        Premature rupture of membranes
        Tight cord around the neck
        Paracervical block anesthesia
    b. Mildly significant conditions
        Intrapartum fever
        Toxemia of pregnancy
        Maternal hypotension
        Breech (with easy labor and delivery)
        Abnormal sugar tolerance

BIBLIOGRAPHY

Altshuler G, Russel P, Ermocilla R: The placental pathology of small-for-gestational-age infants. Am J Obstet Gynecol 121:351, 1975

Cetrulo CL, Freeman R: Biometric evaluation in intrauterine growth retardation. Clin Obstet Gynecol 20:979, 1977

Crane JP, Kopta MM, Welt SI, Sauvage JP: Abnormal fetal growth patterns; ultrasonic diagnosis and management. Obstet Gynecol 50:205, 1977

Frigoletto FD, Rothchild SB: Altered fetal growth: an overview. Clin Obstet Gynecol 20:95, 1977

Green JN, Paul RH: The value of amniocentesis in prolonged pregnancy. Obstet Gynecol 51:293, 1978

Hobbins JC, Berkowitz RL: Ultrasonography in the diagnosis of intra uterine growth retardation. Clin Obstet Gynecol 20:957, 1977

Jones MD, Battaglia FC: Intrauterine growth retardation. Am J Obstet Gynecol 127:540, 1977

Klapholz H, Friedman EA: The incidence of intrapartum fetal distress with advancing gestational age. Am J Obstet Gynecol 127:405, 1977

Tejani N, Mann LE: Diagnosis and management of the small-for-gestational-age fetus. Clin Obstet Gynecol 20:943, 1977

Tulchinsky D: Endocrine evaluation in the diagnosis of intrauterine growth retardation. Clin Obstet Gynecol 20:969, 1977

Vorherr H: Placental insufficiency in relation to postterm pregnancy and fetal postmaturity. Am J Obstet Gynecol 123:67, 1975

42.

Preterm Labor

Preterm labor may be defined as the onset of regular uterine contractions accompanied by cervical effacement and/or dilatation and fetal descent in a gravid woman whose period of gestation is less than 37 completed weeks (less than 259 days) from the first day of the last menstrual period.

An infant of low birth weight is one that weighs less than 2,500 g (5 pounds, 8 ounces) at birth. The average period of gestation for an infant weighing 2,500 g is 34 weeks. Although only 7 to 8 percent of pregnancies end before 37 weeks, the majority of perinatal deaths fall into this group.

ETIOLOGY

Iatrogenic

1. Repeat cesarean section performed too early.
2. Premature termination of the pregnancy on the basis that the fetus is better off in the nursery than in the uterus. Included here are such conditions as maternal diabetes, hypertensive disease of pregnancy, erythroblastosis, and intrauterine growth retardation.

Spontaneous

1. Idiopathic. Cause of the premature labor unknown in 50 percent of cases
2. Premature rupture of the membranes
3. Incompetent cervix
4. Placental insufficiency
5. Uterine overdistension
   a. Multiple pregnancy
   b. Polyhydramnios
   c. Large fetus

6. Bleeding in the third trimester
    a. Placenta previa
    b. Abruptio placentae
    c. Vasa previa
7. Uterine abnormalities, preventing expansion
    a. Hypoplastic uterus
    b. Septate or bicornuate uterus
    c. Intrauterine synechiae
    d. Leiomyomas
8. Trauma
    a. Falls
    b. Blows on the abdomen
    c. Surgical procedures
9. Medical illness in the mother, such as toxemia, anemia, chronic renal disease, and acute febrile illnesses
10. Associated factors
    a. Low socioeconomic status
    b. Certain ethnic groups
    c. Small women
    d. Smoking
    e. Bacteriuria
    f. Poor prenatal care

DIAGNOSIS

The high incidence of false labor makes the accurate diagnosis of true preterm labor difficult. In one-third of cases the so-called labor ceases without treatment or after the administration of a placebo.

The usual criteria of preterm labor include:

1. The cervix is at least 2 cm dilated or 75 percent effaced.
2. There is progressive change in the cervix during a period of observation.
3. The occurrence of regular, painful contractions less than 10 minutes apart suggests that the patient is in labor.

PREVENTION OF PRETERM LABOR

General Measures

1. Prenatal care, diet, vitamins, and hygiene are applied.

2. Activity (work, travel, coitus) is restricted for patients with a history of premature labor.
3. Acute febrile illnesses must be treated promptly and actively.
4. Medical conditions such as toxemia and diabetes need careful control.
5. Elective abdominal surgery and extensive dental work are postponed.

Specific Measures

1. Patients with multiple pregnancy should be at bed rest from weeks 28 to 36 or 38.
2. Uterine fibromyomas, when symptomatic, are managed by bed rest and analgesia. Surgery is avoided as long as possible.
3. Placenta previa is treated by confinement to bed and blood transfusion to delay the birth of the baby until it has reached a viable size. Profuse hemorrhage, of course, calls for immediate surgery.
4. The incompetent cervix should be sutured during the early part of the second trimester, as long as all precepts have been fulfilled.
5. Elective and repeat cesarean section is done only when one is certain that the child is of good size. The danger of too early operation is the delivery of a small baby that does not survive.
6. Drugs may be used to stop labor.

PHARMACOLOGIC CONTROL (INHIBITION) OF PRETERM LABOR

Pharmacologic agents can stop contractions in the prelabor phase or in the early part of the first stage of labor. However, once the active phase of labor has been established, the cervix is dilating, or the membranes have ruptured, it is unlikely that the progress of labor can be halted. The prime goal of therapy aimed at inhibiting labor is to prolong pregnancy to 37 weeks to obtain fetal maturity. Since the developing fetus gains 25 g/day during the last trimester, any delay of labor and delivery may be advantageous. In addition, an interval of 72 hours will make possible the use of corticosteroids to accelerate the development of fetal pulmonary maturity.

It is often difficult to know whether a patient is really in labor. In some cases bed rest and a placebo work well. In other instances preterm labor is nature's best option, and the baby may be better out of the uterus.

INDICATIONS AND CONDITIONS

1. The fetus should be normal and healthy.
2. There must be no maternal or fetal contraindications to prolonging the pregnancy.
3. The degree of prematurity should be such that intervention is warranted. To a point this depends upon the ability of the nursery to care for small babies. As a general rule the limits are 35 weeks gestation and 2,500 g as the estimated weight.
4. The cervical dilatation is less than 5 cm.
5. The membranes are intact.
6. There is no bleeding.

CONTRAINDICATIONS

1. Maternal or fetal conditions where termination of the pregnancy is indicated. These include hypertension, preeclampsia, diabetes, and erythroblastosis associated with Rhesus incompatibility.
2. Dead or malformed fetus.
3. Gestation over 35 weeks and estimated fetal weight over 2,500 grams.
4. Intrauterine growth retardation.
5. Abruptio placentae and placenta previa.
6. Amnionitis.
7. Premature rupture of the membranes or the membranes bulging through the cervix into the vagina.
8. Cervix dilated over 5 cm.

Inhibitory Agents

BETA-MIMETIC DRUGS
The myometrium contains alpha and beta receptors. Stimulation of the former increases and stimulation of the latter inhibits uterine contractions.

Isoxsuprine Isoxsuprine is given as an intravenous drip; 80 mg of the drug is mixed in 500 ml of 5 percent glucose in water. The initial rate of infusion is 10 drops per minute. If there are no side effects, the rate is increased gradually to 40 drops per minute, or until the contractions cease. The average effective dose is 0.25 to 0.50 mg per minute. When there have been no contractions for 24 hours the change is made to oral dosage of 30 to 80 mg every 3 hours. After 3 to 4 days this is reduced to every 6 hours for up to 25 days, as necessary.

There are no fetal complications. Maternal complications include a rise in the pulse rate in 50 percent of cases or a fall of systolic blood pressure of 10 to 20 mm Hg. Should hypotension develop, the infusion must be stopped.

Ritodrine The formula of this drug is similar to that of isoxsuprine. The solution is made by adding 250 mg of ritodrine to 450 ml of 5 percent dextrose in water (526 mg per liter). The patient lies on her side and the intravenous infusion is initiated at a rate of 50 μg per minute. The rate is increased by 50 μg every 10 minutes until uterine relaxation is achieved. The maximal dose is 600 μg per minute. The drip is run for 12 hours. Thirty minutes before the infusion is discontinued, oral therapy is instituted on a schedule of 10 mg q2h for 24 hours, 10 mg q3h for 24 hours, and then 10 mg q8h until the 38th week of gestation. If labor begins before then, the whole regimen is begun again. There may be moderate maternal tachycardia, but no hypotension. Marked fetal tachycardia has been observed, but the babies were born in good condition. If palpitations or maternal tachycardia over 120 beats per minute occur, the speed of the infusion is reduced. Ritodrine is an effective inhibitor of uterine contractions. The only significant side effect is maternal tachycardia.

Salbutamol This drug, whose main use is as a bronchodilator in asthma and chronic bronchitis, has the ability to suppress uterine contractions. It is administered intravenously and, once labor has ceased, orally. Side effects include maternal tachycardia, a drop in the diastolic blood pressure, and nausea. Salbutamol appears to be a useful and effective agent in inhibiting labor.

Salbutamol is given as a continuous infusion of 500 ml of 5 percent dextrose to which 5 ml of salbutamol have been added. The concentration is 10 μg/ml. The infusion is started at 20 drops per minute and increased by increments of 10 drops per minute every 10 minutes until contractions cease. The maximum rate of infusion is 80 drops per minute. Indications for slowing or discontinuing the medication include a maternal pulse rate of over 140 beats per minute, distressful palpitations, and hypotension. Once the contractions have stopped, the infusion is maintained at the successful level for 6 hours and then decreased gradually. Treatment is continued with oral salbutamol, 4 mg four times daily, for at least 48 hours after contractions have ceased.

ETHANOL
This alcohol inhibits the release of vasopressin and oxytocin from the hypophysis. There may be a direct effect on the myometrium as well. Ten percent ethanol is given in an intravenous infusion. The dosage schedule is as follows: 7.5 ml/kg/hour for 2 hours; then 1.5 ml/kg/hour

for 10 hours. If the contractions recur, one or two additional courses of therapy can be employed. The infusion of 1 g per minute results in a blood level of 7 to 9 mg of ethanol per 100 ml. Some women develop symptoms of intoxication or headache, but serious complications are uncommon. Alcohol does have an initial dramatic effect in decreasing uterine contractions. Prolongation of this phenomenon is not universal. Because some patients become uncooperative and are difficult to nurse, because of the questionable long-term efficacy of ethanol, and because other drugs are more effective, the use of ethanol in this area has been given up by most physicians.

ANTIPROSTAGLANDINS

Indomethacin (Indocin)   The dose is 100 mg given as a rectal suppository, followed by 25 mg orally every 6 hours until there have been no uterine contractions for 24 hours. Should labor begin again the treatment is repeated. Some physicians prefer using the suppository twice daily instead of the oral dose. There is no effect on the maternal blood pressure or pulse, and none on the fetal heart rate.

Indomethacin appears to be an effective inhibitor of uterine contractions. However, the question of its safety for the fetus remains unresolved. There have been warnings against the use of indomethacin in pregnancy because of the ability of prostaglandin synthetase inhibitors to bring about premature closure of the ductus arteriosus. A few cases have been reported. On the other hand, pregnant women who have used indomethacin on a long-term basis as an antirheumatic agent have given birth to normal children. However, because the possibility of damage does exist, the drug must be used with caution.

Aspirin   Aspirin, 20 mg, also has an antiprostaglandin effect. The patient can take this at home before she leaves for the hospital. However, long term medication is dangerous for mother and fetus.

MANAGEMENT OF PRETERM LABOR AND DELIVERY

The overall survival rate of infants weighing between 700 and 1,500 g is, today, around 50 percent. Hence, it is no longer justifiable to ignore the small fetus and to base management on maternal considerations alone. Every attempt must be made to save these babies. The birth should take place in hospitals equipped with special intensive care nurseries; postnatal transfer to tertiary care centers is a less than satisfactory approach.

The principle that the premature breech is delivered best by cesarean section is based upon two observations. First, in relation to the body, the premature fetus has a proportionately larger head than the fetus at term. The body passes through the cervix and pelvis, but the maternal soft parts are insufficiently dilated to make room for the head, and arrest may occur. Secondly, there is statistical evidence that premature breeches do better when delivered by cesarean section.

Labor

Gentleness is of paramount importance. The premature baby, with its soft skull and low resistance, withstands trauma poorly. When possible, excessively strong contractions and precipitate labor should be avoided. Unfortunately neither the baby nor the uterus is prepared for normal labor. Often an unripe cervix adds to the difficulties. Continuous monitoring of the fetal heart rate is important.

Analgesia and Anesthesia

The premature baby is hypersensitive to drugs given to the mother for relief of pain. Even a small dose may so depress the vital centers that the onset of respiration is delayed and asphyxia results. During labor it is wisest to avoid narcotics of any kind. Delivery is safest under local infiltration or pudendal block. If more anesthesia is necessary a conduction technique such as epidural block is used.

Delivery

1. Birth should be gentle and slow to avoid rapid compression and decompression of the head.
2. Oxygen is given to the mother by mask during the delivery.
3. The membranes should not be ruptured artificially. The bag of waters acts as a cushion for the soft premature skull with its widely separated sutures.
4. An episiotomy reduces pressure on the baby's cranium.
5. Low forceps may help in dilating the maternal soft parts and in guiding the head over the perineum. We prefer spontaneous delivery when possible.
6. Breech extraction should not be performed. An added danger in

premature births is that the buttocks may not dilate the birth canal enough to make room for the relatively large head.

7. Precipitous and unattended births are dangerous for the premature baby.
8. A neonatologist should be present at the delivery.

Care of Preterm Infant

1. The head-down position (at an angle of about 30°) is maintained to promote drainage of the respiratory tract. If there is suspicion of intracranial hemorrhage the baby should lie in the horizontal plane.
2. The secretions are aspirated from the throat and nose by gentle suction.
3. An incubator is useful so that the temperature, humidity, and oxygen can be controlled. A warm atmosphere is best. To prevent retrolental fibroplasia the oxygen concentration should be below 40 percent.
4. The apneic infant must be oxygenated within 1 to 2 minutes of birth. Adequate ventilation is essential. We have found the bag and mask technique to be efficient and safe.
5. Resuscitation measures must be gentle. Slapping and rubbing are to be discouraged. The least amount of handling is best.
6. Occasionally laryngoscopy is necessary to remove debris from the respiratory tract and intubation to get oxygen in.
7. Persistent labored respiration may indicate a pneumothorax or a diaphragmatic hernia.
8. When the baby has been narcotized by drugs administered to the mother, Nalline is given to the infant to counteract the effects of the depressing drugs. The dose is 0.2 mg into the umbilical vein. If the baby weighs less than 1,000 g the dose is 0.1 mg. Stimulatory drugs are not used.
9. While there is disagreement as to whether the umbilical cord should be clamped early or the baby should be held below the level of the placenta until the cord pulsations cease, there is agreement that the cord should not be milked toward the infant, as the sudden extra blood infused into the circulation may overload it and put a strain on the heart.
10. Because of the association of prematurity with congenital malformation, the baby should be examined thoroughly.
11. When possible a pediatrician should attend the birth.
12. A separate premature nursery with a specially trained staff is invaluable.

PROGNOSIS OF PREMATURITY

1. Prematurity is today the most frequently recurring factor involved in infant death and morbidity. Most babies who die within the first 28 days of life weighed less than 2,500 g at birth.
2. Anoxia is 12 times more common in premature infants.
3. Respiratory distress causes 44 percent of deaths that occur at less than 1 month of age. If the fetus weighs under 1,000 g this figure rises to 74 percent.
4. Because of the softness of the skull bones and the immaturity of the brain tissue, the premature infant is more vulnerable to compression of the head.
5. Intracranial hemorrhage is five times more frequent in the premature than in the term infant. Much of this results from anoxia.
6. Cerebral palsy is more common in premature infants.
7. The prognosis in low-birth-weight infants for physical and intellectual health is not clear despite numerous investigations. There seems to be a higher incidence of organic brain damage in premature babies (although many men and women of genius were born before term).

PREVENTION OF THE RESPIRATORY DISTRESS SYNDROME

Babies born with immature lungs are prone to develop RDS. This condition is the commonest cause of morbidity and mortality in premature infants. As a rule the fetal lungs mature at 35 weeks of gestation. There is a large increase in surfactant in the lungs and the L/S ratio in the amniotic fluid reaches 2.0.

Some observers have noted that in cases in which premature rupture of the membranes has led to the birth of a premature infant, the incidence of RDS is less when the membranes have been ruptured for more than 16 hours as compared with infants in whom the latent period was less than 16 hours. It is postulated that the rupture of the membranes causes stress to the infant, who responds by an increased production of corticosteroids. In some way this increases the rate of production of pulmonary surfactant, and causes an increase in the L/S ratio, induction of pulmonary maturity, and a reduction in the incidence and severity of RDS.

Accelerated maturation occurs in a number of stress-producing situations such as (1) maternal hypertension, (2) diabetes, types D to F, (3) placental insufficiency, and (4) amnionitis.

Liggins and others have shown that the maturation of the fetal lungs can be accelerated by the administration of glucocorticoids to the mother. The placenta is relatively permeable to these substances, which reach the fetus and lead to the liberation of surfactant and an increase in the L/S ratio. The incidence of RDS is reduced. To be effective the corticosteroids must be given at least 24 hours before delivery. If possible, labor should be stopped for that period of time. Treatment of the fetus after birth is of no value.

Dosage schedules vary. Some workers advise giving 12 mg of betamethasone intramuscularly and, if delivery does not take place in 24 hours, then giving another 12 mg; delivery is delayed for 48 hours if possible. Others feel that 12 mg in two doses of 6 mg repeated in 12 hours, 24 hours before delivery, is sufficient and safer.

The levels of serum and urinary estriol in women treated with corticosteroids are reduced. Therefore, in these cases low or falling estriols do not have the same significance as in untreated patients.

Therapy with betamethasone is effective in reducing the incidence of RDS only when the period of gestation is less than 32 weeks. Once that stage is reached betamethasone should not be used.

In patients in whom the membranes have been ruptured for more than 24 hours, betamethasone therapy does not reduce significantly the incidence of RDS in the newborns.

Before administering betamethasone the L/S ratio should be measured. If it is 2.0 or higher it signifies that the lungs are mature and there is nothing to be gained by giving glucocorticoids prior to delivery.

Contraindications to betamethasone include: (1) hypertensive disorders of pregnancy, (2) diabetes, (3) placental insufficiency, and (4) infection.

Although Liggins reported no observable ill effects in his study of infants at 1 year of age, there are not enough data available regarding long-term effects to warrant the use of glucocorticoids indiscriminately.

This form of therapy has certain hazards:

1. In some animals the administration of corticosteroids brings on labor.
2. In patients with hypertension or proteinuria, there is an increase in perinatal mortality.
3. Resistance to infection may be lowered in both mother and child.
4. Decreased growth in weight and length has been noted.
5. Increase in electroencephalographic and gross neurologic abnormalities are seen.
6. Increased incidence of intraventricular hemorrhage has occurred.

Gluck has warned that more and more we are recognizing that properly a fetus's place is in the womb for as long as possible; premature delivery is to be avoided except when the fetus's or mother's life is in jeopardy. At the moment it would appear more physiologic to inhibit labor, prevent delivery, and retain the fetus in utero as long as it is safe, in order to grant the fetus as much developmental endowment as is possible. Already one can see mounting abuse of the fetus as licence is taken in delivering premature infants early because they have been "protected" by corticosteroids. Remember: there is no advantage in being born or delivered prematurely.

PREMATURE RUPTURE OF MEMBRANES

The spontaneous rupture of the membranes 1 hour or more before the onset of labor is defined as premature rupture (Fig. 1).

Incidence and Etiology

The incidence is between 10 and 12 percent. In about 20 percent the infant is premature.

In most cases the etiology is not known. In 20 percent rupture of the membranes is the first sign of impending onset of labor.

Onset of Labor

Between 50 and 70 percent of the patients with premature rupture go into labor spontaneously within 48 hours. The length of the latent period (between rupture of membranes and onset of labor) is influenced by the following:

1. Gestational age is important.
   a. Near term, labor begins within 24 hours in 80 to 90 percent.
   b. Before 36 weeks, labor starts by 24 hours in 35 to 50 percent.
   c. A latent period of over 14 days occurs in only 10 percent of the premature group.
2. The latent period is shorter when the fetus is large.
3. Primigravidas tend to have a longer latent period.
4. Intrauterine infection decreases the latent period.

Risks of Premature Rupture of Membranes

MATERNAL DANGER

In most cases the problem of infection in the mother is not serious and responds promptly to antibiotic therapy and evacuation of the uterus.

FETAL COMPLICATIONS

1. Prematurity: Some 20 percent of babies born after premature rupture of the membranes weigh less than 2,500 g.
2. Infection: The leading cause of fetal death is infection. The longer the latent period, the longer the first stage of labor and the greater the incidence of infection. The incidence rises significantly after a latent period of over 48 hours. The fetus can be infected even when there are no signs of sepsis in the mother. The commonest site is the respiratory tract. Most pneumonias during the first 2 weeks of life have an intrauterine origin.
3. Malpresentation: This is common, particularly breech.
4. Prolapse of the umbilical cord: This accident is frequent, especially in premature infants.
5. Perinatal mortality: The overall figure is 5 percent; in premature babies it is 30 percent. The longer the latent period, the higher the mortality. Malpresentation increases the mortality, and intrauterine infection worsens the prognosis.

FETAL PROGNOSIS

This depends on:

1. Fetal maturity: Babies weighing under 2,500 g do less well than larger ones.
2. Presentation: Breeches have a worse prognosis, especially when premature.
3. Intrauterine infection increases fetal mortality.
4. The longer the pregnancy is carried with ruptured membranes, the higher the incidence of infection.

Management

The problem of prematurity must be weighed against the danger of the long latent period and potential infection. In marked prematurity the gestational age transcends other considerations, and maintaining the pregnancy may give the infant a better chance. Ultrasonic studies

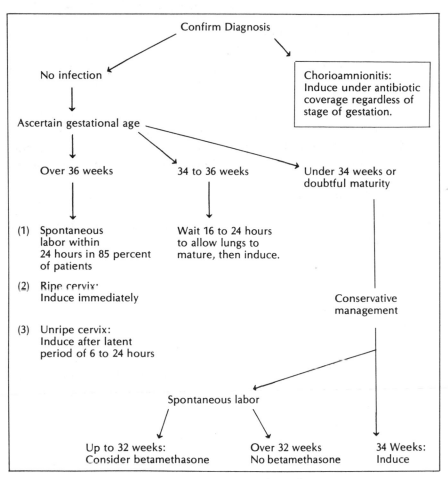

FIG. 1. Premature Rupture of Membranes

have provided evidence that under good conditions and modified bed rest, the fetus can grow at an appropriate rate.

DIAGNOSIS

History and Inspection   When large amounts of fluid are flowing out of the vagina the diagnosis is clear. Occasionally there is doubt, and further steps must be taken.

Sterile Speculum Examination   Under sterile conditions a speculum is inserted into the vagina. Then:

1. The cervix is observed.
2. Escape of fluid from the cervix is seen, spontaneously or following pressure on the abdomen.
3. Nitrazine test: If the vaginal fluid is acid, the membranes are intact. If the fluid is alkaline the membranes are probably ruptured.
4. The microscopic examination of a dried drop of vaginal fluid will show a ferning pattern if it is amniotic fluid.
5. A dried drop of the fluid is stained with Nile Blue. The presence of orange cells, from fetal skin, indicates that the membranes are ruptured.
6. At the same time a high vaginal swab is taken and sent for culture.

Digital Vaginal Examination This procedure increases the risk of infection and should be avoided if possible.

Fetal Heart Careful auscultation or monitoring is important. Abnormalities might be an indication of prolapsed cord.

DETERMINATION OF GESTATIONAL AGE

It is essential to ascertain, as closely as possible, the stage of maturity of the fetus. The following parameters are useful:

1. History and date of the last menstrual period, the length of the cycle, recent use of oral contraception prior to conception, and the induction of ovulation.
2. Date of quickening, 18 to 20 weeks.
3. Date of first stethoscopic auscultation of the fetal heart: 18 to 20 weeks.
4. Fundal height.
5. Ultrasonic measurement of the biparietal diameter.
6. X-ray of distal femoral epiphysis (36 weeks) and proximal tibial epiphysis (38 weeks). This is used only when ultrasound is unavailable.
7. Amniotic fluid examination for L/S ratio, creatinine, fat cells, and bilirubin.

CHORIOAMNIONITIS

The symptoms and signs include maternal fever, tachycardia, leukocytosis, purulent vaginal discharge, and, sometimes, abdominal pain. In this situation the pregnancy must be terminated as soon as possible, but within 8 hours. Cervical and blood cultures are taken and the patient is given wide-spectrum antibiotics. Labor is induced. Vaginal delivery is the preferred method. If induction fails cesarean section may be necessary.

NO CLINICAL INFECTION

Gestation Over 36 Weeks
1. Because 80 to 90 percent of patients near term will go into spontaneous labor within 24 hours, some obstetricians prefer expectant management during this period.
2. If the cervix is ripe, there is no advantage to delay, and labor should be induced.
3. If the cervix is unripe, a latent period of up to 24 hours is permissible before labor is induced.

Gestation 34 to 36 Weeks   In this group there is an increased risk of morbidity and mortality of the infant from the respiratory distress syndrome. There is some evidence that when the membranes have been ruptured for a long time the incidence of RDS is reduced. Therefore, induction of labor is delayed for 16 to 24 hours to allow the lungs to mature.

Gestation Less Than 34 Weeks   In these babies the risks of prematurity, especially those of RDS, are high. In general, conservative management is carried on as long as there is no infection or signs of fetal distress. Should spontaneous labor set in before 32 weeks, the administration of betamethasone to the mother has been suggested to stimulate the process of maturation of the fetal lungs. Because one of the actions of exogenous glucocorticoid is inhibition of the normal inflammatory response and an increased susceptibility to infection, there is danger in using these drugs when the membranes are ruptured. Some authorities advise against the use of betamethasone in this situation. There is some evidence that premature rupture of the membranes alone may enhance pulmonary maturity. After 32 weeks betamethasone is not indicated.

If labor does not start spontaneously, induction is considered at 34 weeks or when the L/S ratio indicates pulmonary maturity. In the absence of a neonatologist and an intensive care nursery it may be better to leave the fetus in utero until it attains greater maturity.

CONSERVATIVE MANAGEMENT IN HOSPITAL
The purpose is to allow the fetus to reach a stage of maturity at which it can survive outside of the uterus. The procedure is as follows:

1. Bed rest as long as there is leakage of fluid.
2. Temperature and pulse q4h.
3. Daily white blood cell count.
4. Daily estriol measurements.
5. Ultrasound weekly.

6. No vaginal examination.
7. Vaginal culture twice weekly.
8. No prophylactic antibiotics. The administration of antibiotics to the uninfected mother has not reduced fetal morbidity. The danger of using these drugs lies in the possible development of resistant bacteria.
9. If infection occurs the uterus must be emptied.

CONSERVATIVE MANAGEMENT AT HOME

If the patient's home situation is good, she may be allowed to go home under the following conditions:

1. Parameters are stable.
2. There is no excessive loss of amniotic fluid.
3. No coitus, douches, or vaginal tampons.
4. Temperature at 8, 16, and 20 hours. If fever develops, she returns to hospital.

MODE OF DELIVERY

Vaginal delivery is preferred. Cesarean section is performed when indicated.

MANAGEMENT OF NEONATE

If there is amnionitis, the following steps are taken:

1. Culture. Swabs are taken from nose, throat, and external ear canal.
2. Gastric aspirate for microscopy and culture.
3. Cultures of blood, urine, and cerebrospinal fluid.
4. Complete blood count and differential white blood examination.
5. Chest x-ray.
6. Treatment with appropriate antibiotics.

If there is no amnionitis and the membranes have been ruptured over 24 hours:

1. The same workup is carried out with the exception of the x-ray and CSF culture.
2. If the infant is under 36 weeks gestation, antibiotics are given until the results of the culture are known. If these are negative and the baby is well, the antibiotics are discontinued.

INCOMPETENT INTERNAL CERVICAL OS

Some women with a history of repeated midtrimester abortions have an incompetent cervix. The internal os undergoes painless dilatation and is unable to maintain the pregnancy.

Etiology

The exact etiology is not known. The condition may be congenital, but most women have a history of previous pregnancy, dilatation of the cervix beyond the ability of the internal os to remain intact, or cervical amputation.

Clinical Picture

The first sign is usually spontaneous rupture of the membranes. The cervix shortens and dilates, and a part of the membranes bulges through and eventually ruptures. Rapid labor often follows.

Diagnosis

1. Historical data such as previous midtrimester loss, cervical trauma, abortion, and clinical evidence of old cervical lacerations are suggestive.
2. In the nonpregnant state the ability to pass a No. 8 Hegar's dilator through the internal os is indicative.
3. Traction test. If a Foley catheter containing 1 ml of water can be pulled through the internal os of the nonpregnant patient, using less than 600 g of pull, the diagnosis is probable.
4. X-ray hysterography may demonstrate that the diameter of the internal os is wider than 8 mm.
5. The finding of progressive, painless cervical effacement and dilatation in the second trimester is suggestive; bulging of the membranes clinches the diagnosis.

Treatment

1. Tracheloplasty is performed in the nonpregnant state; it involves a reconstruction of the internal os.

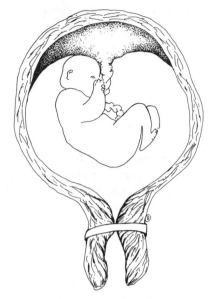

FIG. 2. Cervical cerclage

2. Bed rest reduces pressure on the cervix.
3. Vaginal pessary. This changes the inclination of the cervical canal and redistributes the weight of the growing conceptus away from the internal os of the cervix.
4. Cervical cerclage.

Cervical Cerclage

TECHNIQUE
A suture of fascia or mersilene is placed around the cervix near the internal os to constrict the canal, thereby preventing the descent and rupture of the bag of water (Fig. 2).

1. *Shirodkar Procedure* Incisions are made in the mucosa of the cervix and the suture is placed around the cervix under the mucosa.
2. *McDonald Technique* A purse string suture is placed extra-mucosally. Four or five bites are taken and the suture is tied tightly.

During the procedure minimal anesthesia should be administered to the mother. In the postoperative period broad-spectrum antibiotics, betamimetic drugs to reduce myometrial activity, and progesterone have been used. None is absolutely necessary.

INDICATIONS FOR CERCLAGE

1. Previous premature delivery or midtrimester abortion without obvious cause
2. Visual evidence of previous surgical or obstetric trauma to the cervix
3. History of painless premature labor and rapid delivery
4. Progressive dilatation or dilatation greater than 2 cm on initial examination during midtrimester
5. Previous diagnosis of cervical incompetence and previous cerclage

CONTRAINDICATIONS
Included are infection, ruptured membranes, labor, and bleeding per vaginam.

TIMING OF CERCLAGE
Originally the procedure was performed between the 14th and 16th week. At this stage the cervix is not yet so effaced or dilated that the operation is difficult. In addition, after 12 weeks the period of the highest incidence of spontaneous abortion has passed, and one can be reasonably certain that the pregnancy is viable. At the present time, by the use of ultrasound the normality of the pregnancy can be established and the presence of the fetal heart demonstrates fetal life. At this stage of pregnancy the cervix is long and the operation is easier to perform. On this basis some obstetricians carry out the procedure at the 10th or 11th week of gestation. Others prefer to wait until the 14th week.

COMPLICATIONS OF CERCLAGE
Cerclage is a safe operation and complications are rare. These include:

1. Slipping of the suture occurs when the band cuts through the cervical tissue and fails to keep the cervix closed.
2. Postoperative infection requires removal of the suture and antibiotic therapy.
3. Small cervical tears at delivery are common and require no treatment.

4. Bleeding from the site of the operation.
5. Accidental rupture of membranes.
6. Premature labor.

DELIVERY

At 2 to 3 weeks before term the suture is removed and the onset of labor awaited. Vaginal delivery is permitted unless there is some other indication for cesarean section.

BIBLIOGRAPHY

Bauer CR, Stern L, Colle E: Prolonged rupture of the membranes associated with a decreased incidence of respiratory distress syndrome. Pediatrics 53:7, 1974

Block MF, Kling OR, Crosby WM: Antenatal glucocorticoid therapy for the prevention of respiratory distress syndrome in the premature infant. Obstet Gynecol 50:186, 1977

Caspi E, Schreyer P, Weintraub, et al: Prevention of the respiratory distress syndrome in premature infants by antepartum glucocorticoid therapy. Br J Obstet Gynaecol 83:187, 1976

Gluck L: Administration of corticosteroids to induce maturation of fetal lung. Am J Dis Child 130:976, 1976

Guilliams S, Held B: Contemporary management and conduct of preterm labor and delivery: a review. Obstet Gynecol Surv 34:248, 1979

Koh KS: Premature labor. Canad Med Assoc J 114:700, 1976

Lauerson NH, Merkatz IR, Tejani N, et al: Inhibition of premature labor: a multicenter comparison of ritodrine and ethanol. Am J Obstet Gynecol 127:873, 1977

Liggins GC, Howie RN. A controlled trial of antepartum glucocorticoid treatment for prevention of the respiratory distress syndrome in premature infants. Pediatrics 50:515, 1972

Niebyl JR, Blake DA, Johnson WC, King TM: The pharmacologic inhibition of premature labor. Obstet Gynecol Surv 33:507, 1978

Renaud R, Irrmann M, Gandar R, Flynn MJ: The use of ritodrine in the treatment of premature labor. J Obstet Gynaec Br Commonw 81:182, 1974

Richter R, Hinselmann MJ: The treatment of premature labor by betamimetic drugs. Obstet Gynecol 53:81, 1979

Toaff R, Toaff ME, Ballas S, Ophir A: Cervical incompetence: diagnostic and therapeutic aspects. Israel J Med Sci 13:39, 1977

Zukerman H, Reiss U, Rubenstein I: Inhibition of human premature labor by Indomethacin. Obstet Gynecol 44:787, 1974

43.

Prolonged Labor

GENERAL INFORMATION

Labor that lasts longer than 24 hours is classified as prolonged. However, when adequate progress is not being made during that period the situation must be assessed immediately. Problems should be recognized and treated before the 24-hour limit has been reached. Most prolonged labors represent extensions of the first stage. Whatever the reason, the cervix fails to become fully dilated within a reasonable length of time.

Onset of Labor

Because it is difficult in many cases to be certain exactly when labor began, there is no unanimously accepted definition of the onset of labor. The definition based on the frequency, regularity, and duration of uterine contractions ignores the fact that patients with dysfunctional labor do have painful though irregular contractions.

The definition that insists on progressive effacement and dilatation of the cervix as an essential feature of real labor fails to recognize the important latent phase or preliminary stage of labor. During this period, despite regular uterine contractions, little recognizable change may take place in the cervix.

Perhaps, therefore, the best definition available may be the imprecise one that defines onset of labor as being the time at which the patient experiences uterine contractions that lead toward the birth of a baby.

Incidence and Etiology

The incidence of prolonged labor varies from 1 to 7 percent. Modern methods of diagnosis and treatment have reduced the frequency of this complication.

The principal causes of prolonged labor are:

629

1. Fetopelvic disproportion
2. Malpresentations and malpositions
3. Inefficient uterine action, including the rigid cervix

Accessory factors are:

1. Primigravidity.
2. Premature rupture of the membranes when the cervix is unef-faced, closed, and hard.
3. Excessive analgesia or anesthesia in the latent phase.
4. The dependent, anxious, frightened girl whose parents accompany her to the hospital is a candidate for prolonged labor. Another type is the masculine, masochistic woman who seems almost to be enjoying her pain.

These factors may act alone or in concert. A marked abnormality of one, or a minor deviation in several, can prevent successful termination of the labor. Whereas normal delivery is impossible in the presence of absolute cephalopelvic disproportion, a mild disparity between the size of the pelvis and that of the fetus can be overcome by strong and effective uterine contractions. The pelvis may be sufficiently large to accommodate an occipitoanterior presentation but too small for an occipitoposterior one. It is a matter of balance.

Rupture of the membranes in the presence of a ripe cervix and strong contractions never prolongs labor. If, however, the bag of waters breaks when the cervix is long, hard, and closed, there is often a long latent period before progressive labor sets in.

Inefficient uterine action includes the inability of the cervix to dilate smoothly and rapidly, as well as ineffective uterine contractions.

GRAPHIC ANALYSIS OF LABOR

Friedman described a graphic analysis of labor (Fig. 1), correlating the duration of labor with the rate of cervical dilatation. On graph paper the cervical dilatation in centimeters is placed on the ordinate and the time on the abscissa. Joining the points of contact makes a sigmoid curve. The rate of cervical dilatation, as shown by the slope of the curve, is described in centimeters per hour.

The first stage of labor (from the onset of labor to full dilatation of

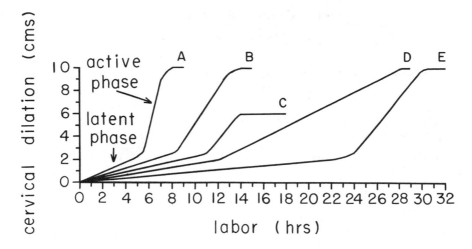

FIG. 1. Normal and abnormal labor during the first stage. A, average multipara. B, average primigravida. C, Secondary arrest of dilation. D, primary dysfunctional labor. E, prolonged latent phase.

the cervix) is divided into two periods, the latent phase and the active phase. By studying a large series, Friedman obtained figures for the lengths of the various phases. The upper normal limits represent the longest time that labor went on and still terminated normally. However, in slow or nonprogressing cases (as shown by a low rate of cervical dilatation) investigation must be instituted long before the maximum time limit has been reached.

Latent Period

This phase begins with the onset of labor and lasts until the beginning of the active phase of cervical dilatation, as shown by the upswing of the curve. The uterine contractions become orientated and the cervix softened and effaced. The slope of the curve is nearly flat, the cervical dilatation averaging only 0.35 cm per hour. At the end of the latent phase the cervix is around 3 cm dilated, well effaced, and soft.

In primigravidas the average length of the latent phase is 8.6 hours, with the upper limit of normal at 20 hours (Table 1). For multiparas the figures are 5.3 and 14 hours. Wide variations occur, and a prolonged latent period does not mean that the active phase will be abnormal.

TABLE 1. Lengths of the Phases of Labor

	Primigravidas		Multiparas	
	Average	**Upper normal**	**Average**	**Upper normal**
Latent phase	8.6 hours	20 hours	5.3 hours	14 hours
Active phase	5.8 hours	12 hours	2.5 hours	6 hours
First stage of labor	13.3 hours	28.5 hours	7.5 hours	20 hours
Second stage of labor	57 minutes	2.5 hours	18 minutes	50 minutes
Rate of cervical dilatation during active phase	Under 1.2 cm/hour is abnormal		Under 1.5 cm/hour is abnormal	

Active Period

The active period lasts from the end of the latent phase to full dilatation of the cervix. The curve changes from the almost horizontal slope of the latent phase to a nearly vertical incline. As the second stage is being reached the curve flattens again. Effective labor begins with the active phase, the period of steady and rapid cervical dilatation.

The vertical linearity of the curve makes possible the early recognition of deviations from the average. Premature flattening of the curve (indicating a reduction in the rate of cervical dilatation) calls for immediate investigation of the cause.

In the primigravidas of Friedman's series the average length of the active phase was 5.8 hours, and the upper limit of normal was 12 hours. The rate of cervical dilatation ranged from 1.2 to 6.8 cm per hour. A rate under 1.2 cm per hour is below normal and suggests dysfunctional labor.

In multiparas the average length of the active phase was 2.5 hours, with the upper normal limit at 6 hours. A rate of cervical dilatation less than 1.5 cm per hour is abnormal.

In the primigravidas the maximum duration of the normal first stage of labor (latent and active phases combined) was 28.5 hours (average 13.3), with the second stage maximum at 2.5 hours (average 57 minutes). In multiparas the figures were 20 hours (average 7.5) for the first stage, and 50 minutes (average 18 minutes) for the second stage.

CLASSIFICATION OF PROLONGED LABOR

Prolonged Latent Phase

A latent phase that exceeds 20 hours in the primigravida or 14 hours in the multipara is abnormal. Causes of a prolonged latent phase include: (1) an unripe cervix at the onset of labor, (2) abnormal position of the fetus, (3) fetopelvic disproportion, (4) dysfunctional labor, and (5) the administration of excessive sedation.

The unripe cervix prolongs only the latent phase, and most cervices open normally once effacement is achieved. Even when the latent phase lasts over 20 hours, many patients advance to normal cervical dilatation when the active phase begins. While a long latent phase is worrisome, it does not endanger the mother or the child.

Prolonged Active Phase in the Primigravida

In the primigravida an active phase longer than 12 hours is abnormal. More important than the length of this phase is the speed of cervical dilatation. A rate less than 1.2 cm per hour is evidence of some abnormality and should alert the attendant.

Prolongation of the active phase is associated with (1) malpositions of the fetus, (2) fetopelvic disproportion, (3) injudicious use of sedation and analgesia, and (4) rupture of membranes before the onset of labor. It is followed by an increase in mid forceps delivery, cesarean section, and fetal damage or death.

The prolonged active period can be divided into two main clinical groups: (1) those in whom there is a progressing albeit slow dilatation of the cervix; and (2) those in whom there is actual arrest of dilatation.

PRIMARY DYSFUNCTIONAL LABOR

The rate of cervical dilatation is less than 1.2 cm per hour. Spontaneous increase in the rate of dilatation occurs rarely, and little can be done to speed up progress.

In the absence of other complications the risk to the mother and child is small. Hence as long as progress is being made and there is no fetal distress, the phenomenon of slow cervical dilatation must be accepted.

Two-thirds of these patients deliver normally, 20 percent require mid forceps, and 10 percent come to cesarean section. A few women go into secondary arrest of dilatation, for which the prognosis is more serious.

SECONDARY ARREST OF DILATATION

During the active phase, previously advancing dilatation of the cervix stops. On the graph there is a flattening of the curve. Two hours of arrest is diagnostic.

There are two subgroups: (1) the uterine contractions become insufficient to maintain progressive dilatation of the cervix; and (2) cervical dilatation ceases in spite of strong and efficient uterine contractions.

While this is a different entity from the primary protracted active phase, both can occur in the same patient and the etiology can be related. Thus either a slowly dilating cervix or one that had been opening normally may stop advancing.

Accurate assessment of the situation and diagnosis of etiology is vital. Keeping in mind that inefficient uterine action is often associated with disproportion and abnormal position of the fetus, one must not blame the lack of progress on poor contractions until mechanical factors have been ruled out.

When ineffective labor (often myometrial fatigue) is the sole cause, half the patients resume progress after no more treatment than rest and an infusion of glucose in water. In this group amniotomy and oxytocin stimulation works well.

When there are complications such as disproportion or abnormal position, the treatment must be aimed in their direction.

Prolonged Active Phase in the Multipara

An active phase in the multipara lasting over 6 hours (average 2.5 hours) and a rate of cervical dilatation of less than 1.5 cm per hour are abnormal. While prolonged labor in a multipara is rare in comparison with the primigravida, it can, because of neglect and a false sense of security, lead to catastrophe. The fact that a normal birth occurred in the past does not mean it will be repeated. Careful observation, avoidance of traumatic vaginal deliveries, and consideration of cesarean section are important in the management of this problem.

The following are characteristics of prolonged labor in the multipara:

1. The incidence is less than 1 percent.
2. Perinatal mortality is higher than in primigravidas with prolonged labor.
3. The number of large babies is significant.
4. Malpresentations present a problem.
5. Prolapse of the umbilical cord is a complication.
6. Postpartum hemorrhage is dangerous.
7. Rupture of the uterus occurs in the grand multipara.
8. Most deliver spontaneously per vaginam.
9. Midforceps extractions are more frequent.
10. Cesarean section rate is high, around 25 percent.

Descent of the Presenting Part

Once active descent begins late in the first stage of labor, it should advance progressively throughout the course of the second stage. Interruption of descent is ominous and suggests that a serious problem exists. Diagnosis is based on the demonstration of there being no change in the station of the fetal presenting part over the period of at least 2 hours. Cephalopelvic disproportion and abnormalities of uterine action are seen often when descent arrests. Cesarean section, midforceps, forceps rotations, and failed forceps are noted frequently in association with this problem. With difficult vaginal operative deliveries maternal and fetal trauma are common.

INVESTIGATION OF PROLONGED LABOR

Graphic Analysis of Labor

By charting the progress of labor on a graph (Fig. 1) we can ascertain whether cervical dilatation is occurring at a normal rate or too slowly, or has ceased altogether. The type of abnormality can be diagnosed, and the point at which detailed investigation should be carried out is indicated.

Fetal Condition

The condition of the baby is evaluated by monitoring the fetal heart and by observing the passage of meconium.

Maternal Status

The patient's general physical and mental condition is assessed with respect to fatigue, morale, hydration, and nourishment.

Vaginal Examination

Vaginal examination is performed under sterile conditions, with the patient in the lithotomy position and the bladder and rectum empty. Sometimes an anesthetic is necessary to ensure adequate assessment.

Rectal examinations have no place in problem cases when a decision must be made as to definite treatment. Errors are made too often as to the condition and dilatation of the cervix, a large caput is mistaken for the skull, and the position and station are diagnosed inaccurately. During the vaginal examination the following points are noted.

STATE OF THE CERVIX

Is it open or closed, soft or hard, effaced or long, dilatable or resistant? Has any progress been made since the last examination? Is an anterior lip caught between the head and the symphysis? In the majority of cases the cervix ceases dilating when it is one-half to three-fourths open. In many of these instances it is erroneously considered to be fully dilated on rectal examination.

STATION OF PRESENTING PART

The station of the bony presenting part is determined. Is it at, above, or below the spines? Has engagement taken place? Is there a caput? Is molding excessive?

POSITION

The position must be diagnosed accurately. In all cases of prolonged labor, malpositions such as brow presentation and occiput posterior should be kept in mind.

FAILURE OF DESCENT

What seems to be holding up the presenting part? Can it be pushed down? Is the cause of arrest in the bony pelvis or is it the cervix? Is the head too big for the pelvis? Or is the problem not the pelvis, the cervix, or the fetus, but in the uterine contractions, and will a few hours of really good labor achieve progress to successful delivery?

Uterine Contractions

The uterine contractions are assessed. Is the basic problem in the type of labor, or is the main problem elsewhere and the poor uterine action a secondary complication? If the contractions are judged to be efficient, then the reason for the failure of progress must be in another field. Since inefficient uterine action is almost entirely a disorder of primigravidas, multiparas with prolonged labors must be investigated for other factors carefully before a diagnosis of poor labor is made. A woman who has delivered a 7-pound baby with no trouble may not be able to do the same with a 9-pound baby.

The strength of the contractions may be assessed manually or by the use of an electronic monitoring system.

X-ray Examination

When diagnosis is difficult and imprecise because of considerable molding and a large caput succedaneum, x-ray may help in determining fetal station and position, as well as pelvic size and shape.

MANAGEMENT OF PROLONGED LABOR

Prevention

1. Good prenatal care and preparation for childbirth reduces the incidence of prolonged labor.
2. Labor should not be induced or forced when the cervix is not ripe. A ripe cervix is less than 1.27 cm (0.5 inch) in length, effaced, patulous to admit at least a finger, and soft and dilatable.
3. False labor is treated by rest and sedation.

Supportive Measures

1. During labor the patient's morale should be bolstered. Encouragement is offered, and remarks that may worry the patient are avoided.
2. A fluid intake of at least 2,500 ml daily is essential. In all prolonged labors this is maintained by intravenous infusions of glucose in water. Dehydration, of which acetone in the urine is a sign, must be prevented.
3. Food taken during labor is not digested well. It remains in the stomach with danger of vomiting and aspiration. Hence in long labors nourishment is given by intravenous feeding.
4. Elimination from bladder and bowel must be adequate. A full bladder and rectum not only cause discomfort and impede progress but are more liable to injury than empty ones.
5. While women in labor must be rested with sedation and relieved of pain by analgesia, this must be administered judiciously. An excessive amount of narcosis may interfere with contractions and can harm the baby.

6. The number of rectal or vaginal examinations should be kept to a minimum. It hurts the patient and increases the risk of infection. Each examination must be done for a definite purpose.
7. Should the findings at examination suggest that progress is being made and that delivery may be expected within a reasonable time, and if there is no fetal or maternal distress, supportive therapy is given and labor allowed to go on.

Prolonged Latent Phase

First the mechanical factors must be ruled out. Further treatment depends on the condition of the cervix.

1. Ripe cervix: effaced, soft, and 2.5 to 3.0 cm dilated.
   a. Amniotomy.
   b. Oxytocin.
2. Unripe cervix: Treatment is supportive. The patient is given nourishment, reassurance, and medication to induce sleep. Following this, one of three courses follows:
   a. The labor ceases (indicating false labor), and the patient is discharged from hospital.
   b. She will go into efficient labor and dilate the cervix.
   c. The original type of labor resumes. In this event oxytocin stimulation often pushes the patient into good labor. Once the cervix ripens the membranes may be ruptured.

The prognosis is good. (1) Most patients proceed into the progressive labor of the active phase leading to vaginal delivery. (2) Some develop dysfunctional labor or secondary arrest of dilatation.

Cesarean section is almost never indicated in the latent stage of labor. Acute fetal distress, absolute cephalopelvic disproportion, and transverse lie are exceptions.

Primary Dysfunctional Labor

Mechanical factors must be ruled out. In some cases there is fetopelvic disproportion, and cesarean section is indicated. For the rest, medical management is carried out as long as the fetus and mother are in good condition. Nothing is done to complicate the situation further. Premature and traumatic vaginal operations are contraindicated. Slow progress is accepted. Support, reassurance, rest, fluids, and electrolytes are provided.

The results of amniotomy are not predictable, nor is there agreement as to whether it is a wise procedure in this situation. In some cases the progress of labor is improved; in others the arrest of labor seems to begin following artificial rupture of the membranes; and in many, amniotomy has no effect on the course of labor. In prolonged labor the incidence of ascending infection is increased once the membranes are ruptured; this danger must be kept in mind when amniotomy is being considered.

Reports concerning the value of an oxytocin infusion vary. Many workers feel it is ineffective in improving the progress of labor. However, we have had good results in some cases and feel it should be given a trial in managing this problem.

Results of medical treatment are as follows:

1. Two-thirds of the patients dilate the cervix slowly and proceed to vaginal delivery spontaneously or with the help of low forceps.
2. About 20 percent require mid forceps.
3. Some 10 percent come to cesarean section because of arrest of progress or fetal distress.

Secondary Arrest of Dilatation

1. It is vital that mechanical factors be ruled out carefully. These include malpositions and malpresentations as well as disproportion.
2. In a large group there is disproportion, and cesarean section must be performed.
3. A few women are exhausted and are given support, rest, fluids, and electrolytes.
4. The majority of patients in whom there is no disproportion and no fetal distress are given an oxytocin infusion and the membranes are ruptured artificially. One of four courses follows:
   a. Rapid progress to full dilatation and vaginal delivery.
   b. Slow progress to full dilatation and vaginal delivery.
   c. Too slow progress so that after 4 to 6 hours cesarean section is done.
   d. No progress at all. At the end of 2 hours cesarean section is carried out.

Failure of Descent

1. Disproportion calls for cesarean section. With the decline of the use of difficult forceps deliveries the fetal results have improved.
2. No disproportion. The use of epidural anesthesia to relieve pain and promote relaxation often results in progress. If descent does not take place, stimulation by an oxytocin infusion, monitored by continuous recording of the FHR and the intrauterine pressure, will often bring about steady progress to vaginal delivery. If this treatment fails, cesarean section is performed.

Fetal and/or Maternal Distress

1. Fetal or maternal distress calls for early intervention.
2. If the cervix is fully dilated, the presenting part is low in the pelvis, and there is no disproportion, the baby should be delivered by forceps if the presentation is cephalic and by cesarean section if it is a breech.
3. Preparations should be at hand for the treatment of postpartum hemorrhage and fetal distress.

Cervical Dystocia

The cervix may be holding up progress.

1. A thick anterior lip may be caught between the head and the symphysis pubis. This can be pushed over the head during a contraction.
2. There may be a thin, soft rim of cervix. This can also be pushed gently over the head.
3. If the cervix is 7 cm dilated and well effaced, and the fetal head is well below the spines, Dührssen's incisions may be considered. In modern times this procedure is carried out rarely.
4. If the cervix is less than half open, vaginal delivery is impossible at that time. If immediate delivery is indicated, cesarean section may be necessary.

DANGER OF PROLONGED LABOR

Maternal Dangers

Prolonged labor exerts a deleterious effect on both mother and child. The severity of the damage increases progressively with the duration of the labor, the risk rising sharply after 24 hours. There is a rise in the incidence of uterine atony, lacerations, hemorrhage, infections, maternal exhaustion, and shock. The high rate of operative deliveries aggravates the maternal dangers.

Fetal Dangers

The longer the labor, the higher the fetal mortality and morbidity, and the more frequently do the following conditions occur:

1. Asphyxia from the long labor itself.
2. Cerebral damage caused by pressure against the fetal head.
3. Injury as a result of difficult forceps rotations and extractions.
4. Rupture of the bag of waters long before delivery. This may result in the amniotic fluid's becoming infected and in turn may lead to pulmonary and general infection in the fetus.

Even when there is no obvious damage these babies require special care. While any type of prolonged labor is bad for the child, the danger is greater once there has been cessation of progress. This is especially true when the head has been arrested on the perineal floor for a long time, with continual pounding of the skull against the mother's pelvis.

Some workers feel that while prolonged labor increases the risk to the child during labor and the neonatal period, it has little effect on the infant's subsequent development. Others claim to have found that children born after extended labor were deficient intellectually as contrasted with babies born after normal delivery.

PROLONGED LABOR IN THE SECOND STAGE

Once the cervix has reached full dilatation, the period until birth should not exceed 2 hours in a primigravida and 1 hour in a multipara. Experience has shown that after this period fetal and maternal morbidity rises. Should fetal or maternal distress occur, immediate treatment is indicated.

Etiology

1. Fetopelvic disproportion
   a. Small pelvis
   b. Large child
2. Malpresentation and malposition
3. Ineffective labor
   a. Primary inefficient uterine contractions
   b. Myometrial fatigue: secondary inertia
   c. Constriction ring
   d. Inability or refusal of the patient to bear down
   e. Excessive anesthesia
4. Soft tissue dystocia
   a. Narrow vaginal canal
   b. Rigid perineum

Management

DISPROPORTION OR CONSTRICTION RING
Cesarean section is indicated.

NO DISPROPORTION

1. An oxytocin drip improves the uterine contractions.
2. Artificial rupture of the membranes is indicated if the bag of waters is intact.
3. The patient should be placed on the delivery table and urged to bear down with each contraction.
4. Forceps are used to further descent and rotation of the head.
5. An episiotomy overcomes the unyielding perineum.

When these methods of treatment fail or when operative vaginal delivery is considered to be too traumatic for safe delivery, cesarean section is indicated. The detailed descriptions of these procedures are found in the chapters concerned with each problem.

BIBLIOGRAPHY

Barber HRK, Graber EA, Orlando A: Augmented labor. Obstet Gynecol 39:933, 1972
Brenner WE: Abnormal progression of labor. Clin Obstet Gynecol 16:243, 1973

Friedman EA: Disordered labor. Objective evaluation and management. J Family Pract 2:167, 1975

Friedman EA, Sachtleben MR: Station of the fetal presenting part. Arrest in nulliparas. Obstet Gynecol 47:129, 1976

Maltau JM, Andersen HT: Epidural anesthesia as an alternative to cesarean section in the treatment of prolonged, exhaustive labor. Acta Anesthesiol Scand 19:349, 1975

O'Driscoll K, Stronge JM, Minogue M: Active management of labor. Br Med J, 3:135, 21 July 1973

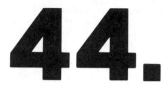

Fetopelvic Disproportion

Fetopelvic disproportion refers to the inability of the fetus to pass through the pelvis. Disproportion may be absolute or relative. It is absolute when under no circumstances can the baby pass safely through the birth canal. Relative disproportion is present when other factors contribute to the problem. Minor degrees of pelvic contraction can be overcome by efficient uterine contractions, dilatability of the soft tissues, favorable attitude, presentation, and position of the fetus, and moldability of the fetal head. On the other hand, poor contractions, rigid soft parts, abnormal positions, and inability of the head to mold properly can make vaginal delivery impossible.

THE PASSAGE

Pelvic Size

While the important question is the relationship between a given pelvis and a particular fetus, in some cases the contraction of the pelvis is such that no normal fetus can pass through. The reduced size may be at any level: the inlet, midpelvis, or outlet. Sometimes the pelvis may be small in all planes—the generally contracted pelvis.

INLET CONTRACTION
Inlet contraction is present when the anteroposterior diameter (obstetric conjugate) is less than 10 cm or the transverse diameter is less than 12 cm. Inlet contraction may result from rickets or from generally poor development.
Effects on the fetus are:

1. Failure of engagement
2. Increase in malpositions
3. Deflexion attitudes

4. Exaggerated asynclitism
5. Extreme molding
6. Formation of a large caput succedaneum
7. Prolapse of the umbilical cord. This becomes a complication since the presenting part does not fit the inlet well.

Effects on labor include:

1. Dilatation of the cervix is slow and often incomplete.
2. Premature rupture of the membranes is common.
3. Inefficient uterine action is a frequent accompaniment.

MIDPELVIC CONTRACTION

Midpelvic contraction is basically a reduction in the plane of least dimensions, the one that passes from the apex of the pubic arch, through the ischial spines, to meet the sacrum usually at the junction of the fourth and fifth segments.

When the distance between the ischial spines is less than 9.0 cm, or when the sum of the interspinous (normal is 10.5 cm) and the posterior sagittal (normal is 4.5 to 5.0 cm) distances is less than 13.5 cm (normal is 15.0 to 15.5 cm), contraction of the midpelvis is probably present. To obtain accurate measurement of these diameters x-ray pelvimetry is essential. Clinical suspicion of a small midpelvis is aroused by the finding on manual examination of a small pelvis, the palpation of large spines that jut into the cavity, and the observation that the distance between the ischial tuberosities is less than 8.5 cm.

Midpelvic contraction is a common cause of dystocia and operative delivery. It is more difficult to manage than inlet contraction, for if the fetal head cannot even enter the inlet there is no doubt that abdominal delivery is necessary. However, once the head has descended into the pelvis, one is loath to perform cesarean section, hoping that the head will come down to a point where it can be extracted with forceps. A danger here is that with molding and caput formation the head may appear lower than it actually is. Instead of the projected midforceps delivery, one is engaged in a high forceps operation, often with disastrous results for both mother and infant.

Midpelvic contractions may prevent anterior rotation of the occiput and may direct it into the hollow of the sacrum. Failure of rotation and deflexion attitudes are associated frequently with a small pelvic cavity.

OUTLET CONTRACTION

Outlet contraction is present when the distance between the ischial tuberosities is less than 8 cm. Dystocia may be expected when the sum of the intertuberous diameter and the posterior sagittal diameter is much less than 15 cm. Diminution of the intertuberous diameter and the subpubic angle forces the head backward, and so the prognosis depends on the capacity of the posterior segment, the mobility at the sacrococcygeal joint, and the ability of the soft tissues to accommodate the passenger. The sides of the posterior triangle are not bony. While outlet contraction causes an increase in perineal lacerations and a greater need for forceps deliveries, only rarely is it an indication for cesarean section. Because the bituberous diameter can be measured manually, however, and since it may warn us that there is contraction higher in the pelvis, it should always be assessed as part of the routine examination.

Delay at the outlet may be caused by a rigid perineum. The tissues do not stretch well; and when they tear, a large uncontrolled laceration results. Treatment is by mediolateral episiotomy as soon as the problem is recognized.

DWARFISM
Dwarfism is defined as a height of less than 4 feet 10 inches at maturity. Vaginal delivery is possible in women with proportionate dwarfism. Respiratory embarrassment in the latter part of pregnancy may make it impossible to await the onset of labor. Most patients are delivered by cesarean section between 35 and 37 weeks. The babies are often of good size, around 2,600 g.

Influence of Pelvic Shape

The obstetric capacity of the female pelvis is governed by its size and shape or configuration. By radiologic techniques accurate classification by shape is more reliable than precise measurement of diameters. Hence, with the exception of cases of extreme contraction, we feel that in attempting prognosis the type of pelvis is more important than the size. These factors complement each other. A poor class of pelvis may be compensated for by being large, or a relatively small pelvis may function well because of a favorable shape.

GYNECOID The gynecoid or normal female pelvis offers the best diameters in all three planes for the uncomplicated passage of the fetus.

ANDROID The android or male pelvis has a bad obstetric reputation. With reduced posterior segments in all pelvic planes, the occiput has a tendency to enter the inlet posteriorly, is impeded in rotation in the midpelvis, and is forced posteriorly at the outlet. The results are arrest of descent, failure of rotation, and lacerations of the perineum and rectum.

ANTHROPOID In the anthropoid pelvis the reduced transverse measurements in the various planes are only relative and are compensated for by large anteroposterior diameters. The head descends often in the occipitoposterior position with surprising ease and is born frequently face to pubis. In general the prognosis is better than that of the android or platypelloid types.

PLATYPELLOID In the platypelloid pelvis there is interference with entry of the presenting part into the inlet, and there may be difficulty at the lower levels as well. In this group is found the highest incidence of cesarean section.

MIXED There are also mixed types of pelves. A gynecoid or anthropoid pelvis may have an android-like narrowing at the midpelvis or the outlet. Thus the head enters the pelvis but becomes arrested lower down. Minor forms of funneling are common and are frequent causes of forceps extractions. In these situations the size of the fetal head, the degree of flexion, and the capacity for molding are critical factors. Even a slight variation in the presenting dimensions makes a great difference in the ease or difficulty of the delivery.

Abnormal Pelves

There are numerous varieties of grossly abnormal pelves associated with deformity and contraction. Fortunately these are not common and do not play a prominent part in the problem of fetopelvic disproportion.

KYPHOSCOLIOSIS The incidence of kyphoscoliosis complicating pregnancy is low, occurring in but 1:6,000 labors in America. In South Africa the rate was reported as 1:2,400 pregnancies. The etiology includes tuberculosis (most frequent), osteomalacia, rickets, poliomyelitis, trauma, and congenital abnormality. When the lesion is in the thoracic area there is little or no reduction of pelvic capacity, but the enlarging uterus may decrease cardiopulmonary function. These patients tolerate pregnancy and labor fairly well as long as there are no significant problems prior to the pregnancy, and a number deliver vaginally. Dorsolumbar and lumbosacral kyphoses, on the other hand, are accompanied by marked pelvic deformity. Cesarean section is required in most of these cases because of pelvic contraction and cephalopelvic disproportion. Women with impaired cardiopulmonary reserve should not become pregnant. If they do, abortion is considered.

BONY DISEASE OF THE FEMURS AND ACETABULA By causing abnormal pressures on the pelvis during development, such disease may result in asymmetry and reduction of pelvic capacity.

FRACTURED PELVIS This may also cause difficulties. Automobile accidents are the main cause. The effect on the pregnancy is twofold: (1) In women who were pregnant at the time of the mishap, fetal loss is the more frequent complication. (2) In pregnancies subsequent to the fracture, cesarean section is more common because the contracted and grossly misshapen pelvis causes disproportion. Cesarean section is a better method of long-term management than orthopedic surgery to try and correct the pelvic deformity.

Rare Abnormalities

NAEGELE PELVIS The absence or imperfect development of one wing of the sacrum leads to an obliquely contracted pelvis. It was described by Naegele in 1803. He discussed six features of the deformity: (1) complete fusion of one sacroiliac joint; (2) absent or imperfect development of one-half of the sacrum with narrowing of the anterior sacral foramina on the side corresponding to the ankylosis; (3) ipsilateral narrowing of the hip bone and its sciatic notch; (4) apparent displacement of the sacrum to the ankylosed side with rotation of its anterior surface to the same side, plus contralateral displacement of the pubic symphysis; (5) ipsilateral flattening of the lateral wall of the pelvis; and (6) the other side of the pelvis not being more spacious than a normal pelvis. The incidence is about 1:2,500 in Hong Kong. In most cases the deformity is of congenital origin. The diagnosis is made on x-ray examination. Vaginal delivery by means of difficult forceps operation is hazardous, and cesarean section gives the best results.

ROBERT PELVIS Robert described the symmetrically transversely contracted pelvis caused by the absence of both sacral alae in 1842. It is extremely rare, fewer than 20 being reported. It is believed to be a congenital anomaly. The sacral alae are absent, and the innominate bone is positioned medially so that there is transverse contraction at the inlet, midpelvis, and outlet. Diagnosis is by radiologic examination. The method of delivery is cesarean section. Vaginal birth is impossible.

SPLIT PELVIS There is failure of union between the pubic bones. This is often associated with nonunion of the walls of the bladder and the anterior abdomen.

ASSIMILATION PELVIS This is an elongated pelvis in which the last lumbar or first coccygeal vertebra resembles a sacral vertebra and seems to be part of the sacrum rather than the lumbar spine or the coccyx.

OSTEOMALACIC PELVIS There is softening of the bones that bend into the cavity of the pelvis. This reduces all the diameters greatly.

SPONDYLOLISTHETIC PELVIS The last lumbar vertebra is displaced forward and downward over the sacral promontory. Symptoms such as pain in and weakness of the back begin in the second and third trimester and become worse in succeeding pregnancies. The sheering force applied to the lower lumbar vertebrae is increased by the protruberant pregnant uterus and, in association with the relaxation of the pelvic ligaments, is responsible for precipitating the symptoms.

MANAGEMENT OF SPONDYLOLISTHESIS

1. During pregnancy corsets and braces help.
2. Prolonged labor and abnormal fetal positions are seen frequently, and an assessment of progress must be made carefully after 8 to 12 hours.
3. Mid forceps and cesarean section are necessary often.
4. The lithotomy position is harmful; the legs should be held in the horizontal position.

Soft Tissues

While poor dilatability of the muscles and fascia of the pelvis rarely causes severe disproportion in itself, in cases of borderline bony disproportion or poor uterine action it may make the difference between vaginal delivery or cesarean section. The rare case has been reported of a septum in the vagina causing obstruction. It must be excised before the baby can be born.

Neoplasms

Uterine fibromyomas or ovarian cysts may block the birth canal and prevent passage of the fetus through the pelvis. A large fibromyoma of the vagina can block passage of the child. It should be removed before or during the pregnancy. If this is not feasible, cesarean section is necessary.

THE PASSENGER

Fetal Size

Fetal size is important. Rarely is a baby too large for any pelvis. The essential problem is the relationship of the child to the pelvis. The question that must be answered is: Can this baby pass through this pelvis?

Oversized Fetus

The excessively large fetus is defined as one weighing either 4,500 g (9 pounds 15 ounces) or 10 pounds (4,545 g).

INCIDENCE AND ETIOLOGY
The incidence varies between 0.5 and 1.8 percent.
The following factors are associated with the oversized fetus:

1. It is more common in white women.
2. There is a familial tendency.
3. In 80 percent the patient is multiparous.
4. There is a slightly higher incidence in older women.
5. Maternal weight gain is often excessive.
6. The incidence of overt or subclinical diabetic mothers is high.
7. Toxemia of pregnancy is a little more common.
8. Often the pregnancy is longer than 40 weeks.
9. Two-thirds of the babies are male.
10. The patient has had a previous large baby.
11. The father is at least 10 years older than the parturient.

DIAGNOSIS
While there is no absolutely accurate way of determining fetal size in utero, estimation by palpation is often correct to within a pound. Ultrasonic measurement of the biparietal diameter of the fetal head and of the thorax and abdomen reduce greatly the margin of error.

LABOR

1. In over 90 percent the presentation is cephalic.
2. The total length of labor is not prolonged, but the second stage is.
3. There is usually no trouble delivering the head.
4. Shoulder dystocia occurs frequently.

DELIVERY

1. Many babies are born spontaneously or by low forceps.
2. There is an increased incidence of mid forceps, cesarean section, and operations to relieve shoulder dystocia.
3. Destructive operations (craniotomy and cleidotomy) were used many years ago, but with modern diagnosis and x-ray pelvimetry cesarean section has obviated the need for these procedures.
4. To improve maternal and fetal results cesarean section may be performed more often.

MATERNAL COMPLICATIONS

1. Lacerations of the genital tract
2. Postpartum hemorrhage from uterine atony and lacerations
3. Separation of the pubic symphysis

FETAL COMPLICATIONS

1. Infant mortality is increased.
2. There is a higher incidence of serious injury.
3. Among central nervous system complications are fractured skull, intracranial hemorrhage, and brain damage by compression.
4. Peripheral neurologic damage includes Erb's and brachial palsy, as well as nonspecific paralyses.
5. Fractures of the humerus, femur, and clavicle are seen.
6. Severe depression is common.
7. Follow-up revealed an increased incidence of medical illness and death during infancy and childhood.

Attitude and Position

In borderline pelves a well flexed head in a good occipitoanterior position may deliver normally, while face presentation or an occipitoposterior becomes arrested.

Moldability

Moldability of the fetal head may be critical. The ability of the head to change its shape to fit the pelvis may enable it to negotiate the birth canal safely. Excessive molding can damage the brain, and this must be considered in deciding whether vaginal delivery is to be awaited. A reduction of more than 0.5 cm in the biparietal diameter is considered dangerous.

Fetal Abdominal Enlargement

This rare condition may cause dystocia. The diagnosis is made after the head is born and the trunk cannot be delivered. The fetal mortality is high because: (1) intrauterine death may take place, (2) the causal condition is incompatible with extrauterine life, and (3) the trauma of a difficult birth may be lethal.

There are several varieties:

1. Generalized edema of all organs and cavities. This is associated with diabetic mothers, erythroblastosis, and toxemia of pregnancy.
2. Ascites (3 to 4 liters) is often associated with abnormalities of the urinary tract and is more common in males. Perforation of the abdomen or thorax is usually necessary before birth can be effected.
3. There may be distention of the urinary tract caused by vesical neck obstruction.
4. Polycystic kidneys may cause dystocia.
5. Fluid collection in and distention of the female genital tract may result from vaginal atresia.
6. Cystic or tumorous liver may be present.

UTERINE CONTRACTIONS

Strong uterine contractions should not be allowed or relied upon to push a baby through a pelvis when there is absolute disproportion. In borderline cases, however, when there are minor degrees of disproportion, uterine efficiency may be the essential difference between success and failure.

INVESTIGATION OF DISPROPORTION

In attempting to determine whether a given baby can be born per vaginam without serious injury to itself or to the mother, the following investigative procedures are carried out: history, abdominal palpation, vaginal examination, radiologic studies, and trial labor.

History

To an extent the information sought varies with the parity of the patient. If there have been previous pregnancies and labors the details of these are of great help in determining the prognosis. In primigravidas other information is elicited to aid in making the decisions.

MULTIPARAS

1. The number of children and the number of pregnancies.
2. The size of the babies at birth, especially the largest. Many women tend to have progressively larger babies, and the knowledge that a 6-pound child was delivered with no difficulty does not guarantee the same success with an 8-pound baby.
3. The condition of the children at birth, including any damaged children or intrapartum deaths.
4. Length of labor.
5. Method of delivery.
6. Maternal lacerations.

Most labors and deliveries subsequent to the first are easier. The pelvic joints and soft tissues, once stretched, offer less resistance.

PRIMIGRAVIDAS

1. The age of the patient: For the purpose of childbearing a woman is said to be as old as her cervix. While some clinics consider that a woman is not an elderly primigravida until she reaches 40, in many institutions 35 years of age is taken as the dividing line. Many elderly primigravidas ripen the cervix well, push the presenting part into the pelvis even before labor has started, and have an easy, spontaneous delivery. An equal number, however, have difficulties. Hence all older women who are pregnant for the first time merit careful investigation.
2. Type of menstrual cycle: This is important. Women whose menses were late in starting, irregular, and attended with severe dysmenorrhea have a tendency toward difficult labor.
3. Sterility: Women with a history of involuntary sterility for 7 or 8 years often have worrisome labors with uterine dysfunction, soft tissue dystocia, and operative deliveries.
4. Familiar history: Information about the patient's mother and sisters are important. A history of dystocia with injured or dead babies calls for an especially careful investigation.

Failure of Engagement

While any doubt as to pelvic adequacy must be resolved by thorough examination, one of the most common problems is the unengaged head in the primigravida near term. In the majority of primigravidas with normal pelves the head engages about 3 weeks before term. Breeches, on the other hand, often do not engage until good labor has set it.

In about 5 percent of primigravidas the head is unengaged at term. Since most of these deliver per vaginam there is no need to panic, but the persistence of nonengagement is an indication for complete study to determine the cause for the failure of descent. In many cases the high station is related to the cervix and uterus being unprepared. The head cannot enter the pelvis until the lower uterine segment is formed.

ABDOMINAL PALPATION

The patient lies on her back on the examining table in as relaxed a condition as possible. First the position is ascertained. Then with one hand the examiner presses the head gently but firmly into the pelvic brim. The fingers of the other hand are applied to the area of the abdomen above the pubic symphysis. As pressure is being applied the examiner determines whether the head will enter the inlet of the pelvis or whether it overrides the pubis and fails to enter the superior strait. If the head can be pushed into the pelvis it suggests that there is no disproportion at the inlet. If it does not go in, further investigation must be carried out.

Causes of failure to descend or overriding include:

1. Disproportion
2. Malpresentation or malposition
3. Underdeveloped lower uterine segment
4. Polyhydramnios
5. Placenta previa
6. Soft tissue tumor blocking the pelvis
7. Full bladder or rectum
8. Patient not close enough to term, a situation often associated with an underdeveloped lower segment

VAGINAL AND COMBINED ABDOMINOPELVIC EXAMINATION

This is the most important procedure in the assessment of fetopelvic disproportion. The patient should be positioned on a table in the lithotomy position to ensure adequate examination. Sometimes the discomfort is such that a short anesthetic is necessary. (See Chap. 9 for details of procedure.)

The inner walls of the inlet, cavity, and outlet of the pelvis are palpated to estimate their capacities and to search for abnormalities. The length, dilatation, and consistency of the cervix are determined. The elasticity of the soft tissues (muscles, fascia, and ligaments) are checked to see whether they are likely to stretch or prevent the head from descending.

The position of the presenting part is noted, as well as its ability to flex. Extreme asynclitism is a bad sign. Pressure is applied to the presenting part over the pubis and to the fundus of the uterus to see whether it can be forced down to the level of the ischial spines, or further. If this can be accomplished by manual pressure, then it can be assumed that strong uterine contractions will have no difficulty in doing the same.

These examinations should allow the patient to be placed into one of three categories:

1. No disproportion is present. This infant should go through this pelvis.
2. There is absolute fetopelvic disproportion.
3. The fetopelvic relationship is borderline. A trial of labor is indicated.

RADIOGRAPHIC EXAMINATION

In doubtful cases x-ray pelvimetry is performed to obtain additional information.

Trial Labor

This is a clinical attempt to evaluate the extent of cephalopelvic disproportion. The patient is allowed to labor under close supervision to see if the natural forces of labor can overcome real or suspected disproportion. It is also an excellent measure of the labor mechanism, which often determines the success or failure of the trial.

First a careful study is made of the pelvic adequacy in the light of the size and presentation of the baby. If gross disproportion is encountered cesarean section should be elected.

It is preferable that the patient go into labor spontaneously. Induction is carried out only in special cases, but augmentation of labor by artificial rupture of membranes or an infusion of oxytocin is permissible once labor is well under way.

During the labor the following factors are evaluated:

1. Mental and physical condition of the mother
2. Fetal heart rate as well as other signs of fetal distress, such as the passage of meconium

3. Force and coordination of the uterine contractions
4. Dilatation of the cervix
5. Descent of the presenting part
6. Degree of molding and the formation and size of the caput succedaneum

There are no satisfactory arbitrary time limits for trial labor. It may last 6 to 18 hours, rarely 24 hours. This is sufficient time to decide the degree of disproportion and, equally important, to demonstrate the effectiveness of the uterine mechanism. Good labor often overcomes small degrees of disproportion. The exact length of a trial labor for a specific case is a matter of judgment and can be determined only by the attending obstetrician and his consultant.

Needless rectal or vaginal examinations should be avoided. They are painful and predispose to infection. At the end of a reasonable period of labor a careful vaginal examination is made under aseptic conditions to evaluate the state of the cervix, the fetal position and presentation, and the station of the presenting part. On the basis of these findings the decision is made as to the success or failure of the trial.

Favorable progress of cervical effacement and dilatation, descent of the head into the pelvis, and the demonstration that the lower part of the pelvis is adequate are the criteria for continuing the trial. A poor labor mechanism with irregular, desultory, and ineffective contractions, the lack of effacement and progressive dilatation of the cervix, and failure of the head to enter the inlet and descend to the ischial spines serve as evidence that the trial of labor has failed and that other means of delivery should be sought.

The old-time test of labor, which is no longer used, lasted long enough for the cervix to become fully dilated, followed by a sufficiently long second stage with the membranes ruptured to demonstrate beyond a doubt that the head would not progress down the pelvic canal. Common complications were infection of the amniotic cavity, formation of a pathologic contraction ring, and uterine rupture. The fetal loss was 25 percent. Fetal and maternal damage could never be evaluated accurately. Thus while a patient should be given the opportunity to achieve a safe vaginal delivery, the trial of labor must not be carried to a dangerous extreme.

Augmentation of Labor

The hypothesis is that many patients who do not make good progress in labor fail to do so because of unrecognized inefficient uterine action. On this basis a trial of augmentation of labor by an infusion of oxytocin has been suggested before a diagnosis of disproportion is made and operative measures employed. The trial is carried out under careful monitoring of the fetal heart and the uterine contractions. This is a test of the functional capacity of the pelvis and the ability of the cervix to dilate. There is no intention of forcing the head through the pelvis. With this approach no patient should be in hard labor for more than 12 hours.

If the head does not descend well, if the rate of cervical dilatation is less than 1 cm per hour, and if delivery does not take place within the allotted time, cesarean section is considered. The achievement of an easy vaginal delivery excludes disproportion and avoids cesarean section.

CONTRAINDICATIONS

1. Fetal distress
2. Malpresentations
3. Disproportion
4. Existence of effective uterine contractions
5. Previous cervical scarring
6. Previous myomectomy, hysterotomy, or cesarean section
7. Parity over 5
8. Bicornuate uterus
9. Lack of adequate monitoring

TREATMENT OF FETOPELVIC DISPROPORTION

Cesarean Section

Cesarean section is the method of choice when a marked degree of disproportion is present. The low transverse incision in the uterus is preferred by most.

Forceps Delivery

When the disproportion is minor, when the arrest is caused by failure of flexion or rotation, and when the obstetrician has experience, low or mid forceps may be used to effect delivery. If, however, extraction by forceps would entail a difficult and traumatic procedure, it is wiser to turn to cesarean section.

Induction of Premature Labor

Induction of premature labor, to try to deliver the baby while it is smaller, was once a popular procedure to overcome disproportion. The drawbacks are:

1. Prematurity with its attendant complications
2. Poorly formed lower uterine segment with its resistant tissues
3. Unripe cervix
4. Inefficient function of the uterus, which is stimulated into labor before its polarity and coordinate action have been established.
5. Prolonged labor

For these reasons we feel that it is preferable to allow the patient to have a trial of labor at term and to perform cesarean section if necessary, rather than induce labor prematurely.

Craniotomy

Craniotomy has no place in the planned treatment of disproportion. It is permissible only for dead babies in situations in which the fetus is not deliverable intact. Its aim is to spare the mother an operative abdominal delivery.

Symphysiotomy

Performed first in 1777 by Signault, symphysiotomy was abandoned because of the frequency of complications and the growing safety of cesarean section. In 1920 Zarate resurrected the procedure in Argentina, and Seedat and Crichton, working in Africa, published their modified technique in 1962. Symphysiotomy widens the space between the pubic bones, enlarges the pelvic capacity permanently, and is, in certain situations, an alternative to cesarean section. In some areas of the world cesarean section, especially when the indication is cephalopelvic disproportion, is associated with a high incidence of uterine rupture because the patient does not return to hospital for consideration of repeat cesarean section with subsequent pregnancies.

ADVANTAGES

1. It takes only 5 minutes to perform.
2. It can be done anywhere.

TREATMENT OF FETOPELVIC DISPROPORTION

3. Local anesthesia is adequate.
4. The uterus is unscarred.
5. The pelvis is enlarged permanently; the next delivery will be easier.

INDICATIONS

1. Moderate cephalopelvic disproportion. Symphysiotomy is an alternative to cesarean section or a difficult forceps delivery.
2. Difficulty with the aftercoming head in a breech presentation.
3. Patients who are poor surgical risks.

PREREQUISITES

1. Effective uterine action, spontaneous or induced by oxytocin
2. Less than 80 percent of the fetal head above the pelvic brim
3. Cervical dilatation of at least 8 cm

CONTRAINDICATIONS

1. Inefficient uterine contractions.
2. Cervical dilatation less than 8 cm.
3. Previous cesarean section.
4. Fetal head more than 80 percent above the pelvic brim, especially if the membranes are ruptured.
5. True conjugate less than 8 cm.
6. Severe disproportion.
7. Malpresentation such as transverse lie or brow.
8. Suspected uterine rupture.
9. Deformity of the pelvis, back, or hips.
10. Marked obesity. The excessive weight puts too great a strain on the pelvis.
11. Baby estimated to weigh over 8 pounds.

TECHNIQUE

With the patient in the lithotomy position and a Foley catheter in the bladder, the skin and subcutaneous tissue over the symphysis are infiltrated with a local anesthetic (Fig. 1). A 2-cm incision is made in an anteroposterior direction. The left hand is placed in the vagina to displace the urethra and catheter to one side and to prevent the knife from penetrating too deeply. The scalpel is positioned vertically with the cutting edge pointing inferiorly. The pubic joint is entered at the junction of the upper and middle thirds, and the lower two-thirds of the joint is incised. The knife is then turned 180° and the upper one-third of the joint is cut. The separation of the symphysis should be less than 2.5 cm.

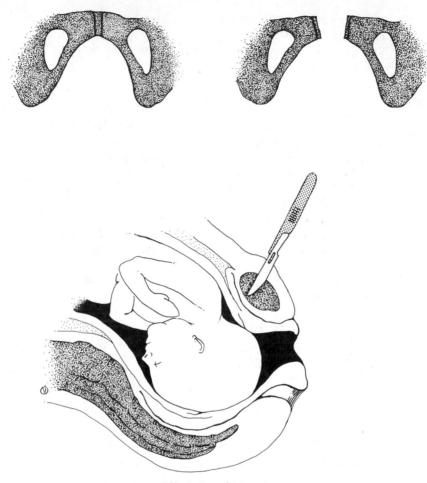

FIG. 1. Symphisiotomy

During delivery the patient's legs must be controlled to prevent excessive separation of the symphyseal joint. The fetal head is pressed posteriorly, away from the anterior vaginal wall. The vacuum extractor may be used, but forceps should be avoided. Episiotomy increases the room posteriorly. After delivery the skin is closed with a single stitch.

DELAY IN DELIVERY
This may be caused by

1. Inadequate uterine contractions
2. Insufficient separation of the joint
3. Inadequate episiotomy

4. Excessive residual disproportion
5. Fetal abnormality

POSTOPERATIVE CARE

1. The Foley catheter is left in the bladder for 5 days.
2. A belt around the trochanters makes the woman more comfortable.
3. The patient remains in bed, preferably on her side, for 3 to 4 days.
4. She sits up out of bed on the 5th day, walks with the help of a cane on the 6th, and by the 10th day no longer needs the belt.
5. Undue muscular effort is avoided for 6 weeks.

COMPLICATIONS

1. Urinary tract.
   a. Infection is the most common.
   b. Vesicovaginal and urethrovaginal fistula.
   c. Stress incontinence is rare.
2. Hemorrhage.
   a. Venous bleeding in the incisional area is controlled by pressure.
   b. Postpartum hemorrhage.
3. Tears of the anterior vaginal wall.
4. Instability of the symphyseal joint occurs occasionally when the separation was excessive.
5. There may be temporary difficulty in walking, but most women are able to resume previous physical activity.

PREGNANCY IN PATIENTS UNDER 15 YEARS OF AGE

A study of pregnant girls under 15 years of age was made and the findings compared with a paired group between the ages of 19 and 25. Only two complications occurred more often in the youngsters, namely, pregnancy-induced hypertension and pelvic contraction, especially at the inlet. It is probable that the bony pelvis had not reached its potential size at the time of delivery. A trial of labor is indicated, but the incidence of cesarean section is higher than average. There is no expected increase in maternal or infant mortality and morbidity.

GRAND MULTIPARITY

The definition varies, but parity of 6 seems to be an acceptable figure. During pregnancy the grand multipara has an increased incidence of

1. Anemia
2. Toxemia of pregnancy
3. Placenta previa
4. Abruptio placentae

COMPLICATIONS OF LABOR AND DELIVERY

1. Malpresentations, such as transverse lie and breech
2. Postpartum hemorrhage
3. Disproportion caused by a large baby
4. Rupture of the uterus
5. High incidence of midforceps

MANAGEMENT

1. Confinement in hospital is essential.
2. Careful monitoring of labor and fetal heart is needed.
3. Oxytocin should be used rarely and with great care.
4. Cesarean section is performed when there is failure of progress or suspicion of disproportion.
5. Postpartum oxytocin drip is given to prevent hemorrhage from uterine atony.

Despite her problems the grand multipara can go through pregnancy, labor, and delivery safely. However, there must be no false sense of security.

BIBLIOGRAPHY

Chau W, Kee KH: Kyphosis complicating pregnancy. J Obstet Gynaecol Br Commonw 77:1098, 1970

Duenhoelter JH, Jimenez JM, Baumann G: Pregnancy performance of patients under fifteen years of age. Obstet Gynecol 46:49, 1975

Hartfield VJ: A comparison of the early and late effects of subcutaneous symphysiotomy and of lower segment cesarean section. J Obstet Gynaecol Br Commonw 80:508, 1973

Kopenhager T: A review of 50 pregnant patients with kyphoscoliosis. Br J Obstet Gynaecol 84:585, 1977

Speer DP, Peltier LF: Pelvic fractures and pregnancy. J Trauma 12:474, 1972

Tyson JE, Barnes AC, McKusick VA, et al: Obstetric and gynecologic considerations of dwarfism. Am J Obstet Gynecol 108:688, 1970

45.

Cesarean Section

Cesarean section is an operation by which the child is delivered through an incision in the abdominal wall and the uterus. The first professional cesarean was performed in the United States in 1827. Before 1800 cesarean section was performed rarely and was usually fatal. In London and Edinburgh in 1877, of 35 cesareans performed 33 resulted in the death of the mother. By 1877 there had been 71 cesarean operations in the United States. The mortality rate was 52 percent, mainly because of infection and hemorrhage.

INDICATIONS FOR CESAREAN SECTION

Indications for cesarean section are absolute or relative. Any condition that makes delivery via the birth canal impossible is an absolute indication for abdominal section. Among these are extreme degrees of pelvic contraction and neoplasms blocking the passage. With a relative indication, vaginal birth is possible but the conditions are such that cesarean section is safer for the mother, the child, or both.

The rate of cesarean section has risen steadily from an incidence of 3 to 4 percent 15 years ago to the present 10 to 15 percent. The latter figure is probably acceptable and correct. Not only has the operation become safer for the mother, but the number of infants damaged by prolonged labor and traumatic vaginal operations has been reduced. In addition, concern for the quality of life and intellectual development of the infant has widened the indications for cesarean section.

Pelvic Contractions and Mechanical Dystocia

FETOPELVIC DISPROPORTION Fetopelvic disproportion includes the contracted pelvis, the overgrown fetus, or a relative disparity between the size of the baby and that of the pelvis. Contributing to the problem of disproportion are the shape of the pelvis, the presentation of the fetus and its ability to mold and engage, the dilatability of the cervix, and the effectiveness of the uterine contractions.

MALPOSITION AND MALPRESENTATION These abnormalities may make cesarean section necessary when a baby in normal position could be born per vaginam. A great part of the increased incidence of cesarean section in this group is associated with breech presentation. Probably one-third of breech presentations should be delivered abdominally. Not only are the immediate fetal results of vaginal birth worse with breech than with cephalic presentation, but there is evidence that there are long-term effects even when the birth is without untoward incident. There is the feeling that viable premature breeches and footling breeches are delivered best by cesarean section.

UTERINE DYSFUNCTION Uterine dysfunction includes incoordinate uterine action, inertia, constriction rings, and inability of the cervix to dilate. Labor is prolonged and progress may cease altogether. These conditions are often associated with disproportion and malpresentations.

SOFT TISSUE DYSTOCIA Soft tissue dystocia may prevent or make difficult normal birth. This includes such conditions as scars in the genital tract, cervical rigidity from injury or surgery, and atresia or stenosis of the vagina. Forceful vaginal delivery results in large lacerations and hemorrhage.

NEOPLASMS Neoplasms that block the pelvis make normal delivery impossible. Invasive cancer of the cervix diagnosed during the third trimester of pregnancy is treated by cesarean section followed by radiation therapy, radical surgery, or both.

FAILURE TO PROGRESS In this group are included such conditions as cephalopelvic disproportion, ineffective uterine contractions, poor pelvis, large baby, and deflexion of the fetal head. Often an exact diagnosis cannot be made and is academic in any case. The decision in favor of cesarean section is made on the failure of the labor to achieve cervical dilatation and/or fetal descent regardless of the etiology.

Previous Uterine Surgery

CESAREAN SECTION The current practice in most areas is that once a cesarean procedure has been performed, all subsequent pregnancies should be terminated in the same way. It is felt that the danger of rupture through the site of the previous uterine incision is too great. However, there is evidence that, under certain conditions, a trial of labor is permissible, with possible vaginal delivery. When successful, both maternal morbidity and length of stay in hospital are reduced.

HYSTEROTOMY Pregnancy in a uterus in which a previous gestation was terminated by hysterotomy is attended by danger of uterine rupture. The risk is similar to that of classical cesarean section. Hysterotomy should be avoided whenever possible, keeping in mind that the next pregnancy might necessitate cesarean section.

EXTENSIVE MYOMECTOMY Myomectomy in the past is an indication for cesarean section only if the operation was extensive, the myometrium disorganized, and the incision extended into the endometrial cavity. The previous removal of pedunculated or subserous fibromyomas does not call for cesarean section.

SUTURE In some cases where there has been a previous cervical suture or repair of an incompetent os, cesarean section is performed.

TRIAL OF LABOR AFTER PREVIOUS CESAREAN SECTION

Prerequisites

1. A single previous low cervical transverse uterine incision.
2. Indication for the first procedure was not disproportion.
3. Expectation of an easy labor and delivery.

Contraindications

1. Previous vertical incision of any kind.
2. Type of incision unknown.
3. More than one previous cesarean section.
4. Advice by the surgeon who did the first operation against a trial of labor.
5. Contracted pelvis.
6. Abnormal presentation, such as transverse lie, brow, or breech.
7. Urgent medical indication for delivery, including diabetes, toxemia, and placenta previa.

Guidelines for Management of the Trial

1. A staff physician should be present.
2. Blood must be cross-matched and available.
3. Personal and electronic maternal and fetal monitoring.
4. The trial continues until vaginal delivery occurs or cesarean section is performed.

5. The main indications for cesarean section are arrest of progress, fetal distress, and suspicion that the scar in the uterus may be giving way.
6. Oxytocin may be used to augment labor in selected cases.
7. Manual exploration of the uterine scar must be performed after delivery.

A recent report of 634 patients who had one previous cesarean section indicated that 83 percent were allowed to have a trial of labor and 17 percent had an elective cesarean section in the present pregnancy. Of those having a trial of labor, 60 percent achieved vaginal delivery and 40 percent were delivered by cesarean section. There were 4 uterine ruptures (0.5 percent), 3 in the trial of labor group and 1 in the elective cesarean section group. There were no maternal deaths. It would appear that, providing certain criteria are observed, vaginal delivery after previous cesarean section is possible. The trial of labor must not go on too long if good progress is not being made.

Hemorrhage

PLACENTA PREVIA Cesarean section for central and lateral placenta previa has reduced fetal and maternal mortality. The final decision is made by vaginal examination in the operating room using a double setup. Blood is cross-matched and available. The operating team stands by in readiness. If central or partial placenta previa is found on vaginal examination, cesarean section is performed immediately.

ABRUPTIO PLACENTAE Abruptio placentae occurring before or during early labor may be treated by rupture of the membranes and oxytocin drip. When the hemorrhage is severe, the cervix hard and closed, or uteroplacental apoplexy suspected, cesarean section may be necessary to save the baby, to control hemorrhage, to prevent afibrinogenemia, and to observe the condition of the uterus and its ability to contract and control the bleeding. In some cases hysterectomy is necessary.

Toxemia of Pregnancy

These states must be considered:

1. Preeclampsia and eclampsia
2. Essential hypertension
3. Chronic nephritis

Toxemia of pregnancy may require termination of the pregnancy before term. In most cases induction of labor is the method of choice. When the cervix is not ripe and induction would be difficult, cesarean section is preferable.

Fetal Indications

DISTRESS   Fetal distress, as indicated by severe bradycardia, irregularity of the fetal heart rate, or late patterns of deceleration, sometimes necessitates emergency cesarean section. The rate of cesarean section is high in monitored patients. This is not surprising since the main indications for monitoring are those which predispose to fetal hypoxia. However, fetal distress is not the prime reason for the increasing rate of cesarean section. Problems associated with dystocia are the main indications for abdominal delivery. A new indication for cesarean section is described as fetal intolerance of labor. This is seen in patients who have desultory labors. Stimulation by oxytocin results in abnormalities of the FHR. Cesarean section is performed and a normal baby with no evidence of distress is delivered.

PREVIOUS FETAL DEATH OR DAMAGE   Especially in older women who have given birth to more than one dead or damaged baby, cesarean section may be elected.

PROLAPSE OF THE UMBILICAL CORD   Prolapse of the umbilical cord in the presence of an undilated cervix is managed best by cesarean section, provided the baby is in good condition.

PLACENTAL INSUFFICIENCY   In cases of intrauterine growth retardation or postterm pregnancy, when clinical examinations and various tests suggest that the baby is in jeopardy, delivery may be necessary. If induction is not feasible or fails, cesarean section is indicated. There is an increased ability of pediatricians to salvage small babies and, when the need exists, cesarean section may offer these infants the best chance for survival and a good chance for normal development.

MATERNAL DIABETES   The fetus of the diabetic mother is inclined to be larger than normal, and this can lead to difficult labor and delivery. Although these infants are large they behave like prematures and do not withstand well the rigors of a long labor. Death during labor and the postnatal period is common. In addition, a number of babies die in utero before term is reached. Because of these dangers to the fetus and because a high proportion of pregnant diabetics develop toxemia, the pregnancy may require termination before term. When conditions are favorable and a rapid and easy labor is anticipated, induction of labor can be carried out. However in primigravidas and in multiparas with a long, closed cervix or a bad obstetric history, cesarean section is the method of choice.

RHESUS INCOMPATIBILITY When a fetus is becoming progressively damaged by the antibodies of a sensitized Rh-negative mother and when induction and delivery per vaginam would be difficult, the pregnancy may be terminated by cesarean section in selected cases for fetal salvage.

POSTMORTEM CESAREAN Rarely, a live baby can be obtained if rapid cesarean section is performed immediately after the death of the pregnant woman.

HERPES VIRUS HOMINIS INFECTION OF THE GENITAL TRACT This is a cause of serious, often fatal, infection of the newborn infant. When herpes virus is present in the birth canal at the time of delivery, at least 50 percent of the infants will be infected, and half of these will be damaged seriously, if not fatally, by the herpetic infection. The greatest hazard exists when the primary genital infection occurred 2 to 4 weeks prior to delivery. Transplacental transmission is far less important than direct contact during labor and delivery. In the latter event there is contamination of the child's eyes, scalp, skin, umbilical cord, and upper respiratory tract.

MANAGEMENT OF PATIENTS WITH GENITAL HERPES:

1. If the genital culture is repeatedly negative, vaginal delivery is indicated.
2. When the genital culture is positive, amniocentesis is performed and the fluid cultured. Positive culture of the amniotic fluid signifies that fetal infection has already occurred and that cesarean section would accomplish nothing.
3. When genital culture is positive and amniotic fluid culture is negative, repeated cultures of the vaginal lesions and the cervix are carried out to determine whether infectious herpes is present. If infectious herpes is present at or near parturition, and if the membranes have been ruptured for less than 4 hours, cesarean section is performed.
4. If the membranes have been ruptured for longer than 4 hours, it is too late to save the fetus by cesarean section.

Miscellaneous

ELDERLY PRIMIGRAVIDITY Elderly primigravidity is difficult to define. While the age varies from 35 to 40 years, other factors are equally important. These include the presence or absence of a good lower uterine segment, elasticity or rigidity of the cervix and the soft tissues of the birth canal, ease of becoming pregnant. number of abortions, fetal presentation, and coordination of the uterine powers. When all these points are favorable vaginal delivery should be considered. When the adverse factors are present cesarean section may be the wiser and safer procedure.

PREVIOUS VAGINAL REPAIR Fear that vaginal delivery will cause a recurrence of cystocele, rectocele, and uterine prolapse may lead to an elective cesarean section.

CONGENITAL UTERINE ANOMALY Not only does an abnormal uterus often function badly, but in the case of anomalies such as a bicornuate uterus one horn may block the passage of the baby from the other. In such cases cesarean section must be performed.

POOR OBSTETRIC HISTORY When a previous delivery has been difficult and traumatic with extensive injury to the cervix, vagina, and perineum, or when the baby has been injured, cesarean section may be selected for subsequent births.

FAILED FORCEPS Failed forceps is an indication for cesarean section. It is wiser to turn to abdominal delivery than to drag a baby through the pelvis by force.

CONTRAINDICATIONS

Cesarean section should not be performed when the following conditions exist.

1. When the fetus is dead or in such bad condition that it is unlikely to survive. There is no point in submitting the patient to a needless serious operation.
2. When the maternal birth canal is grossly infected, and facilities for extraperitoneal cesarean are not available.
3. When the operator is inexperienced, when conditions are unfavorable, or when proper assistance is not available.

TYPES OF CESAREAN SECTION

Lower Segment: Transverse Incision

Because it permits safe abdominal delivery even when performed late in labor and even when the uterine cavity is infected, the lower segment transverse incision (Fig. 1) has revolutionized obstetric practice in the following respects:

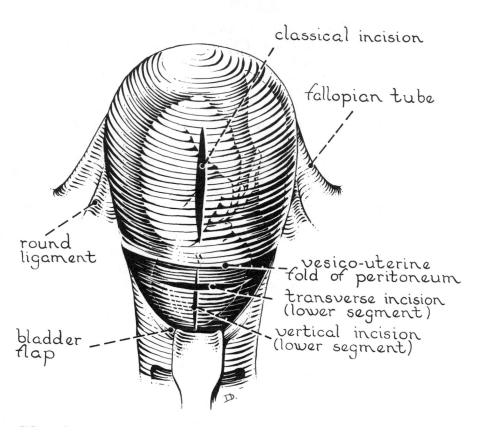

FIG. 1. Cesarean section: composite illustration to demonstrate the three most frequently used incisions. The bladder flap is shown dissected off the lower uterine segment and held out of the way by a retractor. The fetal position is ROT.

1. It allows the obstetrician to change his mind.
2. It has resulted in the concepts of trial of labor, trial of oxytocin stimulation, and trial forceps.
3. The need for traumatic forceps delivery has been virtually eliminated.
4. The indications for cesarean section have been widened.
5. Maternal morbidity and mortality are lower than with upper segment procedures.
6. The uterus is left with a stronger scar.

In our opinion this is the procedure of choice. The abdomen is opened and the uterus exposed. The vesicouterine fold of peritoneum (bladder flap), which lies near the junction of the upper and lower uterine segments, is identified and incised transversely; it is dissected off the lower segment and, with the bladder, is pushed downward and retracted out of the way. A small transverse incision is made in the lower segment of the uterus and is extended laterally with the fingers, stopping short of the area of the uterine vessels. The fetal head, which in most cases lies under the incision, is extracted or expressed, followed by the rest of the body and then the placenta and membranes. The transverse incision is closed with a single or double layer of continuous catgut. The bladder flap is then sewn back to the wall of the uterus so that the entire incision is covered and closed off from the general peritoneal cavity. The abdomen is closed in layers.

ADVANTAGES

1. The incision is in the lower segment of the uterus. However, one must be certain it is in the thin lower segment and not in the inferior part of the muscular upper segment.
2. The muscle is split laterally instead of being cut; this leads to less bleeding.
3. Incision into the placenta is rare.
4. The head is usually under the incision and is extracted easily.
5. The thin muscle layer of the lower segment is easier to reapproximate than the thick upper segment.
6. The entire incision is covered by the bladder flap, thus reducing spill into the general peritoneal cavity.
7. Rupture of the transverse scar is a smaller threat to the life of the mother and the fetus:
   a. The incidence of rupture is lower.
   b. This accident occurs rarely before term. Hence the patient is in the hospital under close observation.
   c. The loss of blood from the less vascular lower segment is less than from the corpus.
   d. Rupture of the low transverse incision is followed only rarely by expulsion of the fetus or by a separation of the placenta, so that there is a chance to save the baby.

DISADVANTAGES

1. If the incision extends too far laterally, as may occur if the baby is very big, the uterine vessels can be torn, causing profuse hemorrhage.
2. The procedure is not advisable when there is an abnormality in the lower segment, such as fibroids or extensive varicosities.
3. Previous surgery or dense adhesions which prevent easy access to the lower segment make the operation onerous.

4. When the lower segment is not well formed, the transverse operation is difficult to perform.
5. Sometimes the bladder is adherent to a previous scar, and it may be injured.

Lower Segment: Vertical Incision

The exposure is the same as with the transverse incision. The vertical incision (Fig. 1) is made with the scalpel and is enlarged with blunt scissors to avoid injury to the baby.

The vertical incision has an advantage in that it can be carried upward when necessary. This may be needed when the baby is large, when the lower segment is poorly formed, when there is a fetal malposition such as transverse lie, or when there is fetal anomaly such as conjoined twins. Some obstetricians prefer this incision for placenta previa.

One of the main disadvantages is that since the muscle is cut there is more bleeding from the incised edges; often, too, the incision extends inadvertently into the upper segment, and the value of a completely retroperitoneal closure is lost.

Classical Cesarean Section

A longitudinal midline incision (Fig. 1) is made with the scalpel into the anterior wall of the uterus and is enlarged upward and downward with blunt-nosed scissors. A large opening is needed since the baby is often delivered as a breech. The fetus and placenta are removed and the uterus is closed in three layers. In modern times there is almost no justification for classical cesarean section. Technical difficulty in exposing the lower segment is the only indication for the upper segment procedure.

INDICATIONS

1. Difficulty in exposing the lower uterine segment
   a. Large blood vessels on the anterior wall
   b. High and adherent bladder
   c. Myoma in the lower segment
2. Impacted transverse lie
3. Some cases of anterior placenta previa
4. Certain uterine malformations

DISADVANTAGES

1. Thick myometrium is cut, large sinuses are opened, and bleeding is profuse.
2. The baby is often extracted as a breech with greater aspiration of amniotic fluid.
3. Should the placenta be attached to the anterior wall of the uterus the incision cuts into it and may lead to dangerous loss of blood from the fetal circulation.
4. The incision lies uncovered in the general peritoneal cavity, and there is greater chance of seepage of infected uterine contents with resultant peritonitis.
5. There is a higher incidence of adhesion of abdominal contents to the line of closure in the uterus.
6. There is a higher incidence of uterine rupture in subsequent pregnancies.

Extraperitoneal Cesarean Section

The extraperitoneal operation was devised to obviate the need for hysterectomy in neglected and grossly infected cases by preventing general and often fatal peritonitis. There are several methods, such as those of Waters, Latzko, and Norton.

The technique of this procedure is relatively difficult, accidental entry into the peritoneal cavity is frequent, and there is an increased incidence of injury to the bladder. Better prenatal care, reduction in the incidence of neglected cases, and the availability of blood and antibiotics have reduced the need for the extraperitoneal technique. This method should not be abandoned but kept in reserve for the occasional case.

Cesarean Hysterectomy

This is the performance of a cesarean section followed by removal of the uterus. Whenever possible total hysterectomy should be performed. However, since the subtotal operation is easier and can be done more quickly, it is the procedure of choice when there has been profuse hemorrhage and the patient is in shock, or when she is in poor condition for other reasons. In such cases the aim is to finish the operation as rapidly as possible.

INDICATIONS

1. Hemorrhage from uterine atony after failure of conservative therapy
2. Uncontrollable hemorrhage in certain cases of placenta previa and abruptio placentae
3. Placenta accreta
4. Gross multiple fibromyomas
5. In certain cases of cancer of the cervix or ovary
6. Rupture of the uterus, not repairable
7. As a method of sterilization when continuation of menstruation is undesirable for medical reasons
8. In neglected and infected cases when the risk of generalized peritonitis is not warranted by the advantage of preserving the uterus—e.g., in a woman who has several children and is not anxious to have more
9. Defective uterine scar
10. Extension of incision into the uterine vessels resulting in bleeding that cannot be stopped by ligature.

COMPLICATIONS

1. Morbidity rate of 20 percent
2. Increased loss of blood
3. Damage to urinary tract and intestines including fistula formation
4. Psychologic trauma due to loss of the uterus

AS A METHOD OF STERILIZATION

When used for sterilization this procedure has certain advantages over tubal ligation, including a lower rate of failure and the removal of an organ that may cause trouble later on. However, the complications are such that cesarean hysterectomy is not recommended as a routine procedure for sterilization.

MORTALITY AND MORBIDITY FOLLOWING CESAREAN SECTION

Maternal Mortality

The gross uncorrected mortality rate in the United States and Canada is approximately 30:10,000 cesarean sections. In many clinics the rate is much lower, well under 10:10,000. However, Evrard and Gold found the risk of maternal death associated with cesarean section to be

26 times greater than with vaginal delivery. They noted a tenfold increase in the risk of maternal death inherent in the operation itself. The increasing use of cesarean section to protect the baby may lead to a higher danger for the mother.

Factors that add to the risk include:

1. Age over 30
2. Grand multiparity
3. Obesity, over 200 pounds
4. Prolonged labor
5. Prolonged period of ruptured membranes
6. Numerous vaginal examinations
7. Low socioeconomic status

CAUSES OF MATERNAL DEATH

1. Hemorrhage
2. Infection
3. Anesthesia
4. Pulmonary embolism
5. Renal failure following prolonged hypotension
6. Intestinal obstruction and paralytic ileus
7. Heart failure
8. Toxemia of pregnancy
9. Rupture of uterine scar
10. Miscellaneous causes not related to the operation, e.g., cancer

REASONS FOR A DECLINE IN MORTALITY RATE

1. Adequate blood transfusion
2. Use of antimicrobial drugs
3. Improved surgical methods
4. Better anesthetic techniques and specially trained anesthesiologists
5. The realization that patients with heart disease do better with vaginal delivery than with cesarean section
6. Basic treatment of toxemia of pregnancy by medical rather than by surgical methods

Maternal Morbidity

Maternal morbidity is defined as a temperature of 100.4 F (38 C) or over occurring on any 2 of the first 10 days post partum, exclusive of the first 24 hours. It is more common after cesarean section than after normal delivery, the incidence being between 15 and 20 percent. Antimicrobials, blood transfusions, better surgical technique, use of the lower segment operation, and improved anesthesia have all contributed to the decrease in postcesarean maternal morbidity.

Almost half of the patients undergoing cesarean section develop operative or postoperative complications, some of which are serious and potentially lethal. It must be accepted that cesarean section is a major operation with the attendant risks. Standard morbidity for cesarean section is around 20 percent.

SERIOUS COMPLICATIONS

1. Hemorrhage
   a. Uterine atony
   b. Extension of uterine incision
   c. Difficulty removing the placenta
   d. Hematoma of the broad ligament
2. Infection
   a. Genital tract
   b. Incision
   c. Urinary tract
   d. Lungs and upper respiratory tract
3. Thrombophlebitis
4. Injury, with or without fistula
   a. Urinary tract
   b. Intestines
5. Intestinal obstruction
   a. Mechanical
   b. Paralytic

PREVENTION OF INFECTION

While our experience has not confirmed the impression, several reports suggest that the incidence of infection can be reduced by using antibiotics prophylactically. One regimen is as follows:

1. A loading dose of 2 g of cephalothin is given in a 15-minute intravenous infusion 15 to 30 minutes before cesarean section.
2. This is followed by 1 g intravenously every 6 hours for 36 hours.
3. Then the patient is given Oral Keflex, 500 mg every 6 hours until the 5th postoperative day.

Concern that the indiscriminate use of prophylactic antibiotics might be harmful to the fetus and the mother has led to the suggestion that their use be confined to patients at high risk for postoperative morbidity.

High Risk Factors

1. Labor prior to cesarean section, especially when prolonged, when the membranes have been ruptured, and when there have been numerous pelvic examinations
2. Anemia, hematocrit under 30 percent
3. Obesity

Fetal Mortality

While fetal mortality associated with cesarean section has declined steadily, it is, at about 5.5 percent, double that of vaginal delivery. Reasons for the higher incidence with cesarean section include the following factors.

1. Conditions such as toxemia of pregnancy, erythroblastosis, and placenta previa that require treatment by cesarean section result in premature, small infants.
2. There are sometimes errors in estimating fetal size and maturity in elective or repeat cesareans when the patient is thought to be at term.
3. While respiratory complications such as atelectasis and hyaline membrane disease and the respiratory distress syndrome are more common in premature infants, the incidence is much higher when the premature baby is born by cesarean section.
4. Conditions such as placenta previa, abruptio placentae, diabetes, preeclampsia, eclampsia, essential hypertension, chronic nephritis, and prolapse of the umbilical cord result in babies whose general condition and powers of resistance and recuperation are low. When these conditions need treatment by cesarean section fetal mortality is increased.
5. In general, cesarean section does not give as good a prognosis for the infant as does the normal vaginal delivery.
6. To prevent the delivery of a premature infant ultrasonic examination and measurement of the L/S ratio should be carried out before elective or repeat cesarean section is performed.

There has been a decline in the mortality rate of infants born both by cesarean section and by vaginal delivery. The great majority of fetal deaths are associated with prematurity. On the one hand cesarean section has reduced the number of babies damaged by traumatic vaginal procedures. On the other hand a number of babies are born alive who have congenital defects incompatible with continuing or reasonable existence.

BIBLIOGRAPHY

Baker DA, Plotkin SA: Genital herpes simplex virus (HSV) isolation during pregnancy. Obstet Gynecol 53:9S, 1979

Carswell W: The current status of classical cesarean section. Scot Med J 18:105, 1973

Case BD, Corcoran R, Jeffcoate N, et al: Cesarean section and its place in modern obstetrics. J Obstet & Gynaecol Br Commonw 78:203, 1971

Clou WM, Crompton AC: The wounded uterus: pregnancy after hysterotomy. Br Med J 10 Feb 73:321, 1973

Evrard JR, Gold EM: Cesarean section and maternal mortality in Rhode Island. Obstet Gynecol 50:594, 1977

Green SL, Sarubbi FA: Risk factors associated with post cesarean section febrile morbidity. Obstet Gynecol 49:686, 1977

Hanshaw JB: Herpes virus hominis in the fetus and newborn. Am J Dis Child 126:546, 1973

Hibbard LT: Changing trends in cesarean section. Am J Obstet Gynecol 125:798, 1976

Hughey MJ, LaPata RE, McElin TW, Lussky R: The effect of fetal monitoring on the incidence of cesarean section. Obstet Gynecol 49:513, 1977

Jones OH: Cesarean section in present day obstetrics. Am J Obstet Gynecol 126:521, 1976

Merrill BS, Gibbs CE: Planned vaginal delivery following cesarean section. Obstet Gynecol 52:50, 1978.

Moro M, Andrews M: Prophylactic antibiotics in cesarean section. Obstet Gynecol 44:688, 1974

Ranney B, Stanage WF: Advantages of local anesthesia for cesarean section. Obstet Gynecol 45:163, 1975

46.

Dystocia: Uterine Abnormalities

PROLAPSE OF THE UTERUS

Prolapse of the uterus during pregnancy is rare but troublesome. As a rule the uterus rises out of the pelvis by the end of the 4th month. Occasionally it fails to do so. In most cases it is only the cervix, with or without an associated hypertrophic elongation, that protrudes through the vagina. Occasionally the whole uterus is involved. No pregnancy has carried to term with the uterus completely out of the vagina.

Complications

ANTE PARTUM

1. Abortion and premature labor
2. Cervical edema, ulceration, and sepsis
3. Urinary retention and infection
4. Need for prolonged bed rest

INTRA PARTUM

1. Cervical dilatation may begin outside the vagina, offering resistance to progress.
2. The edema and fibrosis may cause cervical dystocia.
3. Lacerations of the cervix are common.
4. Obstructive labor may lead to uterine rupture.
5. Fetal mortality is higher.

POST PARTUM
Puerperal infection is increased.

Treatment

ANTE PARTUM

1. Bed rest in Trendelenberg position to reduce edema and permit repositioning of the uterus
2. Local antiseptics to the cervix
3. Pessary to maintain the position of the uterus

DURING LABOR

1. Most patients have a normal vaginal delivery, but arrest of progress may ensue.
2. If cervical dystocia develops, several procedures may be considered:
    a. Dührssen's incisions of the cervix.
    b. Pitocin augmentation of labor.
    c. Cesarean section.

POST PARTUM

A pessary should be inserted to elevate the uterus and support the ligaments.

ANOMALIES OF THE UTERUS

Diagnosis

During pregnancy a uterine anomaly may be suspected when the following conditions are present:

1. Notching and broadening of the uterine fundus
2. Abnormal lie
3. Recurring breech
4. Trapped or retained placenta
5. Prolonged third stage of labor
6. Habitual abortion
7. Axial deviation of the uterus
8. Flanking of the fetal limbs
9. Cervix located in the lateral fornix of the vagina
10. Presence of a vaginal septum

In any suspicious case hysterography should be performed post partum.

Labor and Delivery

Many women will deliver their babies vaginally, so a trial of labor is indicated. Failure of progress is treated by cesarean section.

Complications

1. Breech presentation.
2. Transverse lie; the fetus often assumes the hammock position with the head in one horn and the feet in the other.
3. Incoordinate uterine action is common and failure of progress is treated best by cesarean section.
4. Premature rupture of membranes.
5. Placenta previa.
6. Obstruction of descent of the fetus by the nonpregnant horn.
7. Postpartum hemorrhage.
8. Obstruction by a thick vaginal septum.

Bicornuate Uterus

Diddle reviewed 90 pregnancies in 33 women with bicornuate uteri (bicornis uteri unicollis, uterus arcuatus, and uterus subseptus). The diagnosis was made by palpation, postpartum exploration of the uterine cavity, during curettage, by hysterosalpingography, and at hysterectomy. Abortion occurred in one-third of the pregnancies. Premature labor and premature rupture of the membranes was more common than in normal uteri, and there was a higher incidence of incompetent cervix. Twenty percent of viable infants presented by breech or in transverse lie.

Labor proceeds to vaginal delivery in most cases. Cesarean section is indicated only for obstetric reasons and not because of the anomaly per se. Dystocia may be caused by uterine inertia, obstruction by the nongravid horn, and hypertrophy of a septum. Occasionally the nonpregnant horn may rupture during labor.

Retained placenta requiring manual removal occurred in 20 percent of the confinements in Diddle's study. Postpartum hemorrhage was usually associated with placental retention.

Double Uterus

Complete duplication of the female reproductive tract is not rare. Incidences of 1:1,500 to 1:15,000 have been reported in pregnant women. Many have normal vaginal deliveries.

Ineffectual contractions, desultory labors, and slowly dilating cervices are common during the first stage of labor. Postpartum atony leading to hemorrhage is observed often. Sloughing of a decidual cast from the nonpregnant uterus can cause excessive bleeding. The cervix of the nongravid uterus may interfere with descent and rotation of the fetal presenting part, and may so obstruct progress that cesarean section is necessary.

TORSION OF PREGNANT UTERUS

Uterine torsion is defined as rotation of the uterus on its long axis of more than 45°. Torsion of the pregnant uterus is rare. It was first reported in animals in 1662, and in the human 200 years later. The exact cause is unknown, but some uterine malformation or tumor is present in many instances.

Most pregnant uteri show a slight degree of rotation, to the right in 80 percent and toward the left in 20 percent. In most abnormal situations the rotation has been 180°, although a case was reported of a 540° torsion associated with uterine necrosis.

In 20 percent of cases no causative factor is apparent. Predisposing conditions include:

1. Malpresentation, especially transverse lie
2. Uterine myomas
3. Anomalies of the uterus
4. Pelvic adhesions
5. Ovarian cyst
6. Uterine suspension
7. Abnormal pelvis
8. Placenta previa

Preoperative diagnosis is rare. The picture is one of an acute abdominal crisis, including pain, shock, bleeding, obstructed labor, and symptoms referable to the intestinal and urinary tracts. The most serious complication is uterine rupture.

Acute torsion results in compromise of the uterine circulation. The overall maternal mortality rate, around 13 percent, increases as term is approached and is directly proportional to the degree of torsion. The perinatal mortality rate of 30 percent also varies with the degree of rotation of the uterus.

Treatment at or near term is by cesarean section. Before viability of the fetus has been reached laparotomy is performed, the uterus is rotated to its normal position, and the pregnancy is allowed to continue to term.

SACCULATION OF THE UTERUS

Sacculation of the uterus (Fig. 1), a rare entity, defined as a diffuse ballooning of a portion of the wall, may be primary or secondary to incarceration of the retroverted uterus. In the primary variety, if the sac involves the lower part of the uterus, it will present as a pelvic mass. In sacculation of the retroverted uterus the saccule represents the stretched anterior wall, while the pelvic mass represents the uterine fundus. The saccule is a functional, transitory pouch, contains all layers of myometrium, and is present only during pregnancy. In half of the reported cases the placenta was located in the sacculation; in one-fourth, part of the fetus was in the pouch; and in the remainder the sacculation was empty. The sacculation may be in the anterior or the posterior wall of the uterus.

Etiology

The causation of sacculation is obscure. Hypothetical explanations include:

1. An embryologic abnormality of the uterus, the müllerian ducts having failed to fuse completely.
2. A myometrial defect leading to attenuation of the muscle during gestation. The increased intrauterine pressure makes the thin

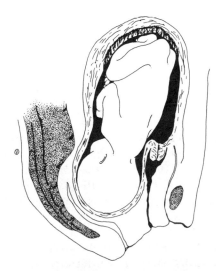

FIG. 1. Sacculation of the uterus.

area bulge out. Once the fetus is expelled the pouch collapses and disappears.
3. Faulty innervation of a segment of the uterus, resulting in a functional disturbance and a ballooning of the affected area.
4. Weakening of part of the uterine wall by trophoblastic digestion, placenta accreta, adenomyosis, curettage, or myomectomy.

Symptoms and Signs

1. There is abdominal pain.
2. The patient experiences a sensation of heaviness.
3. In anterior sacculation the presenting part is felt in front of and above the pubic symphysis.
4. The cervix is often high.
5. Dysuria, caused by an elongation of the urethra and compression of the neck of the bladder, is present.

Diagnosis

Diagnosis is difficult, having been achieved preoperatively in only two of 38 reported cases. In most situations the diagnosis is made at laparotomy performed during the first trimester for suspected ectopic pregnancy, and at cesarean section in treating dysfunctional labor. An x-ray of the abdomen may help. Amniography has been useful in establishing the true state of affairs. Postpartum hysterosalpingography may show a defect, but in most cases a normal picture is seen.

Retroverted Uterus

In most cases a pregnant retroverted uterus will correct its position and grow out of the pelvis; the pregnancy will proceed normally. If this does not happen one of three events may occur: (1) The uterus will contract and expel its contents. (2) The uterus continues to grow until, at 14 to 16 weeks' gestation, the retroverted gravid uterus becomes incarcerated in the pelvis. (3) In the rare case of incarceration a part of the uterine corpus remains imprisoned in the pelvis, while the anterior wall expands into the abdomen to accommodate the growing fetus. This sacculation was described by Oldham in 1860.

Examination will reveal a large, cystic, tender mass (the body of the uterus) which fills the posterior cul de sac and often bulges into the vagina. The cervix is displaced upward above the symphysis pubis and is hard to see or reach.

Course of Labor

In primary sacculation the uterine fundus is in the correct position, polarity is maintained, and there is a chance for vaginal delivery. Rupture of the uterus is rare in progressing cases. In some situations, especially when the presenting part is in the sacculation, the cervix does not dilate but is displaced more and more upward as the sac is pushed down. In neglected cases prolonged labor may lead to fetal and even maternal death as a result of infection, necrosis of the sac, and rupture of the uterus. Retained placenta is common.

In sacculation secondary to retroversion the uterine forces are misdirected and the cervix fails to dilate even in the presence of strong contractions. Cesarean section is the procedure of choice. Once the baby is delivered the uterus corrects its position and no abnormality is evident. If diagnosed in the early part of pregnancy, the position of the retroverted uterus can be corrected and the pregnancy can proceed normally.

Management

1. During the first trimester nothing need be done since the pregnancy will go to term.
2. At term a trial of labor is permissible, as vaginal delivery may occur especially if the pouch is empty.
3. At term, when labor is prolonged or progress has ceased, cesarean section is the treatment of choice.
4. Sacculation secondary to retroversion requires cesarean section. Vaginal delivery is impossible.

BIBLIOGRAPHY

Fadel HE, Misenhimer HR: Incarceration of the retroverted uterus with sacculation. Obstet Gynecol 43:46, 1974

Koh KS, Bradford CR: Uterine torsion during pregnancy. Can Med Assoc J 117:501, 1977

Lavery JP, Boey CS: Uterine prolapse with pregnancy. Obstet Gynecol 42:681, 1973

Semmons JP: Congenital anomalies of the female genital tract. Obstet Gynecol 19:328, 1962

47.

Embryotomy:
Destructive
Operations
on the Fetus

INDICATIONS

The purpose of destructive operations on the unborn child is to reduce
its size (head, shoulder girdle, or body) and so enable the vaginal delivery of a baby which is too large to pass intact through the birth canal.
This procedure is tolerable only on a fetus that is dead or so deformed
that survival is impossible. The risk of abdominal delivery to the mother
has decreased to the point where embryotomy on the living normal child
is never justified. Indeed the operation is so unpleasant and the dangers
to the mother are such that destructive procedures are rarely performed
today. After delivery the birth canal must be examined thoroughly to be
certain that no injury has been caused by the instruments or the sharp
edges of the skull bones.

CONTRAINDICATIONS

1. Living normal fetus
2. Markedly contracted pelvis
3. Cervix less than three-fourths dilated (full dilatation preferable)
4. Neoplasms obstructing the pelvis

DANGERS

1. Lacerations of the vagina, cervix, and uterus, as well as fistulas
   in the bladder or rectum

2. Uterine rupture, especially through the thinned-out lower segment, when labor has been obstructed
3. Hemorrhage from lacerations and uterine atony
4. Infection
5. Risks attendant on prolonged deep anesthesia

CLASSIFICATION OF DESTRUCTIVE OPERATIONS

Living Fetus

1. Needle drainage in hydrocephaly
2. Fracture of the clavicle or arm
   a. Shoulder dystocia
   b. Breech with nuchal arms

Dead Fetus

1. Craniotomy
   a. When delivery of the intact head is impossible
   b. Hydrocephaly
2. Decapitation
   a. Neglected transverse lie
   b. Interlocked twins
3. Cleidotomy
   a. Shoulder dystocia
   b. Breech with nuchal arms
4. Spondylectomy
   a. Breech with hydrocephaly
5. Evisceration or morcellation
   a. Hydrops fetalis with marked ascites
   b. Monsters

TYPES OF EMBRYOTOMY

CRANIOTOMY Craniotomy is the opening of the skull. This can be done by perforating the head with Smellie scissors, evacuating the brain, and delivering the head by applying scalp traction with a tenaculum. Sometimes following craniotomy the head is crushed and extracted by special instruments (cranioclast, basiotribe).

The purpose of the operation is to reduce the bulk of the head. The only indication acceptable today is hydrocephalus. The excess cerebrospinal fluid can be removed, even in a live infant, by inserting a large-bore needle (16 to 18 gauge) through the scalp. The size of the head is reduced and its delivery made possible.

The most direct approach to encephalocentesis is via the vagina. The needle is inserted into the cranial cavity through a fontanelle or suture, avoiding the sagittal sinus. If necessary, the needle can be pushed through one of the cranial bones. When the presentation is breech, drainage can be achieved by spondylectomy or, if the head is accessible, by direct entry into the ventricles beneath the occipital plate or behind the ear.

When the head cannot be reached through the vagina, an alternative route is the transabdominal one. The needle is passed through the abdominal and uterine walls, and through the fetal cranial bones into the interior of the skull.

SPONDYLECTOMY Spondylectomy is the transection of the spine of the delivered thorax. In a breech presentation this may allow drainage of cerebrospinal fluid. It is done when the back is anterior and the head and neck are out of reach. In cases of hydrocephalus when there is communication between the ventricles and the spinal cord, the fluid may drained from the brain in this way, thus obviating the need for craniotomy.

DECAPITATION Severing the head from the body may be done for neglected transverse presentations when the child is dead and version and extraction or cesarean section are contraindicated. It may be done also when twins have become interlocked, chin to chin. A blunt hook is placed over the neck to steady the fetus, and decapitation is performed with scissors. The fingers of the other hand are used to protect the mother's soft tissues. After decapitation the body is extracted by pulling on an arm or a lower limb. The head is delivered either by forceps or by inserting a finger in the mouth and exerting traction on the jaw. This must be done slowly.

CLEIDOTOMY Cleidotomy is indicated when there is shoulder dystocia and a dead fetus. One or both clavicles are cut with scissors. The shoulder girdle then collapses, and delivery is accomplished.

EVISCERATION Evisceration is the removal of organs from the abdomen and thorax to reduce the body size of the fetus.

MORCELLATION Cutting the fetus into pieces is necessary on rare occasions before vaginal delivery can be accomplished.

BIBLIOGRAPHY

Smale LE. Destructive operations on the fetus. Am J Obstet Gynecol 119:369, 1974

48.

The Newborn

ASPHYXIA NEONATORUM

The normal healthy infant should breathe within 0.5 to 1.0 minute of birth. Asphyxia of the newborn (mild or severe) is a syndrome in which apnea is the principal clinical manifestation. In severe cases the infant is flaccid, there is bradycardia, the color is blue to white, and the response to stimulation is poor or nonexistent. Frequently the baby is covered with meconium, a sign of intrauterine distress. The infant is hypoxic, and if the oxygen-deficient state is prolonged, permanent brain damage occurs. Such brain damage may be gross and demonstrable by obvious neurologic signs, or it may be subtle and affect the child's mental ability, leading to late manifestations of retardation or backwardness.

There are two large groups:

1. Central nervous system failure resulting from
   a. Narcosis by maternal sedatives, analgesics, and anesthesia
   b. Prenatal or paranatal anoxia
   c. Intracranial trauma or hemorrhage
   d. Congenital anomalies
2. Peripheral respiratory difficulty
   a. Respiratory distress syndrome
   b. Aspiration of meconium and amniotic fluid
   c. Pneumonia
   d. Congenital anomalies

In the first group the children are either born with apnea or the breathing ceases after a few ineffectual gasps. In the second category the breathing begins fairly promptly but is or soon becomes labored and inadequate. The central nervous system seems to function, but the grunting, retraction, and cyanosis point to disturbances in the peripheral respiratory apparatus. This is the more common of the two groups.

Etiology

DURING PREGNANCY

1. Maternal causes
   a. Anemia
   b. Hemorrhage and shock
   c. Cardiorespiratory disease
   d. Toxemia of pregnancy
   e. Age of mother over 40 years
   f. Grand multiparity
2. Placental causes
   a. Placental diseases (syphilis, infarction)
   b. Hemorrhage (placenta previa, abruptio placentae)
3. Umbilical cord causes
   a. Prolapse
   b. Knots and entanglements
   c. Compression
4. Fetal causes
   a. Congenital anomalies
   b. Prematurity
   c. Premature rupture of the membranes leading to infection, especially pneumonia
   d. Prolonged gestation

LABOR AND DELIVERY

1. Anoxia from uterine contractions that are too strong and last too long
2. Narcosis from excessive analgesia and anesthesia
3. Maternal hypotension from spinal anesthesia
4. Obstruction of the airway by aspiration of blood, mucus, and vaginal debris
5. Prolonged labor
6. Difficult delivery (with or without forceps) causing cerebral hemorrhage or damage to the central nervous system

Diagnosis

ANTE PARTUM

1. Nonstress fetal heart monitoring: abnormal (nonreactive) pattern
2. Contraction stress test: late deceleration pattern

INTRA PARTUM

1. Bradycardia under 100 beats per minute between uterine contractions, or abnormal patterns of deceleration.
2. Gross irregularity of the fetal heart.
3. Tachycardia, over 160. This is not of great significance by itself; however, when it alternates with periods of bradycardia it is an ominous sign.
4. Late deceleration pattern of fetal heart rate.
5. The passage of meconium in a cephalic presentation. This indicates relaxation of the sphincter ani, a result of insufficient oxygenation.

POST PARTUM

Apgar elaborated a method of grading newborns: 0, 1, or 2 points are awarded for each of five signs, depending on their presence or absence (Table 1). The grading is done at 1 minute after birth and may be repeated at 5 minutes. Most children are normal and fall in the 7 to 10 point range. A score of 4 to 6 indicates mild to moderate depression. When the Apgar score is 0 to 3 the infant is severely depressed.

TABLE 1. Apgar Scoring of Newborns

Sign	0 Points	1 Point	2 Points
Heart rate	Absent	Under 100	Over 100
Respiratory effort	Absent	Slow, irregular	Good, crying
Muscle tone	Limp	Flexion of extremities	Active motion
Reflex irritability: response to catheter in nostril	No response	Grimace	Cough or sneeze
Color	Blue-white	Body pink, extremities blue	Completely pink

Treatment

1. Gentleness in handling the infant is of paramount importance. It is either in a state of shock or close to it.
2. The correct temperature and humidity must be maintained. This is achieved best in an incubator. The baby should be kept warm, but excessive heat is contraindicated.
3. A clear airway to the lungs must be established.
   a. Except in cases in which cerebral hemorrhage is suspected, the baby should be postured head down, at an angle of about 30° with the horizontal.
   b. Mucus and debris are sucked out of the nose and throat by means of a soft rubber catheter.

c. When simple methods are not successful, direct endotracheal intubation is performed. This must be done carefully to avoid damage to the larynx and trachea. The tube is available for both aspiration of secretion and administration of oxygen.

4. The most important principle of therapy is to supply oxygen to the fetal lungs and to maintain pulmonary ventilation until the respiratory center can take over this function. Oxygen is the essential therapeutic agent, the physiologic stimulant to the anoxic respiratory center. It can be administered in the incubator, by positive pressure mask, or by mouth to mouth breathing when better methods are unavailable.

5. When the infant has been narcotized by the administration of analgesics to the mother, Nalline (N-allyl-nomorphine) can be given to counteract the effects of certain drugs. Effective in combating respiratory depression caused by morphine, codeine, Demerol, Pantapon, Dilauded, Nisentil, and heroin, Nalline is of no value against the barbiturates, the anesthetic gases, or other causes of respiratory failure. It may act as a respiratory depressant when given to nonnarcotized infants. Repeated administration is of no value and may be harmful. It can be given to the narcotized mother intravenously (5 to 10 mg) 15 minutes before delivery. The most effective route is by injection into the umbilical vein of the infant in the dose of 0.2 to 0.4 mg diluted in 2 ml of saline. Another drug used for the same purpose is Lorfan Tartrate (0.05 to 0.10 mg), given to the baby. Drugs such as alpha-lobeline, Coramine, caffeine, and Metrazol are of no value as respiratory stimulants, may cause convulsions, and are no longer used.

6. Especially in babies born by cesarean section the stomach should be aspirated to remove the large amounts of fluid.

7. Antibiotics are given to combat possible pneumonia.

8. The baby should be kept in an incubator under close observation until its condition is good. In this way the body temperature, humidity, and oxygen concentration can be maintained at proper levels.

Prevention

1. Trauma must be kept to the minimum. Prolonged labor and difficult vaginal operations should be avoided whenever possible.

2. Oxygen is given to the mother for at least 5 minutes before and during difficult deliveries.

3. Excessive narcosis and deep prolonged inhalation anesthesia should not be used. Local or conduction anesthesia is preferable. If inhalation anesthesia must be used, one is chosen that gives the mother and infant the highest oxygen saturation with the least physiologic alterations. Conduction anesthesia sometimes causes hypotension in the mother. Posturing the mother on her left side corrects this problem in most cases.
4. Careful observation is necessary so that fetal distress (fetal brady-cardia, irregular fetal heart rate, passage of meconium in a vertex presentation) can be diagnosed and prompt treatment carried out both during the labor and after birth.

RESPIRATORY DISTRESS SYNDROME

RDS, the respiratory distress syndrome, is a severe disorder of the lungs that is a consequence of the infant's being born before the lungs have reached functional maturity. As such it affects mainly the preterm infant. If the fetus stays in utero long enough for the lungs to develop normally, there will be no hyaline membrane disease after birth.

In the mature lung certain surface-active phospholipids (surfactant) are present in the alveolar lining; these lower the surface tension at the air-liquid interface and stabilize the fine air spaces of the lung. At delivery the first breath requires very high intrathoracic pressures to expand the lungs with air. In the mature lung a large amount of the air inspired with the first breath remains in the lungs as the alveoli coated with surfactant remain expanded with the residual air. Hence, subsequent breaths require far lower inspiratory effort. With continuing respiration the alveoli are ventilated, pulmonary blood flow increases, and gas exchange takes place.

In the immature lung surfactant is absent or inadequate, alveolar stabilization does not occur, the lungs cannot hold residual air, and the alveoli collapse with each expiration. The same high inflating pressure is required at the next breath and again the alveoli collapse on expira-tion. In effect the baby is taking its first breath again and again, and soon becomes exhausted.

The sequence of events is:

atelectasis ⟶ hypoxemia ⟶ acidemia ⟶ constriction of pulmonary blood vessels ⟶ aggravation of hypoxemia and acidemia ⟶ disruption of normal metabolic function of surfactant-producing cells and alveolar epithelium ⟶ atelectasis and transudation of fluid into the alveolar spaces.

The progressive expiratory atelectasis accompanied by pulmonary edema worsens until death. At autopsy the lungs are almost airless, with alveolae lined by hyaline membranes.

Clinical Manifestations

The baby, who is almost always premature and may require resuscitation at birth, begins to breathe normally. Usually within 30 minutes the breathing becomes more difficult, there is retraction of the lower ribs and sternum on inspiration, flaring of the alae nasi, and an audible expiratory grunt.

Several hours later the signs of respiratory distress become more obvious. The rate of breathing increases to 80 to 120 per minute, and each breath requires extra effort. The diaphragm contracts strongly, there is retraction of the ribs and sternum, and the entry of air into the lungs is reduced.

During the next 12 to 24 hours the signs of respiratory distress may abate and complete recovery ensue. Very often, however, the respiratory distress and cyanosis increase. The baby becomes flaccid and unresponsive and begins to have periods of apnea. Once severe apnea sets in the chances of recovery are small. However, any baby who survives the first 96 hours has a reasonable chance of recovery.

Treatment

Therapy is supportive and consists of keeping the baby alive until the lungs can develop a functionally adequate respiratory state. Hypoxemia is treated by increased amounts of atmospheric oxygen; soda bicarbonate is given to normalize the pH of the blood; and assisted ventilation is used both to increase pulmonary ventilation and to decrease the metabolic demands of the work of respiration.

The most recent advances in the management of respiratory distress syndrome are related to prevention of the condition. The functional maturity of the lung can be determined in utero by measurements of the lecithin/sphingomyelin ratio in the amniotic fluid. Lecithin is the main surface-active phospholipid and is most abundant in the alveolar lining of the mature lung. Lecithin and related phospholipids in amniotic fluid appear to arise principally from the fetal lung. When the lecithin/sphingomyelin ratios are equal to or greater than 2:1, the fetal lung has usually achieved functional maturity. This test is of considerable benefit to the obstetrician faced with the decision of when to deliver the infant of a complicated pregnancy, such as infants of diabetic mothers and those with hemolytic disease of the newborn.

When the pregnancy is less than 32 weeks, prenatal administration of betamethasone to the mother may be indicated to stimulate maturity of the fetal lungs.

FETAL INJURY

Skull Fracture

Most fractures of the skull are caused by traumatic vaginal deliveries, often associated with the misuse of forceps. The two more common varieties are: (1) linear fractures, which require no treatment other than observation; and (2) depressed (ping pong) fractures. Here the periosteum is intact, but the bone is bent inward. Often these follow delivery with forceps but may occur in utero, the result of pressure from one of the maternal bones. All should be elevated under local anesthesia within the first week and as soon as the baby's condition is stable.

Intracranial Hemorrhage

ANATOMY

The brain is enclosed in a tough membrane, the dura mater. The falx cerebri and the tentorium cerebelli are extensions of the dura inside the skull and act as scaffolding to support the brain. The falx occupies a vertical plane between the two cerebral hemispheres. The tentorium lies in a horizontal plane separating the cerebral hemispheres above from the cerebellum below. Venous sinuses are enclosed in the margins of the falx and tentorium.

COMPRESSION OF THE HEAD

Excessive compression of the fetal head, either by natural forces or by instruments, can cause hemorrhage or brain damage. Death, mental retardation, epilepsy, or cerebral palsy may follow. Compression of the fetal skull acts in several ways:

1. The pressure is transmitted to the interior of the calvarium and overcomes the intravascular pressure. This leads to arrest of the cerebral circulation, followed by anoxia and then degeneration of the brain cells and blood vessels. The latter become more permeable, and there is bleeding into the brain.

2. The falx and the tentorium may be torn. If the laceration extends into the venous sinuses, extensive hemorrhage occurs.
3. A fractured skull bone may lacerate the underlying brain.

Thus hemorrhage in the fetal brain is the result of mechanical trauma and/or anoxia. It is more common in premature infants. The improvement in general obstetric care and the elimination of heroic vaginal operations have contributed to the reduction in the incidence and severity of cerebral hemorrhage.

ETIOLOGY

1. Prolonged labor, especially when obstructed
2. Cephalopelvic disproportion
3. Difficult forceps deliveries
4. Breech extraction
5. Delivery of preterm infants
6. Unattended deliveries

SYMPTOMS AND SIGNS

The symptoms and signs may not appear for 24 to 48 hours or longer. They include:

1. High-pitched cry
2. Signs of increased intracranial pressure such as bulging fontanelles
3. Irritability or convulsions
4. Spasticity or opisthotonus
5. The circumference of the head may enlarge
6. If there is pressure on the vital centers: possible death
7. Recurrent apnea
8. Congestive heart failure
9. Unexplained hypocalcemia and hypoglycemia

SITES OF BLEEDING

Subdural Hematoma This type of hemorrhage is the result of difficult labor and delivery. The venous sinuses are torn and blood collects between the dura mater and the pia-arachnoid. The intracranial pressure is increased. The cerebrospinal fluid may be xanthrochromic, rarely bloody. Prognosis depends on the associated damage to the brain.

Subarachnoid Hemorrhage The picture is one of focal convulsions, between the 2nd and 10th days, in a previously well infant. Often the delivery was normal. The cerebrospinal fluid is bloody. The prognosis is fairly good. Many infants are normal on follow-up examination.

Intraventricular Hemorrhage   This condition is seen mainly in preterm babies. The signs include agitation, apnea, convulsions, shock, and collapse. The hematocrit falls in the absence of overt hemorrhage. Death occurs within a few hours.

Intercerebral Hemorrhage   The amount of bleeding is small, often petechial. There may be signs of irritation, including seizures, but without evidence of increased intracranial pressure.

Hemorrhage into the Posterior Fossa   The accumulation of blood is gradual and often leads to an increase in the size of the head. The baby becomes irritable and may convulse. Treatment is surgical and is usually successful.

Intracerebral Hemorrhage   This variety occurs during difficult births. The bleeding is directly into the brain and may be gross or petechial. The prognosis depends upon the amount of damage done to the brain.

TREATMENT OF INTRACRANIAL HEMORRHAGE

1. Traumatic deliveries should be avoided and cesarean section performed when there is disproportion.
2. The baby is kept in an incubator.
3. The temperature is controlled.
4. Extra oxygen is given as needed.
5. Secretions are removed from the throat.
6. The baby is handled as little as possible.
7. Vitamin K is administered when indicated.
8. Convulsions are controlled by sedatives.
9. The head should not be lowered, since this may increase the bleeding.
10. If there is suspicion of a subdural collection of blood, lumbar puncture is done to relieve pressure as well as for diagnosis.
11. Prophylactic antibiotics are given.

Cerebral Palsy

Cerebral palsy includes a group of conditions which affect the control of the voluntary motor system, and which have their origin in lesions in various parts of the brain. The incidence of cerebral palsy is

4:1,000 to 7:1,000 births. It is the greatest neurologic crippler of children today. While the reduction of traumatic vaginal deliveries has lowered the incidence of cranial damage, the occurrence of cerebral palsy has not decreased.

Although Little (who gave his name to the disease) believed that asphyxia was the prime etiologic factor, many observers considered that trauma at birth was the main cause. However, most children traumatized at birth do not develop cerebral palsy. Today it is felt that anoxia is, by far, the leading agent in producing permanent cerebral damage, and that prematurity is the greatest contributing factor. Since not every premature infant develops cerebral palsy, it may be that the same factors caused both conditions.

A recent concept is that of an unfavorable intrauterine environment producing hypoxia or anoxia. If this anoxia is compounded by other factors, the requirements for permanent brain damage may be met.

Conditions associated with cerebral palsy include:

1. Maternal age
2. Relative sterility
3. Bleeding during pregnancy
4. Multiple pregnancy
5. Prolonged second stage of labor
6. Fetal distress, as it points to anoxia
7. Abnormal delivery—higher incidence with breech presentation
8. Frequency of poor condition at birth, probably a reflection of previously occurring damage which also caused the palsy
9. Prematurity
10. Traumatic delivery (probably under 10 percent)

Cephalhematoma

The term cephalhematoma refers to a collection of blood outside the bony skull. There are two main types:

SUBGALEAL The galea is an aponeurotic layer attached loosely to the external side of the periosteum. The veins in this area may be torn, resulting in a hematoma containing as much as 250 ml of blood. Anemia and even shock occur. The hematoma is not limited to any specific area.

SUBPERIOSTEAL Because the periosteum is attached to the bony skull at the suture lines, the hematoma is limited to an area bound by the sutures. The amount of blood is less than in the subgaleal variety. Skull fractures may be associated.

ETIOLOGY

Forces acting on the head to produce cephalhematomas include: (1) a tangential force which causes displacement of the soft tissues of the scalp and lacerations of the blood vessels, and (2) a vertical force which draws the scalp away from the underlying bones. Cephalhematoma may occur following spontaneous birth but is more common in association with abnormal positions of the head, forceps deliveries, and vacuum extraction.

CLINICAL PICTURE

1. The incidence of large and significant lesions is less than 1 percent
2. In most cases the hematoma remains static. Occasionally it becomes larger after birth, indicating that bleeding is continuing.
3. The babies have no discomfort.
4. Occasionally anemia and jaundice develop.
5. Generally there is no neurologic disorder.
6. Skull fracture is uncommon.
7. Spontaneous infection sets in only rarely.
8. The blood resorbs in 6 to 12 weeks.
9. Calcification in the clot may take place.

MANAGEMENT

1. No specific treatment is needed other than observation and protection of the head from damage.
2. An x-ray rules out fracture.
3. Blood transfusion is given if severe anemia develops.
4. Aspiration is contraindicated. It introduces infection.
5. Surgical intervention is necessary only when the bleeding is excessive and progressive, leading to enlargement of the hematoma.

Injuries of Facial Nerve

The seventh cranial nerve is involved. Facial palsy is seen after spontaneous delivery, in which case the maternal sacrum may be the source of the injury. The majority follow forceps extractions, the tips of the blades pressing on the stylomastoid foramen, where the nerve leaves the skull. In some instances the nerve is actually torn, partially or totally. In others the loss of function is the result of edema. Occasionally facial palsy follows central nervous system injury.

The facial muscles, including those of the eyelids, are paralyzed. The characteristic sign is the failure of one side of the mouth to move and the eyelid to close. Spontaneous resolution takes place often after the edema subsides. There is some return of function in 2 to 3 weeks (sometimes as soon as 5 to 6 days) and complete recovery in 2 to 3 months. In rare cases the paralysis is permanent with resultant weakness or atrophy of the facial muscles.

Immediate care includes irrigating the eye to maintain moisture and light finger massage of the face. In some cases surgery to relieve pressure on the nerve brings improvement.

Injury to the Spinal Cord

Spinal cord injuries are unusual. The most common site of damage is in the lower cervical area. The type of lesion ranges from localized hemorrhage to complete destruction of the spinal cord at one or more vertebral levels. There is seldom an associated fracture or dislocation of the vertebral body. Vaginal breech delivery is involved in 75 percent of cases, especially when the head is hyperextended.

There are four groups of clinical outcomes:

1. Stillbirth or immediate neonatal death takes place when the damage is extensive.
2. The infant may survive for a short period of time, succumbing in a state of shock and respiratory depression.
3. There may be long-term survival of children who are paralyzed in flaccid diplegia or quadriplegia.
4. Some survive with minimal neurologic symptoms or spasticity, often diagnosed as cerebral palsy.

Damage to Brachial Plexus

Paralysis of the arm from injury to the brachial plexus during birth was described by Smellie in 1764, but it was Erb who, in 1872, localized the most common lesion to the fifth and sixth cervical roots in the upper trunk of the plexus. The incidence is less than 1:1,000 births.

This paralysis is caused by stretching, hemorrhage, or edema of the roots of the brachial plexus. Complete recovery is not unusual. In a few cases there is actual avulsion of the nerve roots; here the damage is permanent.

Brachial palsy occurs during breech delivery when there is difficulty with the arms, and with shoulder dystocia in cephalic presentations when there is excessive flexion of the head obliquely toward one shoulder.

Erb's Palsy (Erb-Duchene)   This involves C-5 and C-6. The arm hangs limply to the side and is rotated internally. The elbow is extended and the wrist flexed with the palm upward in the so-called waiter's tip position. Sensory loss is minimal.

Klumpke's Paralysis   This involves C-8 and T-1. There is weakness and wasting of the muscles supplied by the median and ulnar nerves, including the wrist and finger flexors, and flaccid paralysis of the small muscles of the hand. Sensory deficit is more common than with Erb's palsy and involves the palm of the hand.

Treatment of brachial palsies is symptomatic and supportive, directed toward minimizing the deformity. After 6 months correctional surgery may be considered.

Radial Nerve Palsy

This lesion is usually associated with fractures of the humerus. Prognosis is good with supportive treatment.

Sternomastoid Muscle

This muscle may be damaged during delivery. A hard, painless, nonfluctuant swelling appears in the lower part of the muscle. The underlying pathology is uncertain. Theories include hemorrhage, venous thrombosis, or an exudate from ruptured muscle fibers. Treatment includes local massage and passive stretching of the neck to the opposite side. Occasionally contracture of the muscle takes place, resulting in torticollis (wry neck).

Bony Injuries

This group includes fractures of the clavicle, humerus, and femur. These are seen most often following difficult breech deliveries and shoulder dystocia.

Intraabdominal Trauma

HEMORRHAGE
This is a serious problem. In infants presenting with shock, pallor, anemia, and abdominal distension intraperitoneal bleeding must be considered. Paracentesis is diagnostic.

HEPATIC RUPTURE

The liver is the organ damaged or lacerated most often. A sub-capsular hematoma may develop, increase in size gradually, rupture into the peritoneal cavity, and lead to profound shock. Infants at risk include:

1. Those with hepatomegaly
2. Those with coagulation disorders
3. Those with asphyxia
4. Premature and postmature babies
5. Breech deliveries

SPLENIC RUPTURE

This accident is less common than injury to the liver. Splenomegaly increases the danger of its occurrence, but in most cases the organ is of normal size.

CONGENITAL MALFORMATIONS

Of the many congenital anomalies that may occur, only those that complicate labor and delivery are described.

Anencephalus

Anencephalus is the absence of the vault of the skull with complete or partial absence of the brain. What brain tissue there is is uncovered and unprotected.

The diagnosis is established by ultrasound and x-ray, but suspicion may be aroused by the inability of the attendant to feel the head and by hyperactive movement of the fetus after rectal or vaginal examination. The examining finger abuts against the exposed lower brain tissue and stimulates the fetus to move vigorously. Anencephaly is the most common cause of polyhydramnios and should be suspected in all cases of unexplained excessive amniotic fluid.

Most anencephalics deliver without difficulty. Since the head is small it does not dilate the cervix well, and traction on the head with clamps may be necessary to pull the shoulders through. In general it is better to await the spontaneous onset of labor than to attempt induction through an unripe cervix. It is impossible for an anencephalic monster to survive.

Hydrocephalus

Hydrocephalus is the accumulation of cerebrospinal fluid in the ventricles of the brain. The amount usually varies between 500 and 1,500 ml, although much larger amounts have been reported. The obstetric problem is one of gross disproportion between the head and the pelvis. Breech presentation occurs in about 30 percent of cases. In these cases labor proceeds normally in the early part, and it is often not until the aftercoming head cannot be extracted that the attendant suspects hydrocephaly.

Diagnosis is made by abdominal, vaginal, ultrasonic, and radiologic examination. When the head is extremely large, the abnormality is recognized by palpation. X-ray will confirm the diagnosis in most cases, but sometimes the distortion produced by divergence of the x-rays leads to misinterpretation. Ultrasonic measurement of the biparietal diameter showing it to be over 11.0 cm is strongly suggestive of hydrocephaly. In borderline cases it may be difficult to be certain of the diagnosis and care must be taken to avoid damaging a normal baby by ill-advised procedures.

During labor, when the head is presenting, one notes the enlarged fontanelles, the widely separated sutures, and the cystic consistency of the head. In breech delivery associated anomalies such as spina bifida and talipes are clues.

The danger of hydrocephaly to the mother is uterine rupture during the obstructed labor. Because of the disproportion the lower segment of the uterus becomes distended and thin, and rupture may take place spontaneously or as a result of obstetric manipulations. After labor is in progress, the cervix is dilated, and the baby is diagnosed as dead, the size of the head should be reduced by evacuating the fluid through a large-bore needle. This makes the head smaller and delivery ensues. In breech presentations when the aftercoming head cannot be extracted, the obstetrician must resist the temptation to pull the head through by force since this ruptures the lower uterine segment. The fluid should be drained either by perforating the skull or by transecting the spinal canal in the thoracic region.

Occasionally cesarean section must be performed if there is: (1) a maternal indication, (2) an infant in a transverse lie who cannot be turned easily, (3) a constriction ring dystocia, (4) failure of decompression and/or descent of the head, and (5) doubt of the diagnosis and the baby is alive.

Spina Bifida

Spina bifida cystica is a midline defect of the spine in which there is an external saccular protrusion. When the sac contain meninges and spinal fluid but no neural elements, it is referred to as a meningocele. If spinal cord and nerves are included in the sac it is called a myelomeningocele or myelocele. The latter is often associated with hydrocephalus.

Many of these infants die of infection. Surgical management has raised the survival rate, but many of these have severe locomotor disability, incontinence of urine and feces, and mental retardation.

Amniotic Bands

Amniotic fibrous bands may cause a variety of fetal malformations. The incidence is estimated at from 1:10,000 to 1:5,000 pregnancies. The fetal limbs are affected most often and amputation of part or all of one finger, or even an entire arm, has been reported. The band may encircle or compress the umbilical cord, cutting off the flow of blood to the fetus and resulting in fetal death.

This condition is often associated with oligohydramnios. Two etiologic theories have been advanced. One suggests that the amniotic bands result from defects occurring when the germ disk and the amniotic cavity are being formed. The other claim is that the bands develop as a result of early rupture of the amnion and its partial or complete separation from the chorion.

PERINATAL MORTALITY

Perinatal mortality has been defined as the number of infants dying before birth, during birth, or in the first 7 days of life, and weighing more than 1,000 g at birth. Of the babies who die during the first month, 90 percent do so in the first week.

Death before or during delivery is usually caused by anoxia, preceded frequently by a period of hypoxia. In the 1st week of life most deaths are the result either of damage from intrauterine hypoxia or of inefficient pulmonary ventilation after birth.

Anoxia

There are four kinds of anoxia.

1. Anoxic anoxia is the low uptake of oxygen as a result of insufficient supply from the mother:
   a. Low oxygenation of maternal blood (anemia, intoxication).

  b. Reduction of blood flow through the placenta.

  c. Insufficiency of the placenta, poorly developed and inadequate number of villi, placental degeneration.

  d. Antepartum hemorrhage, mainly abruptio placentae, associated with premature births. This accident occurs as an unexpected emergency 1 to 2 months before term and may result in immediate fetal death. The prognosis is better with placenta previa.

  e. Umbilical cord problems. Actual prolapse of the cord carries a high rate of fetal death. Knots or loops of the cord are considered causes of fetal death only when they are very tight and when no other etiologic factor can be found.

  f. Abnormalities of labor and delivery are included under anoxic causes only when no traumatic lesions can be found. Among these situations are breech presentation and prolonged labor.

  g. Maternal diseases (e.g., diabetes, toxemia) are considered in this group when no other reason for the death can be found.

2. Anemic anoxia signifies inefficient oxygen transport in the fetus and includes:

  a. Fetal anemia (erythroblastosis, umbilical cord hemorrhage)

  b. Carbon monoxide poisoning

  c. Congenital malformations

3. Stagnant anoxia is the poor uptake of oxygen in the tissues and includes conditions such as postnatal shock.

4. Histotoxic anoxia is reduced oxygenation in the cells, as under the effect of narcotics and anesthetics.

Congenital Malformations

Congenital malformations can cause both stillbirth and neonatal death. Included here are abnormalities of the central nervous system (anencephaly, hydrocephaly, myelomeningocele), congenital heart disease, hypoplasia of the lungs, gastrointestinal anomalies, renal agenesis, and diaphragmatic hernia. In some instances the mechanism that resulted in fetal death is not clear. In many cases prematurity is associated.

Fetal Malnutrition

Included here are infants whose birth weights are below the 10th percentile for gestational age. Deaths in these babies are potentially preventable if early diagnosis can be made and proper treatment instituted while the fetus is still in utero.

Respiratory Distress Syndrome

This is a disease of infants born prematurely. It accounts for approximately two-thirds of deaths associated with prematurity. It is almost never responsible for death in infants born after 36 weeks' gestation.

Isoimmunization

These deaths are caused by immunization to the Rh "D" factor. Improved methods of prevention, diagnosis, and treatment are currently reducing the mortality from this condition.

Infection

Infection is an important and serious problem. Most of the infections are acquired in utero, often when the membranes have been ruptured for a long period of time, and with or without clinical evidence of intrauterine infection. Many of these deaths occur in premature infants. While pneumonia is a common problem, septicemia, meningitis, urinary infection, and gastroenteritis are found. In numerous babies the exact site of infection cannot be ascertained.

Trauma During Birth

Fortunately, deaths from this cause are being reduced, especially by the more judicious use of cesarean section. However, ill-advised delivery by forceps and other vaginal manipulations continue to contribute the occasional dead baby.

Etiology

Fetal mortality is increased in the following groups:

1. Maternal factors
   a. Women over 40 years of age
   b. Primigravidas over 35
   c. Grand multiparas
   d. Women of low economic and social strata

2. Factors at birth
   a. The larger the fetus, the greater the risk during birth
   b. The smaller the infant, the higher the danger after delivery
   c. Abnormal presentations
3. Fetal conditions
   a. Multiple pregnancy
   b. Male infants
   c. Premature babies
   d. Dysmature infants

BIBLIOGRAPHY

Brans YW, Cassady G: Neonatal spinal cord injuries. Am J Obstet Gynecol 123:918, 1975

Bresnan MJ: Neurologic birth injuries. Postgrad Med 49:199, 1971

Brown BJ, Gabert HA, Stenchever M: Respiratory distress syndrome, surfactant biochemistry, and acceleration of lung maturity: a review. Obstet Gynecol Surv 30:71, 1975

Chemke J, Graff G, Hurwitz N, Liban E: The amniotic band syndrome. Obstet Gynecol 41:332, 1973

Greesham EL: Birth trauma. Pediatr Clin North Am 22:317, 1975

Gordon M, Rich H, Deutschberger J, Green M: The immediate and long term outcome of obstetric birth trauma. Brachial plexus paralysis. Am J Obstet Gynecol 117:51, 1973

Mayer PS, Wingate MB: Obstetric factors in cerebral palsy. Obstet Gynecol 51:399, 1978

Nelson GH: Relationship between amniotic fluid lecithin concentration and respiratory distress syndrome. Am J Obstet Gynecol 112:827, 1972

Tan KL: Cephalhematoma. Aust NZ J Obstet Gynaecol 10:101, 1970

Index